Tina Bhutani
Wilson Liao · Mio Nakamura
Editors

Evidence-Based Psoriasis

Diagnosis and Treatment

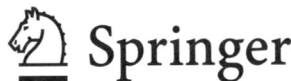

Editors
Tina Bhutani, MD
Department of Dermatology
UCSF Psoriasis Center
University of California
San Francisco, CA, USA

Wilson Liao, MD
Department of Dermatology
UCSF Psoriasis Center
University of California
San Francisco, CA, USA

Mio Nakamura, MD
Department of Dermatology
Psoriasis and Skin Treatment Center
University of California
San Francisco, CA, USA

ISSN 2523-8884   ISSN 2523-8892   (electronic)
Updates in Clinical Dermatology
ISBN 978-3-030-07935-2   ISBN 978-3-319-90107-7   (eBook)
https://doi.org/10.1007/978-3-319-90107-7

Printed on acid-free paper

This Springer imprint is published by the registered company Springer International Publishing AG part of Springer Nature.
The registered company address is: Gewerbestrasse 11, 6330 Cham, Switzerland

Preface

Psoriasis is a chronic, inflammatory condition with an estimated prevalence of 3–4% in the US population. It is a systemic disease with many known serious comorbidities including psoriatic arthritis, cardiovascular disease, and diabetes. In addition, psoriasis is associated with depression, anxiety, and self-consciousness, which causes patients to limit social interactions and prevents them from forming close, intimate relationships with others.

Although there are many other textbooks focusing on dermatologic treatments, there are very few specific books with the aim of guiding physicians through the diagnosis and treatment of psoriasis in a practical and evidence-based manner. Given the multitude of new treatment options for this disease including topicals, phototherapy, oral systemic therapy, and injectable biologics, the treatment of psoriasis has truly become an art of individualizing treatments to each patient based on the available evidence. This book will attempt to pass on this art to practicing physicians in a very practical and easy to use form in the hopes of improving care of psoriasis patients around the world.

San Francisco, CA, USA   Tina Bhutani
                                                            Wilson Liao
                                                            Mio Nakamura

Contents

Contributors

Ladi Afifian, MD Department of Dermatology, UCSF Medical Center, San Francisco, CA, USA

Kristen M. Beck, MD Department of Dermatology, UCSF Medical Center, San Francisco, CA, USA

Tina Bhutani, MD Department of Dermatology, UCSF Psoriasis Center, University of California San Francisco, San Francisco, CA, USA

Leah A. Cardwell, MD Department of Dermatology, Wake Forest School of Medicine, Winston-Salem, NC, USA

Abigail Cline, PhD, MD Department of Internal Medicine, Medical College of Georgia, Augusta, GA, USA

Steven R. Feldman, MD, PhD Department of Dermatology, Wake Forest School of Medicine, Winston-Salem, NC, USA

Department of Pathology, Wake Forest School of Medicine, Winston-Salem, NC, USA

Department of Public Health Sciences, Wake Forest School of Medicine, Winston-Salem, NC, USA

Kayla H. Felix, MS Department of Dermatology, Wake Forest School of Medicine, Winston-Salem, NC, USA

James L. Griffith, MD, MS Department of Dermatology, Henry Ford Hospital, Detroit, MI, USA

Kody Heubach, BS Lumberton, NC, USA

Caleb Jeon, BS Department of Dermatology, UCSF Psoriasis Center, University of California San Francisco, San Francisco, CA, USA

Grace W. Kimmel, MD Department of Dermatology, Icahn School of Medicine at Mount Sinai, New York, NY, USA

John Koo, MD Department of Dermatology, Psoriasis and Skin Treatment Center, University of California San Francisco, San Francisco, CA, USA

Mark Lebwohl, MD Department of Dermatology, Icahn School of Medicine at Mount Sinai, New York, NY, USA

Wilson Liao, MD Department of Dermatology, UCSF Psoriasis Center, University of California San Francisco, San Francisco, CA, USA

Henry W. Lim, MD Department of Dermatology, Henry Ford Hospital, Detroit, MI, USA

Mio Nakamura, MD Department of Dermatology, Psoriasis and Skin Treatment Center, University of California San Francisco, San Francisco, CA, USA

Elias Oussedik, BSc Department of Dermatology, Wake Forest School of Medicine, Winston-Salem, NC, USA

Di Yan, MD Department of Dermatology, UCSF Medical Center, San Francisco, CA, USA

Sahil Sekhon, MD Department of Dermatology, UCSF Psoriasis Center, University of California San Francisco, San Francisco, CA, USA

Eric J. Yang, BS Department of Dermatology, UCSF Psoriasis Center, University of California San Francisco, San Francisco, CA, USA

Allison J. Zarbo, MD Department of Dermatology, Henry Ford Hospital, Detroit, MI, USA

Psoriasis: Overview and Diagnosis

Grace W. Kimmel and Mark Lebwohl

Introduction and Epidemiology

Psoriasis is a common, chronic inflammatory skin disease that is characterized by the formation of sharply demarcated, scaly, erythematous plaques. It is a prevalent disease, both in the USA and globally. According to the large population-based Multinational Assessment of Psoriasis and Psoriatic Arthritis (MAPP) survey, the prevalence of psoriasis ranges from 1.4% in Spain to 3.3% in Canada, with an overall prevalence of 1.9%. The prevalence in the USA is slightly higher than the average at 2.2% [1]. Worldwide, the prevalence has been found to vary both geographically and among different ethnic groups within the same region and is overall reported at higher rates in locations distant from the equator [2, 3].

Psoriasis can present at any age. However, the disease onset appears to follow a bimodal distribution, peaking around 20–30 years of age and again around 50–60 years of age [4]. A family history of the disease is common. Approximately 30% of patients have a first-degree relative with psoriasis, and the risk of psoriasis increases with the number of affected relatives a patient has [5]. Some studies suggest that this bimodal distribution represents two distinct forms of psoriasis; compared to patients whose psoriasis presents later in life, patients with early onset psoriasis are much more likely to possess a genetic marker that is highly associated with psoriasis and to have a parent with psoriasis. Earlier onset psoriasis is also associated with more severe disease [4]. In most cases, the disease waxes and wanes throughout a patient's life, and spontaneous remission without treatment is unlikely [6].

The plaques of psoriasis can be disfiguring and severely pruritic and/or painful. Itching is often the most bothersome symptom of psoriasis [1]. Quality of life can be substantially affected, and many psoriasis patients report a significant social and emotional burden along with the negative impact of psoriasis on their physical well-being [7, 8]. Functional disability due to psoriasis is comparable or even greater compared to those seen in other serious diseases including cancer, depression, and heart disease [9].

In the MAPP survey, there was a 2-year median delay from symptom onset to time of diagnosis. In terms of disease severity, approximately 30% of psoriasis patients and 50% of those with both psoriasis and psoriatic arthritis rated their disease as severe. Despite this, nearly half of psoriasis patients had not seen a physician in the past year, and many were on either no treatment or topical therapy alone. One of the reasons for this undertreatment was lack of tolerability or efficacy of available oral or biologic agents [1]. These statics highlight the importance of improving disease detection and the need for improved therapeutic choices.

G. W. Kimmel (✉) · M. Lebwohl
Department of Dermatology, Icahn School of Medicine at Mount Sinai, New York, NY, USA
e-mail: grace.kimmel@mssm.edu

© Springer International Publishing AG, part of Springer Nature 2018
T. Bhutani et al. (eds.), *Evidence-Based Psoriasis*, Updates in Clinical Dermatology,
https://doi.org/10.1007/978-3-319-90107-7_1

Associated Conditions and Complications

In recent years, the impact of psoriasis has been found to extend beyond the skin, and psoriasis has been found to be associated with a variety of systemic conditions. Approximately 75% of patients will have at least one comorbid condition, and many will have multiple comorbidities [10]. The association is thought to be due to the chronic inflammatory changes and elevated pro-inflammatory cytokines found in psoriasis that lead to a systemic inflammatory state.

The most well-recognized associated condition is psoriatic arthritis, a seronegative inflammatory arthritis. The exact proportion of patients with psoriasis who will develop psoriatic arthritis is unknown but is estimated to be <10 to 40%. Psoriatic arthritis typically occurs in patients who have had preexisting skin findings of psoriasis for 5–12 years; however, approximately 20% of patients will present with joint symptoms first [1, 11]. The most common presentation of psoriatic arthritis is polyarticular peripheral arthritis but can vary widely with peripheral and/or axial, monoarticular, or polyarticular patterns. The severity of psoriatic arthritis can also vary drastically among individuals but does not necessarily correlate with the severity of skin findings. At its most severe, the arthritis can be erosive and deforming (arthritis mutilans) [11]. Even among psoriasis patients without a diagnosis of psoriatic arthritis, 50% report joint pain [10]. Given the high prevalence and disease burden of psoriatic arthritis, it is important to screen for arthritis symptoms in every patient with psoriasis at each visit [11].

Of notable concern, psoriasis is also associated with an increased risk of cardiovascular disease. Psoriasis patients are more likely to have cardiovascular risk factors including diabetes mellitus (especially type 2), obesity, hyperlipidemia, hypertension, and tobacco and alcohol abuse [12–14]. However, psoriasis patients have been found to have an increased risk of myocardial infarction even after controlling for these cardiovascular risk factors, signifying that psoriasis itself may be an independent risk factor for cardiovascular disease. The risk of cardiovascular disease appears to be highest in patients with more severe psoriasis at a younger age [15, 16]. Other significant associated conditions include depression, autoimmune diseases, Parkinsonism, and cancers, such as skin cancers and lymphomas [6, 17, 18].

Overview of Pathogenesis

The pathophysiology of psoriasis is characterized by excessive epidermal growth and altered keratinocyte differentiation. The underlying pathogenesis is multifactorial and complex with genetic, immunologic, and environmental contributions. Certain environmental triggers are thought to disrupt the homeostasis of the skin immune system in genetically predisposed individuals [19]. Medications implicated in the induction and exacerbation of psoriasis include angiotensin-converting enzyme (ACE) inhibitors, angiotensin II receptor blockers (ARBs), antimalarials, lithium, and nonsteroidal anti-inflammatory drugs [20–22]. Despite the association with ACE inhibitors and ARBs, a population-based case-control study found that beta-blockers and other anti-hypertensives are not associated with psoriasis [23]. Other potential triggers include infections (i.e., human immunodeficiency virus [HIV] and streptococcus) and trauma to the skin (the Koebner phenomenon) [20, 24].

In recent years, a variety of genes have been identified that predisposes an individual to psoriasis, many of which involve mediators of immune signaling pathways, emphasizing the importance of the immune system in the pathogenesis of psoriasis [25–28]. Early genetic linkage studies identified a major genetic determinant of psoriasis in the susceptibility-1 locus (PSORS1) of the major histocompatibility complex (MHC). Later, the human leukocyte antigen (HLA)-Cw6 was identified as the diseased allele at PSORS1 [26]. In recent years, genome-wide association studies have identified 63 genes that account for approximately 28% of the heritability of psoriasis. These genes include those of inflammatory interleukins and immune mediators [27]. In particular, a review of single-nucleotide polymorphism (SNP) analyses from multiple studies has shown an association between psoriasis and the loci for the T-helper type 2 (Th2) pathway (including interleukin [IL]-4 and IL-13), the T-helper type 17 (Th17) pathway (including subsets of IL-12 and IL-23), innate immune signaling pathways for nuclear factor kappa-light-chain-enhancer of activated B cells (NFkB) and interferons (IFN), and adaptive immune pathways involving CD8 T cells [28].

Although early research focused on aberrant keratinocyte activity as the primary cause of psoriasis, more recent studies have shown that psoriasis is an immune-mediated disease, as the skin inflammation of psoriasis is dependent on immune cells and their cytokines [29]. This has been supported by the genetic studies mentioned above. Abnormal activation of inflammatory mediators from the innate and adaptive immune systems has been implicated in the pathogenesis of psoriasis. Involved cells include keratinocytes, dendritic cells, and T cells, and important inflammatory mediators include tumor necrosis factor (TNF)-α, IL-17, IL-12, and IL-23 [30]. Recent advances in understanding the underlying inflammatory mechanisms have been pivotal in the development of new and more efficacious targeted therapies such as TNF-α, IL-12 and/or -23, and IL-17 inhibitors.

Diagnosis

Psoriasis is a clinical diagnosis, and a skin biopsy is usually not necessary for classic presentations of the disease. The characteristic lesions are sharply demarcated, scaly, erythematous plaques. The plaques may be pruritic and/or painful. They can be ovoid, round, or irregular in morphology and are often symmetrically distributed. When the xerotic scale is removed with scraping, points of fine bleeding may be seen (the "Auspitz sign"). Lesions may develop at sites of trauma or injury, known as the Koebner phenomenon.

The plaques are most frequently found on the extensor surfaces (elbows and knees), the scalp, and the intergluteal cleft. The palms and soles may be affected in the variants of palmoplantar psoriasis and palmoplantar pustulosis. Other forms of psoriasis include generalized pustular, guttate, erythrodermic, and inverse psoriasis.

The extent and severity of psoriasis can be measured using the Psoriasis Area and Severity Index (PASI), which includes evaluations of body surface area (BSA) involvement, erythema, induration, and scaling. This generates a severity score ranging from 0 to 72 [31]. Although more commonly used in clinical trials than in the context of clinical practice, the PASI can be a useful measurement in assessing response to a given treatment. For example, PASI-75 indicates that the patient's psoriasis has improved by 75% or greater from baseline. The Physician Global Assessment (PGA) is another simplified measurement tool that rates the severity of psoriasis at a single point in time [32]. It is important to note that one of the limitations of the PASI and PGA is that there can be high interobserver variability.

In addition to assessing the severity of psoriasis, it is also important to include evaluations of subjective symptoms and quality of life burden. Furthermore, given the high probability of systemic comorbidities, including arthritis and cardiovascular, metabolic, and psychiatric disorders, patients should be screened for such conditions and have an established primary care physician who can help manage the patient's overall health.

Clinical Characteristics of Psoriasis and Its Variants

Plaque Psoriasis

Also known as psoriasis vulgaris, plaque psoriasis is the most common form of psoriasis, accounting for 80–90% of cases [33]. The lesions are characteristically well-defined, erythematous, scaly plaques and often have the distribution detailed above (elbows, knees, scalp, intergluteal cleft) (Figs. 1.1, 1.2, 1.3, 1.4, and 1.5). The plaques vary in size, and patients may present with only a few lesions or with widely generalized disease. Lesions are often symmetrically distributed. Mild to moderate disease, classified as involving less than 10% of the BSA, represents approximately 80% of cases of plaque psoriasis. The remainder of patients have moderate to severe disease and may have involvement of the majority of the BSA [6].

Palmoplantar psoriasis is characterized by erythematous, desquamative plaques in the acral distribution (Fig. 1.6). Palmoplantar psoriasis can be an isolated entity or may coexist in the context of plaque psoriasis [34].

Guttate Psoriasis

Guttate psoriasis presents with the sudden appearance of many small (1–10 mm) erythematous papules, often covered with fine scale (Figs. 1.7 and 1.8). It is found more commonly in children and young adults and represents less than 2% of psoriasis cases [6]. The lesions of guttate psoriasis are widely disseminated, particularly on the proximal extremities and trunk. Lesions may also be found on the face [35]. Guttate psoriasis can occur in patients with and without a history of plaque psoriasis. It is associated with group A beta-hemolytic streptococcal infections, which often precedes the skin findings by 2–3 weeks [6]. This disease is often self-limiting in nature and can resolve spontaneously or with treatment [17]. Some patients with guttate

psoriasis can go on to develop chronic guttate psoriasis or chronic plaque psoriasis [36].

Generalized Pustular Psoriasis

Generalized pustular psoriasis is characterized by the formation of sterile pustules on a background of erythematous skin, which are widespread and can be generalized (Figs. 1.9 and 1.10). The etiology remains unclear; however, administration of certain medications, including lithium and nonsteroidal anti-inflammatory drugs, may precede the onset of pustular psoriasis [24]. Other precipitating factors include infection and abrupt cessation of systemic corticosteroids [17]. Generalized pustular psoriasis may follow a mild and chronic course or appear severely and acutely (von Zumbusch type). Pustules can coalesce, and the whole body may be involved, including mucosal areas [37].

Given the widespread involvement, these patients can lose the skin's protective function. Loss of the thermoregulatory function of the skin may cause fever or hypothermia. Fluid loss through the skin can result in volume depletion, dehydration, and even shock. There can be significant loss of electrolytes, iron, and protein through the skin. Patients with acute generalized pustular psoriasis often meet systemic inflammatory response syndrome (SIRS) criteria on presentation, and associated lab abnormalities include neutrophilia, leukocytosis up to 30,000 WBC/μL, elevated erythrocyte sedimentation rate (ESR), and elevated liver function tests

Fig. 1.1 Plaque psoriasis: classic morphology characterized by a sharply demarcated, erythematous plaque with silver scale

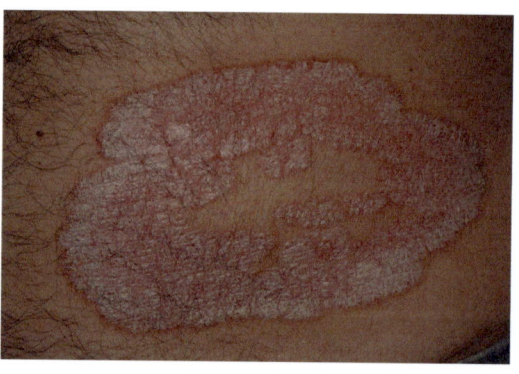

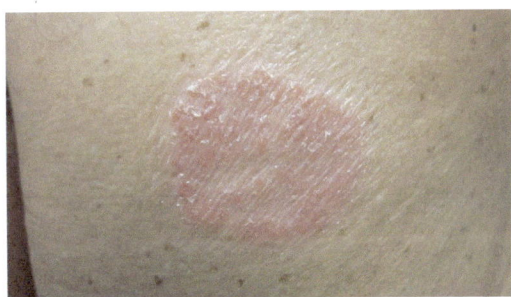

Fig. 1.2 Plaque psoriasis: this lesion is less severe with mild scaling but is diagnostic for psoriasis

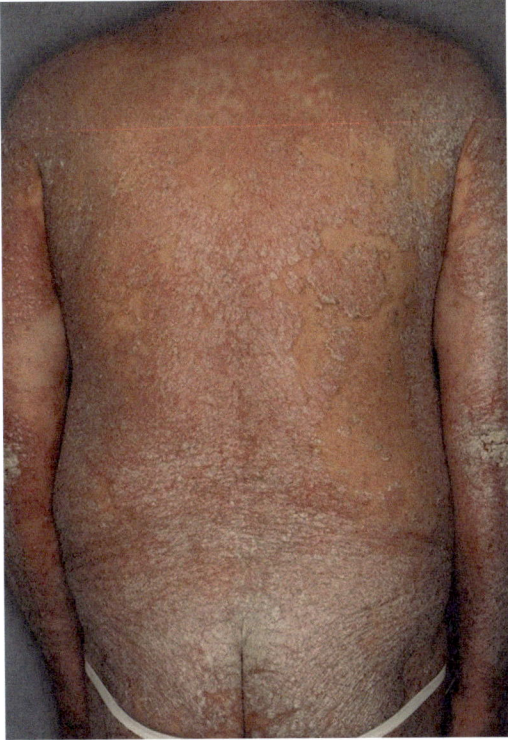

Fig. 1.3 Plaque psoriasis: this patient has widespread involvement of the majority of the body surface area

Fig. 1.4 Scalp psoriasis: scaling is prominent with notable background erythema

[37]. Most importantly, these patients lose the protective function of the skin against the entry of pathogens, leaving them susceptible to bacteremia. There are multiple reports of staphylococcal sepsis and death in patients with generalized pustular psoriasis [38–40]. Another potential fatal complication is the development of aseptic neutrophilic pneumonitis, which can lead to acute respiratory distress syndrome (ARDS) [37]. Severe cases of generalized pustular psoriasis therefore necessitate admission to the burn unit or intensive care unit (ICU). Treatment of generalized pustular psoriasis with rapidly acting agents like cyclosporine can reduce the need for hospitalization.

Palmoplantar Pustulosis

Unlike generalized pustular psoriasis, pustular psoriasis can be limited to the palms and soles, referred to as palmoplantar pustulosis. This disease is characterized by recurrent eruptions of sterile pustules on the palmar and plantar surfaces [34] (Figs. 1.11 and 1.12). Although this form is not life-threatening as in generalized pustular psoriasis, it is a debilitating condition with high morbidity, as patients can have severe pain. Patients with psoriasis on the hands and feet have been found to have a worse quality of life than patients with extensive involvement on the trunk [41, 42]. Palmoplantar pustulosis typically presents between 30 and 40 years of age, and the palmar lesions typically precede plantar involvement by a few months [43]. Notably, the majority of patients are female, with a female to male ratio of 9:1. Palmoplantar pustulosis is also highly asso-

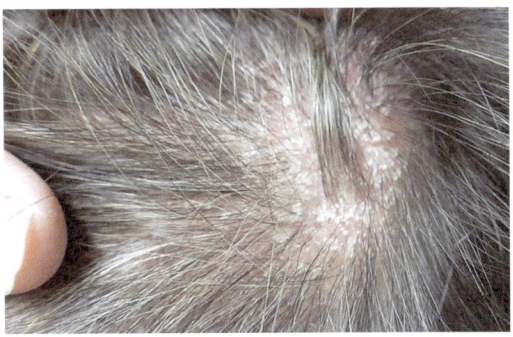

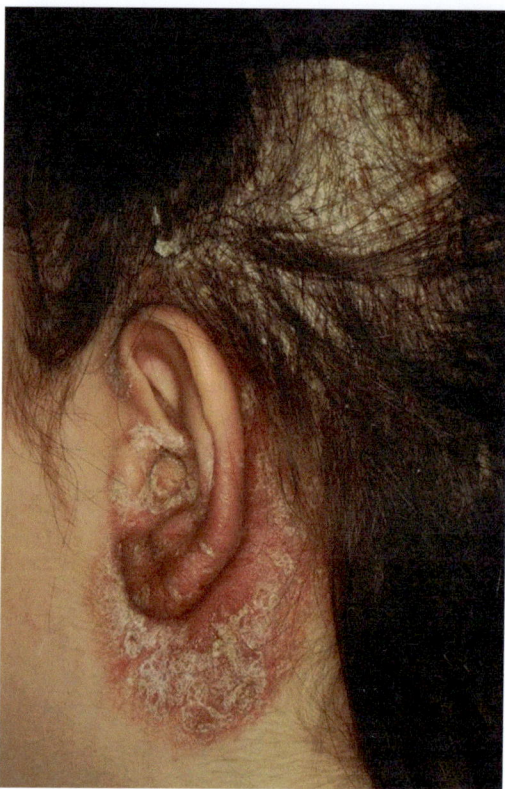

Fig. 1.5 Scalp psoriasis: severe scaling involving the periauricular region

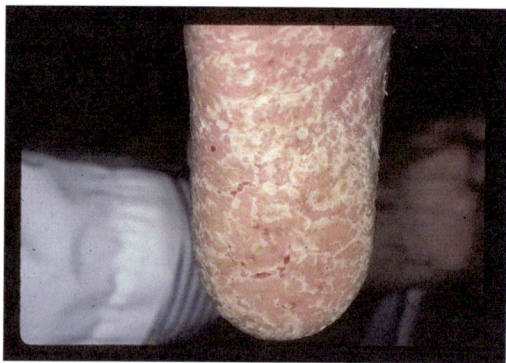

Fig. 1.6 Palmoplantar psoriasis: notable severe scaling and erythema on the palmer surface of the distal finger

ciated with smoking with 95% of patients having a previous or current smoking history [17]. Roughly 25% of palmoplantar psoriasis patients will also have a diagnosis of chronic plaque psoriasis, although genetic studies indicate that they are distinct entities [25].

Erythrodermic Psoriasis

Erythrodermic psoriasis is another potentially life-threatening form of psoriasis associated with the loss of skin function. In addition to being one of the most severe forms of psoriasis, it is also one of the rarest, affecting only 1% of psoriasis patients [44]. Among patients with a history of psoriasis who presents with erythroderma, the erythroderma is due to the preexisting psoriasis in only 20% of patients [45]. Even in patients with known psoriasis, it is important to consider other possible causes of erythroderma, of which there are many (see section "Differential Diagnosis").

In erythrodermic psoriasis, the skin over the entire body surface area is inflamed, erythematous, and scaly. Desquamation may occur (Figs. 1.13, 1.14, and 1.15). Although erythrodermic psoriasis can develop over time in patients with chronic plaque psoriasis, it may also occur suddenly in patients without a previous psoriasis history [6]. It can be precipitated by antimalarial drugs, the rapid discontinuation of either topical or systemic corticosteroids, overexposure to sun or UV light, and infections [35]. As in generalized pustular psoriasis, the loss of thermoregulatory and barrier functions of the skin can lead to fever, hypothermia, fluid loss, dehydration, and shock [6]. Patients are also at a high risk of sepsis and even death, especially staphylococcal sepsis [46].

Inverse Psoriasis

Inverse psoriasis, also known as intertriginous or flexural psoriasis, affects 3–7% of psoriasis patients [47]. It involves the skinfolds, including the axillae, genital regions, and inframammary and inguinal creases. The face can also be involved. These lesions are less likely to be scaly given the high moisture in these areas and mainly present as shiny, erythematous plaques [6] (Fig. 1.16). Fissuring and superimposed bacterial or fungal infections may occur. Histologically, there is no difference between inverse and plaque psoriasis, and thus the two

Fig. 1.7 Guttate psoriasis: widespread small, erythematous papules generalized over the entire body surface area

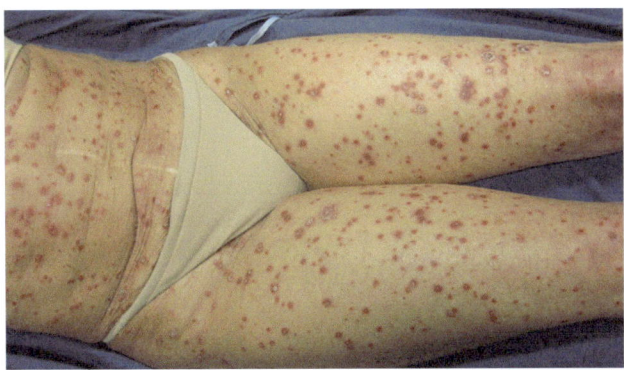

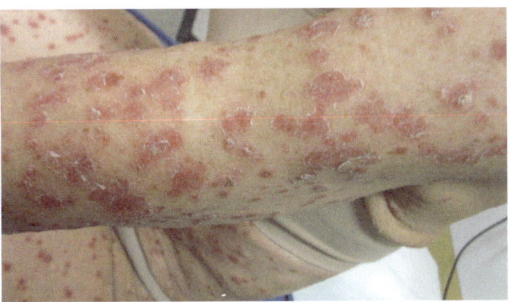

Fig. 1.8 Guttate psoriasis: a close-up image showing the characteristic fine scale

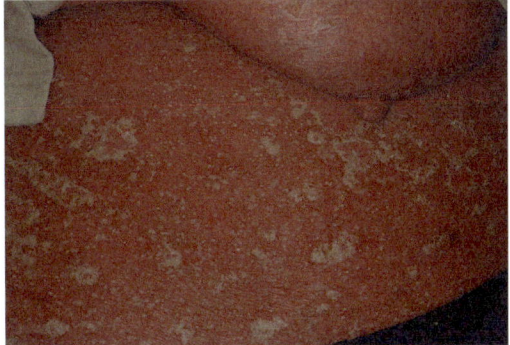

Fig. 1.10 Pustular psoriasis: severe erythema and desquamation are present

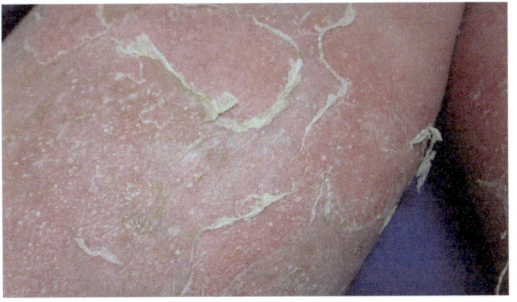

Fig. 1.9 Pustular psoriasis: pustules on a background of erythema. Desquamation is also prominent here

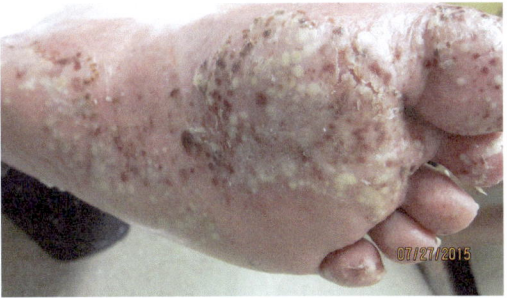

Fig. 1.11 Palmoplantar pustulosis: a severe case on the plantar surface

are differentiated on clinical presentation alone [47]. Notably, psoriasis patients with palmar involvement are approximately five times more likely to have inverse psoriasis than classic plaque psoriasis [48].

Nail Changes

Nail changes can occur in any type of psoriasis. Among patients with psoriasis, fingernail changes occur in 50% of patients and toenail changes occur in 35% of patients. Nail changes are com-

Fig. 1.12 Palmoplantar
pustulosis: a mild case
on the palmar surface

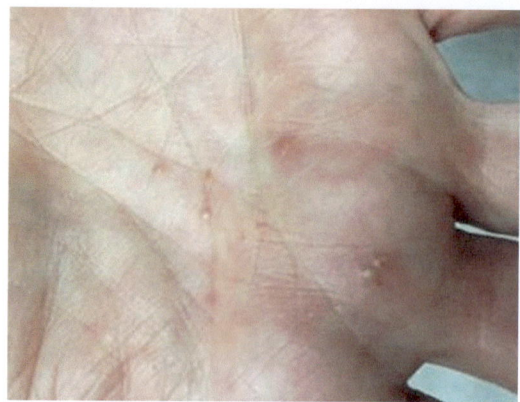

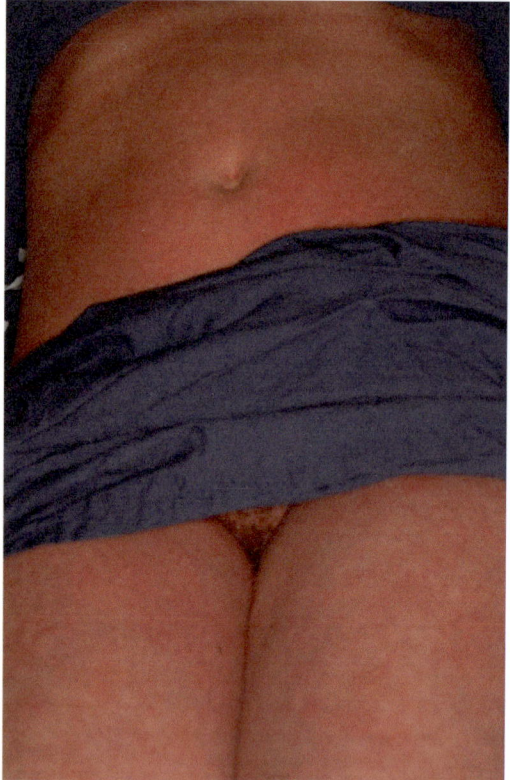

Fig. 1.13 Erythrodermic psoriasis: widespread erythroderma covers the majority of the body surface area

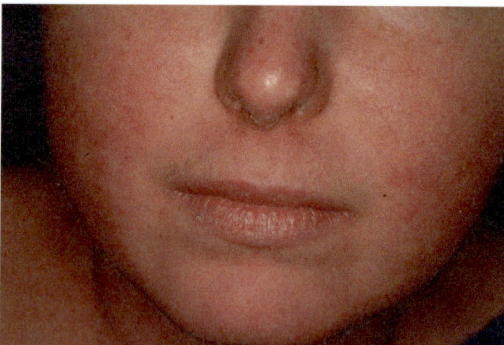

Fig. 1.14 Erythrodermic psoriasis: a close-up of the face
shows erythema with areas of desquamation

mon in psoriatic arthritis patients, occurring in up
to 90% of cases [6]. Many of the structures within
the nail unit can be affected, resulting in a broad
range of clinical presentations, include pitting,
onycholysis, "oil drop" spots, discoloration,
splinter hemorrhages, and subungual hyperkeratosis (Fig. 1.17).

Pitting is the most common nail finding in psoriasis. These superficial depressions in the nail
plate are caused by psoriatic lesions within the nail
matrix, resulting in parakeratotic foci in the nail
plate that slough off upon exposure to the environment. "Oil drop" or "salmon-colored" spots repre-
sent psoriatic lesions that are completely contained
within the nail bed of the affected nail. If the lesion
involves the hyponychium, onycholysis can occur.
Subungual hyperkeratosis results in the raising of
the nail plate off the nail bed secondary to deposits
of cells underneath the nail plate that have not
undergone desquamation. Leukonychia and ony-
chorrhexis (longitudinal ridges and splinting) may
also be seen in the nail plate. Splinter hemorrhages
occur secondary to rupture of capillaries in the
dermis of the nail bed. A variety of other dystro-
phic nail changes may also be found. Nail psoriasis is particularly difficult to treat and is often a
persistent condition [49].

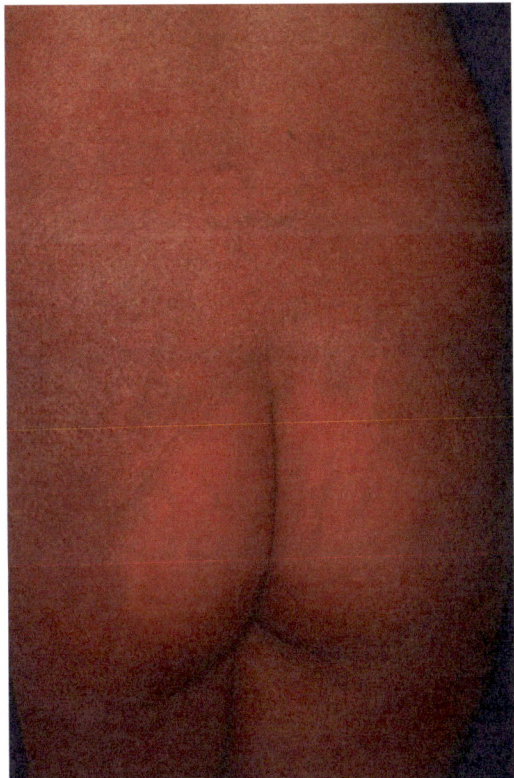

Fig. 1.15 Erythrodermic psoriasis: severe erythema can be observed

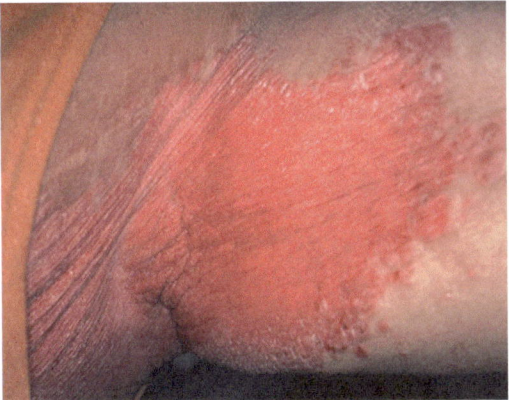

Fig. 1.16 Inverse psoriasis: an erythematous plaque in the axilla with minimal to no scale

Differential Diagnosis

The differential diagnosis of psoriasis is broad, depending on the patient's presentation. When the skin findings are characteristic with erythem-atous, sharply demarcated, scaling plaques found symmetrically on the extensor surfaces, the diagnosis is straightforward. Involvement of the skin in the periumbilical region and gluteal cleft and nail findings are clues to the diagnosis of psoriasis. However, the variants of psoriasis and atypical cases may present more diagnostic difficulty.

Common conditions on the differential diagnosis for plaque psoriasis include atopic dermatitis, nummular dermatitis, lichen simplex chronicus, pityriasis rosea, pitryiasis rubra pilaris, and tinea. If clinical diagnosis is unclear, a biopsy may be helpful. Drug reactions may also result in erythemato-papulosquamous psoriasiform eruptions. If this is a consideration, the presence of bright red lesions with intense pruritus and eosinophilia point more toward a drug eruption [35]. Mycosis fungoides can also present as inflammatory papulosquamous lesions and can be misdiagnosed as psoriasis.

In the differential diagnosis for scalp psoriasis, seborrheic dermatitis or tinea capitis may be considered. The lesions of psoriasis can be distinguished by the findings of well-demarcated, xerotic plaques with silvery scale, which may advance beyond the border of the hairline. Tinea can be distinguished from psoriasis by fungal culture, potassium hydroxide (KOH) preparation of skin scrapings, or histologically if a biopsy is performed [35, 45]. Palmoplantar psoriasis can also be confused with lichen simplex chronicus, lichen planus, secondary syphilis, hand dermatitis, or contact dermatitis. Clinical presentations of these conditions usually have distinct characteristics, but in unclear cases, a biopsy may be necessary to distinguish these conditions [35, 50].

Pustular psoriasis on the palms and the soles can resemble dyshidrotic eczema, irritant dermatitis, folliculitis, or allergic contact dermatitis. Infectious causes should also be ruled out. Work up may include cultures, KOH preparation, PAS or GRAM stains, and patch testing [35, 43]. Generalized pustular psoriasis may be mistaken for Stevens-Johnson syndrome (SJS) or toxic epidermal necrolysis (TEN) given the widespread erythema and desquamation [37]. Another important differential diagnosis is that of acute general-

Fig. 1.17 Onychody-
strophy due to psoriasis:
findings include nail
yellowing, onycholysis,
and subungual
hyperkeratosis

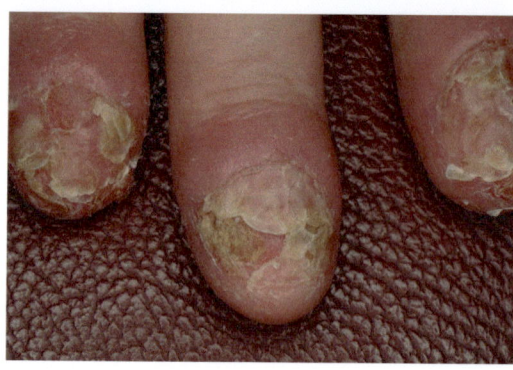

ized exanthematous pustulosis (AGEP), a febrile drug eruption also characterized by small sterile pustules on an erythematous base. The short latency period between drug administration and the skin reaction can help differentiate this from pustular psoriasis. Biopsy findings can also be helpful [35]. Subcorneal pustulosis is another consideration, but clinical and histological clues often help to differentiate the two [35].

The differential diagnosis for guttate psoriasis includes lymphomatoid papulosis, pityriasis rosea, pityriasis lichenoides chronica, tinea versicolor, and secondary syphilis, although these conditions often have distinctive presentations [35].

It is important to distinguish erythrodermic psoriasis from the other causes of generalized erythroderma, including drug reactions, atopic dermatitis, congenital ichthyoses, bullous dermatoses, cutaneous T cell lymphoma, and pityriasis rubra pilaris. If present, a prior personal or family history of psoriasis can be very helpful. Identifying the underlying etiology of erythroderma is difficult, and in many cases, even with biopsies and other tests, the cause is never identified [35].

In cases of inverse psoriasis, the differential diagnosis often includes fungal and bacterial infections. KOH examination of skin scrapings, Wood's lamp examination, and bacterial cultures are useful to rule out infections. Intertrigo secondary to skin friction can also be very similar in appearance to inverse psoriasis. Other causes of intertriginous plaques include Hailey-Hailey disease, flexural Darier disease, extra-mammary Paget's disease, Langerhans cell histiocytosis, and glucagonoma syndrome. These conditions

may be differentiated by clinical and histological findings, lab abnormalities, and systemic symptoms [35, 47].

The nail findings of psoriasis have a broad differential diagnosis. Pitting, a common feature of psoriatic nail disease, can also be seen in alopecia areata and contact dermatitis. However, the pitting seen in psoriasis is usually deeper than that seen in the other conditions. Oil spots can be seen in other inflammatory diseases, including systemic lupus erythematosus (SLE). Subungual hyperkeratosis can be seen in onychomycosis, pityriasis rubra pilaris, contact dermatitis, or with trauma. A positive KOH or nail culture would suggest onychomycosis; however, it is important to note that onychomycosis and nail psoriasis can occur concurrently. Lastly, onycholysis is also a feature of many other systemic, infectious, traumatic, or congenital syndromes [35].

Histopathology

As previously stated, a skin biopsy is not usually necessary to diagnose psoriasis. However, in the event that a biopsy is deemed necessary, certain key features can be seen. Classic histopathological findings of plaque psoriasis include hyperkeratosis, parakeratosis, loss of the granular cell layer, epidermal acanthosis, dilated and tortuous vasculature, and a leukocytic infiltrate [35]. The histology of uninvolved skin will be normal [17].

Hyperproliferation and impaired differentiation of keratinocytes are the two key features that lead to the skin findings of psoriatic plaques. This can be seen histologically as epidermal thicken-

Fig. 1.18 Histological findings of plaque psoriasis: epidermal hyperkeratosis and elongated, clubbed rete ridges are seen

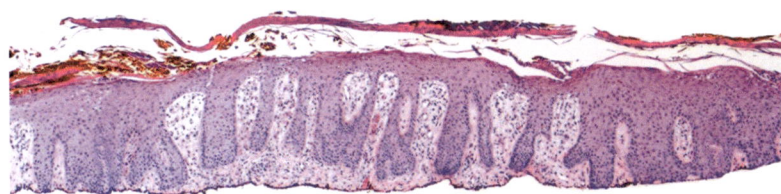

Fig. 1.19 Histological findings of plaque psoriasis: elongated, club-like rete ridges are visualized, along with dilatation and ectasia of the interdigitating dermal capillaries

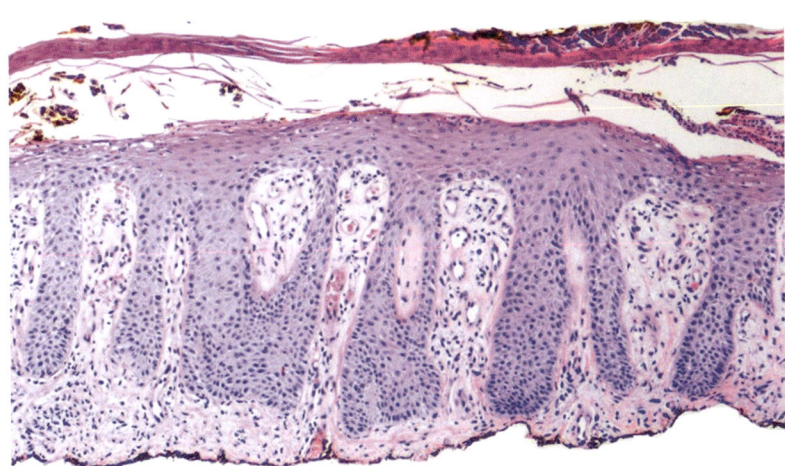

ing (hyperkeratosis) with regularly elongated rete ridges [51]. The rete ridges display increased thickening toward the tips, resulting in a club-like appearance (Fig. 1.18). The capillaries of the interdigitating dermal papillae will be dilated and tortuous (Fig. 1.19). Fine fibrillary collagen bundles can also be seen in the papillae. The suprapapillary plate is thinned, particularly in the stratum spinosum and stratum granulosum [45]. Terminal differentiation begins in the granular cell layer of the epidermis, which is absent in the areas subjacent to the observed parakeratosis. The stratum corneum therefore develops from keratinocytes that have not undergone normal differentiation, leading to the finding of parakeratosis (aberrant retention of nuclei in the stratum corneum) [45, 52] (Fig. 1.20). Orthokeratosis (hyperkeratosis without parakeratosis) is also often seen, alternating with areas of parakeratosis. Another finding related to hyperproliferation includes increased mitoses in the basal and suprabasal layer [45]. A mononuclear leukocytic infil-

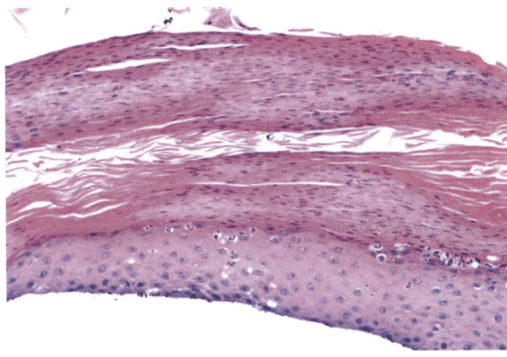

Fig. 1.20 Histological findings of plaque psoriasis: classic findings include hyperkeratosis, acanthosis, and parakeratosis of the epidermis

trate can be seen in the epidermis and dermis consisting of predominately lymphocytes [51].

Two key histological markers of psoriasis are the findings of foci of neutrophils in the parakeratotic stratum corneum, otherwise known as "Munro's microabscesses," and spongiform neutrophilic micropustules in the spinous layer of the

Fig. 1.21 Histological findings of plaque psoriasis: scattered collections of neutrophils are present within the stratum corneum, forming Munro's microabscesses

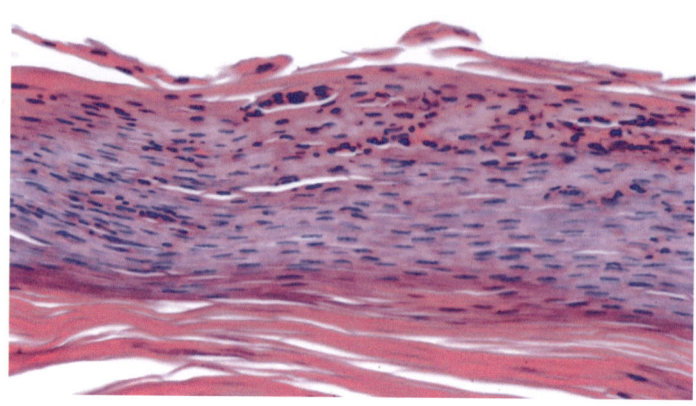

Fig. 1.22 Histological findings of plaque psoriasis: neutrophils replace keratinocytes in the epidermis, forming a classic spongiform pustule of Kogoj

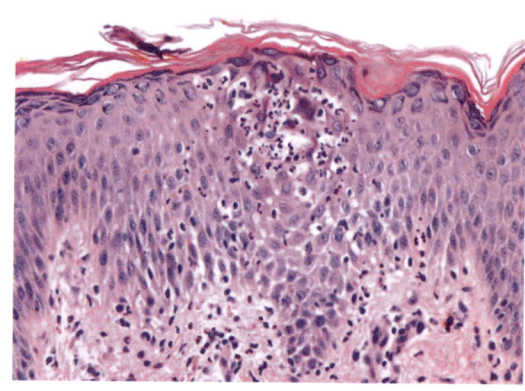

epidermis, termed "spongiform pustules of Kogoj" [45, 51] (Figs. 1.21 and 1.22). Munro's microabscesses are found commonly and can be seen in 75% of cases [45]. These features, along with dilated and tortuous dermal capillaries, are diagnostic for psoriasis, especially when combined with the findings detailed above [45].

It is important to note that the histopathologic features will vary depending on the stage of the lesion that is biopsied, and the histology described above for a typical psoriatic lesion may not be found in all cases. For example, biopsy of a very early lesion may show predominantly dermal changes including a mild perivascular lympho-cytic infiltrate, along with dilation and minimal tortuosity of the vasculature, in a background of a slight edema and spongiosis [45]. Once the lesion evolves, further changes can be seen, including

mild epidermal hyperplasia, mounds of parakera-tosis, ectatic superficial dermal vasculature, neu-trophilic exocytosis, and Munro's microabscesses with nearby hypogranulosis [45]. Conversely, a resolving plaque may show a decrease in neutro-phils, less parakeratosis and orthokeratosis, and a reforming granular cell layer. Key findings that may lead to the correct diagnosis in resolving psoriasis lesions include residual epidermal hyperplasia and dermal capillary dilatation and tortuosity [45] (Fig. 1.23).

The histopathology of pustular psoriasis is characterized by sterile intraepidermal pustules. These are analogous to the spongiform pustules of Kogoj but are larger than those seen in other forms of psoriasis. A mixed inflammatory infiltrate may be seen in the dermis (Figs. 1.24, 1.25, and 1.26). Munro's microabscesses can also form from neu-

Fig. 1.23 Histological findings of a partially treated psoriasis plaque: telangiectasias and ectatic vessels are still present. Thinning of the suprapapillary plate can be seen, along with some residual thickening of the epidermis. The neutrophilic infiltrate is less prominent compared to active psoriasis lesions

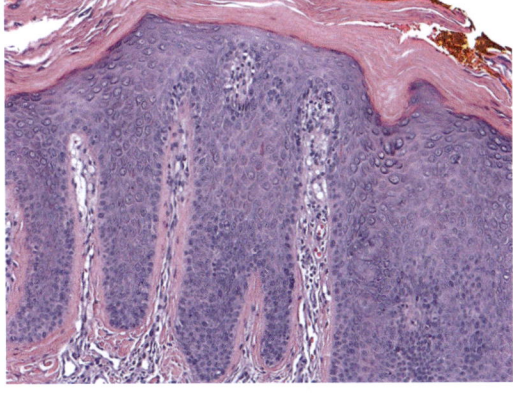

Fig. 1.24 Histological findings of pustular psoriasis with a prominent intraepidermal pustule

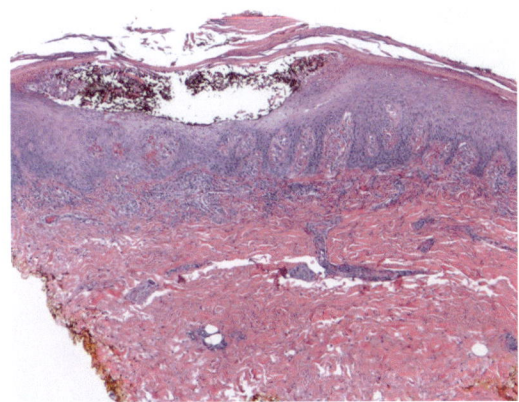

Fig. 1.25 Histological findings of pustular psoriasis: a spongiform pustule of Kogoj is observed near the intraepidermal pustule

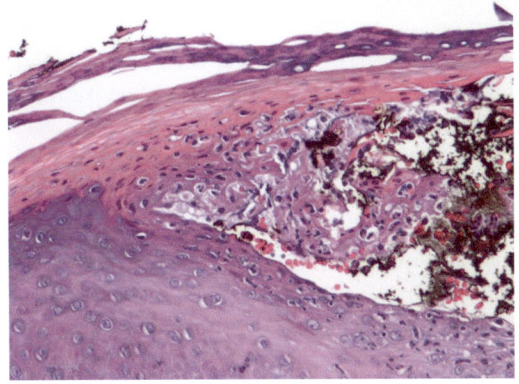

Fig. 1.26 Histological findings of pustular psoriasis: a mixed inflammatory infiltrate is seen in the dermis

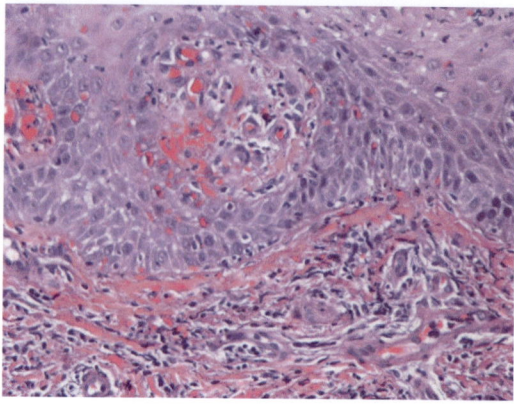

Fig. 1.27 Histological findings of pustular psoriasis: a subcorneal collection of neutrophils is present. A mixed inflammatory infiltrate is seen in the dermis

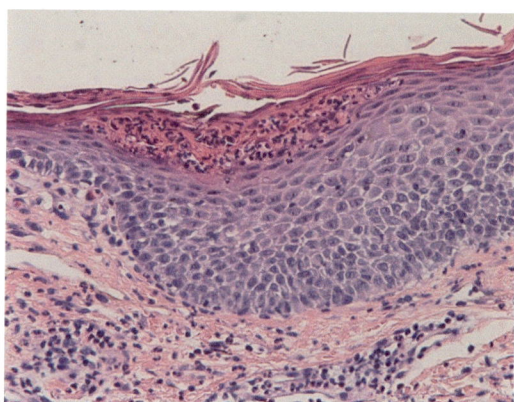

trophils that have made their way up to the stratum corneum (Fig. 1.27). In acute cases, the neutrophilic infiltrate occurs before any epidermal hyperplasia is seen, and thus the histologic changes associated with chronic plaque psoriasis will not be visualized [45].

In erythrodermic psoriasis, common histological changes include absence of the stratum corneum and an even more notable dilation of the dermal vasculature than that seen in plaque psoriasis. Some of the changes seen in early plaque psoriasis lesions may also be visualized. Overall, this is a difficult diagnosis to make, as the histological findings may be nonspecific. Often, multiple biopsies are required [45].

The histology of palmoplantar psoriasis is characterized by multiple foci of alternating parakeratosis and orthokeratosis with an inflammatory infiltrate [50]. Palmoplantar pustulosis

will show similar findings to those seen in generalized pustular psoriasis including epidermal sterile pustules. Other features that are typically seen in plaque psoriasis may also be seen, including mild acanthosis and parakeratosis [43].

References

1. Lebwohl MG, Bachelez H, Barker J, Girolomoni G, Kavanaugh A, Langley RG, Paul CF, Puig L, Reich K, van de Kerkhof PC. Patient perspectives in the management of psoriasis: results from the population-based Multinational Assessment of Psoriasis and Psoriatic Arthritis Survey. J Am Acad Dermatol. 2014;70(5):871–881.e871–830.
2. Rachakonda TD, Schupp CW, Armstrong AW. Psoriasis prevalence among adults in the United States. J Am Acad Dermatol. 2014;70(3):512–6.
3. Parisi R, Symmons DP, Griffiths CE, Ashcroft DM. Global epidemiology of psoriasis: a system-

atic review of incidence and prevalence. J Invest Dermatol. 2013;133(2):377–85.

4. Henseler T, Christophers E. Psoriasis of early and late onset: characterization of two types of psoriasis vulgaris. J Am Acad Dermatol. 1985;13(3):450–6.

5. Andressen C, Henseler T [Inheritance of psoriasis. Analysis of 2035 family histories]. Hautarzt. 1982;33(4):214–7.

6. Menter A, Gottlieb A, Feldman SR, van Voorhees AS, Leonardi CL, Gordon KB, Lebwohl M, Koo JYM, Elmets CA, Korman NJ, et al. Guidelines of care for the management of psoriasis and psoriatic arthritis: Section 1. Overview of psoriasis and guidelines of care for the treatment of psoriasis with biologics. J Am Acad Dermatol. 2008;58(5):826–50.

7. Krueger G, Koo J, Lebwohl M, Menter A, Stern RS, Rolstad T. The impact of psoriasis on quality of life: results of a 1998 National Psoriasis Foundation patient-membership survey. Arch Dermatol. 2001;137(3):280–4.

8. Pariser D, Schenkel B, Carter C, Farahi K, Brown TM, Ellis CN. A multicenter, non-interventional study to evaluate patient-reported experiences of living with psoriasis. J Dermatolog Treat. 2016;27(1):19–26.

9. Rapp SR, Feldman SR, Exum ML, Fleischer AB Jr, Reboussin DM. Psoriasis causes as much disability as other major medical diseases. J Am Acad Dermatol. 1999;41(3 Pt 1):401–7.

10. Lebwohl MG, Kavanaugh A, Armstrong AW, Van Voorhees AS. US perspectives in the Management of Psoriasis and Psoriatic Arthritis: patient and physician results from the population-based multinational assessment of psoriasis and psoriatic arthritis (MAPP) survey. Am J Clin Dermatol. 2016;17:87–97.

11. Gottlieb A, Korman NJ, Gordon KB, Feldman SR, Lebwohl M, Koo JYM, Van Voorhees AS, Elmets CA, Leonardi CL, Beutner KR, et al. Guidelines of care for the management of psoriasis and psoriatic arthritis: Section 2. Psoriatic arthritis: overview and guidelines of care for treatment with an emphasis on the biologics. J Am Acad Dermatol. 2008;58(5):851–64.

12. Sommer DM, Jenisch S, Suchan M, Christophers E, Weichenthal M. Increased prevalence of the metabolic syndrome in patients with moderate to severe psoriasis. Arch Dermatol Res. 2006;298(7):321–8.

13. Herron MD, Hinckley M, Hoffman MS, Papenfuss J, Hansen CB, Callis KP, Krueger GG. Impact of obesity and smoking on psoriasis presentation and management. Arch Dermatol. 2005;141(12):1527–34.

14. Higgins. Alcohol, smoking and psoriasis. Clin Exp Dermatol. 2000;25(2):107–10.

15. Gelfand JM, Neimann AL, Shin DB, Wang X, Margolis DJ, Troxel AB. RIsk of myocardial infarction in patients with psoriasis. JAMA. 2006;296(14):1735–41.

16. Mallbris L, Akre O, Granath F, Yin L, Lindelöf B, Ekbom A, Ståhle-Bäckdahl M. Increased risk for cardiovascular mortality in psoriasis inpatients but not in outpatients. Eur J Epidemiol. 2004;19(3):225–30.

17. Griffiths CEM, Barker JNWN. Pathogenesis and clinical features of psoriasis. The Lancet. 2007;370(9583):263–71.

18. Sheu J-J, Wang K-H, Lin H-C, Huang C-C. Psoriasis is associated with an increased risk of parkinsonism: a population-based 5-year follow-up study. J Am Acad Dermatol. 2013;68(6):992–9.

19. Mahil SK, Capon F, Barker JN. Update on psoriasis immunopathogenesis and targeted immunotherapy. Semin Immunopathol. 2016;38(1):11–27.

20. Basavaraj KH, Ashok NM, Rashmi R, Praveen TK. The role of drugs in the induction and/or exacerbation of psoriasis. Int J Dermatol. 2010;49(12):1351–61.

21. Gilleaudeau P, Vallat VP, Carter DM, Gottlieb AB. Angiotensin-converting enzyme inhibitors as possible exacerbating drugs in psoriasis. J Am Acad Dermatol. 1993;28(3):490–2.

22. Marquart-Elbaz C, Grosshans E, Lipsker D, Lipsker D. Sartans, angiotensin II receptor antagonists, can induce psoriasis. Br J Dermatol. 2002;147(3):617–8.

23. Brauchli YB, Jick SS, Curtin F, Meier CR. Association between beta-blockers, other antihypertensive drugs and psoriasis: population-based case-control study. Br J Dermatol. 2008;158(6):1299–307.

24. Schleicher SM. Psoriasis: pathogenesis, assessment, and therapeutic update. Clin Podiatr Med Surg. 2016;33(3):355–66.

25. Asumalahti K, Ameen M, Suomela S, Hagforsen E, Michaëlsson G, Evans J, Munro M, Veal C, Allen M, Leman J, et al. Genetic analysis of PSORS1 distinguishes guttate psoriasis and palmoplantar pustulosis. J Investig Dermatol. 2003;120(4):627–32.

26. Nair RP, Stuart PE, Nistor I, Hiremagalore R, Chia NVC, Jenisch S, Weichenthal M, Abecasis GR, Lim HW, Christophers E, et al. Sequence and haplotype analysis supports HLA-C as the psoriasis susceptibility 1 gene. Am J Hum Genet. 2006;78(5):827–51.

27. Tsoi LC, Stuart PE, Tian C, Gudjonsson JE, Das S, Zawistowski M, et al. Large scale meta-analysis characterizes genetic architecture for common psoriasis associated variants. Nat Commun. 2017;24(8):15392.

28. Elder JT, Bruce AT, Gudjonsson JE, Johnston A, Stuart PE, Tejasvi T, Voorhees JJ, Abecasis GR, Nair RP. Molecular dissection of psoriasis: integrating genetics and biology. J Investig Dermatol. 2010;130(5):1213–26.

29. Eberle F, Brück J, Holstein J, Hirahara K, Ghoreschi K. Recent advances in understanding psoriasis [version 1; referees: 2 approved]. F1000 Res. 2016:5.

30. Kim J, Krueger JG. The immunopathogenesis of psoriasis. Dermatol Clin. 2015;33(1):13–23.

31. Fredriksson T, Pettersson U. Severe psoriasis—oral therapy with a new retinoid. Dermatology. 1978;157(4):238–44.

32. Langley RG, Ellis CN. Evaluating psoriasis with psoriasis area and severity index, psoriasis global assessment, and lattice system physician's global assessment. J Am Acad Dermatol. 2004;51(4):563–9.

33. Nestle FO, Kaplan DH, Barker J. Psoriasis. N Engl J Med. 2009;361(5):496–509.

34. Raposo I, Torres T. Palmoplantar psoriasis and palmo-plantar pustulosis: current treatment and future prospects. Am J Clin Dermatol. 2016;17(4):349–58.

35. Lisi P. Differential diagnosis of psoriasis. Reumatismo. 2007;59(Suppl 1):56–60.

36. Martin BA, Chalmers RG, Telfer NR. HOw great is the risk of further psoriasis following a single episode of acute guttate psoriasis? Arch Dermatol. 1996;132(6):717–8.

37. Varman KM, Namias N, Schulman CI, Pizano LR. Acute generalized pustular psoriasis, von Zumbusch type, treated in the burn unit. A review of clinical features and new therapeutics. Burns. 2014;40(4):e35–9.

38. Matsubara M, Komori M, Koishi K, Yasuno H, Ueda K, Seto Y, Nonomura K. Generalized pustular psoriasis and bacteremia. J Dermatol. 1983;10(6):525–9.

39. Augey F, Renaudier P, Nicolas JF. Generalized pustular psoriasis (Zumbusch): a French epidemiological survey. Eur J Dermatol. 2006;16(6):669–73.

40. Sharkey MP, Muir JB. Staphylococcal scalded skin syndrome complicating acute generalized pustular psoriasis. Australas J Dermatol. 2002;43(3):199–201.

41. Pettey AA, Balkrishnan R, Rapp SR, Fleischer AB, Feldman SR. Patients with palmoplantar psoriasis have more physical disability and discomfort than patients with other forms of psoriasis: implications for clinical practice. J Am Acad Dermatol. 2003;49(2):271–5.

42. Sampogna F, Tabolli S, Söderfeldt B, Axtelius B, Aparo U, Abeni D, investigators IDIMPRoVE. Measuring quality of life of patients with different clinical types of psoriasis using the SF-36. Br J Dermatol. 2006;154(5):844–9.

43. Yamamoto T. Extra-palmoplantar lesions associated with palmoplantar pustulosis. J Eur Acad Dermatol Venereol. 2009;23(11):1227–32.

44. Goeckerman WH, O'Leary PA. Erythroderma psoriaticum: a review of twenty-two cases. J Am Med Assoc. 1932;99(25):2102–5.

45. Murphy M, Kerr P, Grant-Kels JM. The histopathologic spectrum of psoriasis. Clin Dermatol. 2007;25(6):524–8.

46. Green MS, Prystowsky JH, Cohen SR, Cohen JI, Lebwohl MG. Infectious complications of erythrodermic psoriasis. J Am Acad Dermatol. 1996; 34(5:911–4.

47. Syed ZU, Khachemoune A. Inverse psoriasis. Am J Clin Dermatol. 2011;12(2):143–6.

48. Fransson J, Storgards K, Hammar H. Palmoplantar lesions in psoriatic patients and their relation to inverse psoriasis, tinea infection and contact allergy. Acta Derm Venereol. 1985;65(3):218–23.

49. Jiaravuthisan MM, Sasseville D, Vender RB, Murphy F, Muhn CY. Psoriasis of the nail: anatomy, pathology, clinical presentation, and a review of the literature on therapy. J Am Acad Dermatol. 2007;57(1):1–27.

50. Aydin O, Engin B, Oğuz O, İlvan Ş, Demirkesen C. Non-pustular palmoplantar psoriasis: is histologic differentiation from eczematous dermatitis possible? J Cutan Pathol. 2008;35(2):169–73.

51. Raychaudhuri SK, Maverakis E, Raychaudhuri SP. Diagnosis and classification of psoriasis. Autoimmun Rev. 2014;13(4–5):490–5.

52. Lowes MA, Bowcock AM, Krueger JG. Pathogenesis and therapy of psoriasis. Nature. 2007;445(7130):866–73.

Topical Treatments

Caleb Jeon, Sahil Sekhon, Tina Bhutani,
and John Koo

Introduction

Psoriasis is a chronic inflammatory skin disease that affects 2–4% of the world's population. Approximately 80% of psoriasis patients have limited, localized mild-to-moderate disease where topical therapies serve as the mainstay of treatment. Topical therapies can provide both high efficacy as well as safety in this population. Furthermore, in patients with moderate-to-severe disease, short-term topical treatments may provide symptomatic relief, minimize doses of photo- or systemic therapy, and be of benefit for resistant lesions as part of a combination regimen. The aim of this chapter is to provide an evidence-based concise overview of the available topical treatments for chronic plaque psoriasis.

C. Jeon (✉) · S. Sekhon · T. Bhutani
Department of Dermatology, UCSF Psoriasis Center,
University of California San Francisco,
San Francisco, CA, USA
e-mail: Caleb.Jeon@ucsf.edu; caljeon@hawaii.edu;
sahil.sekhon@ucsf.edu; tina.bhutani@ucsf.edu

J. Koo
Department of Dermatology, Psoriasis and Skin
Treatment Center, University of California San
Francisco, San Francisco, CA, USA
e-mail: john.koo2@ucsf.edu

Topical Corticosteroids

Topical corticosteroids are the primary treatment option for psoriasis in the United States. At least three out of four psoriasis patients are treated with topical corticosteroids [1]. When individualized appropriately to a patient, they are fast-acting, highly effective, and relatively safe compared to other types of therapies (e.g., photo-, systemic, and biologic therapies). There are a great number of topical corticosteroid agents that can be categorized by potency, formulation (e.g., creams, ointments, lotions, sprays, etc.), or the combination of active agents (e.g., betamethasone plus calcipotriene). Thus, understanding the subtle yet dynamic differences of topical corticosteroid potencies and formulations can translate into flexibility and maximum therapeutic benefit to patients.

Mechanism of Action and Pharmacology

The mechanism of action of corticosteroids is both specific and nonspecific and involves modulation of the skin at multiple levels, including anti-inflammatory, immunosuppressive, vasoconstrictive, and antiproliferative effects. The pharmacological effects of topical and systemic corticosteroids are overall similar but differ in the amount of the effective dose of the drug delivered to the target organ and the enhanced effect of systemic corticosteroids

© Springer International Publishing AG, part of Springer Nature 2018
T. Bhutani et al. (eds.), *Evidence-Based Psoriasis*, Updates in Clinical Dermatology,
https://doi.org/10.1007/978-3-319-90107-7_2

on suppressing recruitment of immune cells from the blood and bone marrow [2]. Generally, topical corticosteroids have three essential abilities in the treatment of psoriasis: (1) suppression of localized immune response through local reduction in cytokines, (2) vasodilatory effects, and (3) slowing hyperproliferation of keratinocytes.

A corticosteroid is a fat-soluble molecule that can freely diffuse through the cell membrane and bind to a corticosteroid receptor in the cytoplasm. This complex of corticosteroid and its receptor then enters the nucleus where it alters gene transcription and expression of mRNA. This process leads to alteration in protein expression, including decrease in the production of cytokines (e.g., interleukin [IL]-1, IL-2, IL-6, and interferon [IFN]-α) [3]. Corticosteroids also decrease the production of key vasodilatory substances and consequently lead to vasoconstriction [4]. The ability of corticosteroids to decrease cytokines and vasodilatory substances lead to suppression of localized inflammation and further immune cell recruitment. The antiproliferative effect of topical corticosteroids is mediated by inhibition of DNA synthesis and mitosis and is known to reduce keratinocyte size and proliferation [5].

Topical corticosteroids are made in several formulations with varying potency that are appropriate for use in certain body sites. In the United States, the potency of corticosteroids is scaled I to VII in the Stoughton-Cornell classification based on their ability to cause vasoconstriction [6]. Table 2.1 summarizes the topical corticosteroids available in the United States by potency. While the potency of systemic corticosteroids generally translates into predictable clinical results dependent on their route of administration (e.g., oral or intramuscular injection), topical corticosteroids must penetrate the stratum corneum to reach their target cells. The penetration of the stratum corneum varies according to the body site due to differences in skin thickness and the vascular supply to the area. For example, inflamed, moist, or denuded skin areas have greater penetration than the skin of the scalp, palms, and soles. Therefore, while the inherent potency of topical corticosteroids is ranked based on their vasoconstrictive properties, this does not necessarily accurately predict the ability of a formulation to deliver the medication to a target

area. Furthermore, in addition to the skin barrier, the potency of topical corticosteroids is also affected by its chemical modification, its vehicle formulation, and its application (e.g., patient compliance and application with or without occlusion) (see Special Considerations below).

Efficacy

Superpotent (class I) topical corticosteroids are well established for effective treatment of mild-to-moderate plaque psoriasis [7–10]. Katz et al. showed that clobetasol-17-propionate and betamethasone dipropionate are effective in clearing or markedly improving psoriasis in 75–80% of patients after approximately 3 weeks [11]. Blum et al. demonstrated rapid onset of efficacy of halobetasol propionate 0.05% occurring within 5 days of initiating treatment. There was also clearance or marked improvement in 88% of patients over the course of 4 weeks compared to 64% of patients treated with betamethasone valerate [9]. Studies on the use of highly potent (class II) topical corticosteroids showed less efficacy in that only an average of 50% of patients achieved at least 75% improvement and less than 10% achieved clearance [8, 12, 13, 14].

Betamethasone dipropionate spray (Sernivo™) is a new mid-potent (class IV) formulation of betamethasone dipropionate 0.05% that has been recently approved for the treatment of mild-to-moderate psoriasis in 2016. When assessed using the Investigator's Global Assessment (IGA) and Total Severity Score (TSS) in phase III clinical trials, betamethasone dipropionate spray showed equivalent efficacy to augmented, superpotent formulation (lotion) of betamethasone dipropionate 0.05% and superiority to vehicle at day 15 (19% versus 18.9% and 2.3%, respectively) [15, 16]. These studies also showed superiority of this new medication in terms of its faster onset of action in improving erythema and scaling by day 4. Furthermore, improvements were also seen in locations that are typically difficult to treat such as the knees and elbows. The mid-potency designation suggests its superiority in safety and limited systemic absorption compared to superpotent topical corticosteroids.

Table 2.1 Topical corticosteroids available in the United States

Potency	Corticosteroid	Vehicle form	Trade name (United States)
Class I (superpotent)	Betamethasone dipropionate, augmented	Ointment	Diprolene
		Lotion	Diprolene
		Gel	Diprolene
	Clobetasol propionate	Ointment	Temovate
		Lotion	Clobex
		Gel	Temovate
		Cream	Temovate
		Cream, emollient based	Temovate E
		Foam, aerosol	Olux-E
		Foam, aerosol (scalp)	Olux
		Shampoo	Clobex
		Solution (scalp)	Temovate, Cormax
		Spray (aerosol)	Clobex
	Fluocinonide	Cream	Vanos
	Flurandrenolide	Tape (roll)	Cordran
	Halobetasol propionate	Ointment	Ultravate
		Lotion	Ultravate
		Cream	Ultravate
Class II (high potency)	Amcinonide	Ointment	Cyclocort[a], Amcort[a]
	Betamethasone dipropionate	Ointment	Diprosone
		Cream, augmented	Diprolene, augmented
	Desoximetasone	Ointment	Topicort
		Gel	Topicort
		Cream	Topicort
	Diflorasone diacetate	Ointment	ApexiCon[a], Florone[a]
		Cream, emollient	Apexicon E
	Fluocinonide	Ointment	Lidex[a]
		Gel	Lidex[a]
		Cream, anhydrous	Lidex[a]
		Solution	Lidex[a]
	Halcinonide	Ointment	Halog
		Cream	Halog
Class III (high potency)	Amcinonide	Lotion	Amcort[a]
		Cream	Cyclocort[a], Amcort[a]
	Betamethasone dipropionate	Cream, hydrophilic ointment	Diprosone
	Betamethasone valerate	Ointment	Valisone[a]
		Foam	Luxiq
	Desoximetasone	Cream	Topicort
	Diflorasone diacetate	Cream	Florone[a]
	Fluocinonide	Cream aqueous emollient	Lidex-E[a]
	Fluticasone propionate	Ointment	Cutivate
	Mometasone furoate	Ointment	Elocon
	Triamcinolone acetonide	Ointment	Kenalog[a]
		Cream	Triderm, Aristocort HP[a]

(continued)

Table 2.1 (continued)

Potency	Corticosteroid	Vehicle form	Trade name (United States)
Class IV (medium potency)	Betamethasone dipropionate	Spray	Sernivo
	Clocortolone pivalate	Cream	Cloderm
	Fluocinolone acetonide	Ointment	Synalar[a]
	Flurandrenolide	Ointment	Cordran
	Hydrocortisone valerate	Ointment	Westcort
	Mometasone furoate	Lotion	Elocon
		Cream	Elocon
		Solution	Elocon[a]
	Triamcinolone acetonide	Ointment	Kenalog[a]
		Cream	Kenalog[a]
		Aerosol spray	Kenalog
Class V (lower-mid-potency)	Betamethasone dipropionate	Lotion	Diprosone
	Betamethasone valerate	Cream	Beta-Val, Valisone[a]
	Desonide	Ointment	DesOwen, Tridesilon[a]
		Gel	Desonate
	Fluocinolone acetonide	Cream	Synalar[a]
	Flurandrenolide	Lotion	Cordran
		Cream	Cordran
	Fluticasone propionate	Lotion	Cutivate
		Cream	Cutivate
	Hydrocortisone butyrate	Ointment	Locoid
		Lotion	Locoid
		Lotion, spray	Cortizone 10 maximum
		Cream	Locoid, Locoid Lipocream
		Solution	Locoid
	Hydrocortisone probutate	Cream	Pandel
	Hydrocortisone valerate	Cream	Westcort[a]
	Prednicarbate	Ointment	Dermatop
		Cream, emollient	Dermatop
	Triamcinolone acetonide	Ointment	Kenalog[a]
		Lotion	Kenalog[a]
Class VI (low potency)	Aclometasone dipropionate	Ointment	Aclovate
		Cream	Aclovate
	Betamethasone valerate	Lotion	Beta-Val, Valisone
	Desonide	Lotion	DesOwen, Tridesilon
		Cream	DesOwen, LoKara
		Foam	Verdeso
	Fluocinonide acetonide	Cream	Synalar[a]
		Shampoo	Capex
		Solution	Synalar[a]
		Oil (scalp)	Derma-Smoothe/FS
		Oil (body)	Derma-smoothe/FS
	Triamcinolone acetonide	Lotion	Kenalog[a]
		Cream	Kenalog[a], Aristocort[a]

(continued)

Table 2.1   (continued)

Potency	Corticosteroid	Vehicle form	Trade name (United States)
Class VII (least potent)	Hydrocortisone (base, ≥2%)	Ointment	Hytone
		Lotion	Hytone, ala scalp, Scalacort
		Cream	Hytone[a], Nutracort[a]
		Solution	Texacort
	Hydrocortisone (base, <2%)	Ointment	Cortaid, Hytone, Nutracort
		Lotion	Aquanil HC, Sarnol-HC, Cortizone 10
		Cream	Cortaid, Hytone, Synacort
		Solution	Cortaid, Noble, scalp relief
		Spray	Cortaid
	Hydrocortisone acetate with pramoxine 1% combination	Ointment	Pramosone
		Lotion	Pramosone, Analpram-HC
		Cream	Pramosone, Analpram-HC
		Aerosol foam	Epifoam

[a]Inactive US trade name; the brand may be available outside the United States

Special Considerations

The choice of vehicle can significantly affect the use and penetration of topical corticosteroids and therefore translates to differences in efficacy. Patient compliance to topical therapy can be positively or negatively impacted depending on the topical agent's esthetic appeal. There are numerous types of vehicles including ointment, lotion, cream, shampoo, gel, solution, spray, foam, oil, and tape (see Table 2.1). Different vehicles are indicated for different body sites, but the optimal choice will generally be the vehicle that the patient is most likely to use (e.g., a patient may have a different preference of vehicle [shampoo, gel, solution, spray, or foam versus cream or ointment] for psoriasis on the scalp).

Occlusion of topical corticosteroids can also alter the penetration, thereby altering the effectiveness. For example, a lower-mid-potent (class V) topical corticosteroid, flurandrenolide 0.1%, has been shown to act as a superpotent topical corticosteroid when applied with tape [8].

Application

Generally, for thick psoriasis plaques on the extensor surfaces, super- or high-potency topical corticosteroids (e.g., betamethasone 0.05% or

Table 2.2   Side effects of topical corticosteroids

Cutaneous	Systemic
Irritation	HPA axis suppression
Burning	Cushing syndrome
Pruritus	Glaucoma
Atrophy of the skin	
Striae	
Telangiectasia	
Acneiform eruption	
Rosacea	
Perioral dermatitis	
Folliculitis	
Infection (bacterial, fungal)	
Contact dermatitis	
Hypopigmentation	
Purpura/ecchymoses	
Folliculitis	
Rebound of psoriasis	
Tachyphylaxis	

clobetasol propionate 0.05%) are needed. Low-potency cream (e.g., hydrocortisone 1%) is suitable for the face and intertriginous areas.

Side Effects

The risk of cutaneous and systemic side effects associated with long-term topical corticosteroid use increases with higher potency formulations (see Table 2.2). Thus, it is important to avoid excessive frequency, duration, or application of topical corticosteroids to sensitive areas such as the face or intertriginous areas.

Vitamin D Analogs

The vitamin D analogs include calcitriol and its synthetic derivatives calcipotriene (also called calcipotriol) and tacalcitol. Of these, only calcipotriene and calcitriol are available in the United States. Calcitriol is only available in ointment form, while calcipotriene can be found in solution, cream, ointment, foam, and gel suspension formulations. Calcipotriene is also available in combination with betamethasone in ointment, suspension, or foam formulations.

Mechanism of Action and Pharmacology

Although the mechanism of action of vitamin D analogs is not completely known, binding of these analogs to vitamin D receptors leads to inhibition of keratinocyte proliferation and enhancement of keratinocyte differentiation [17, 18]. In addition, vitamin D analogs have immunosuppressive properties including inhibition of production of several proinflammatory cytokines, including IL-2 and IFN-γ, that may be equally important to their anti-psoriatic effects [19, 20].

Vitamin D analogs are often used in combination with other topical agents including halobetasol propionate, tazarotene, and crude coal tar to maximize efficacy while reducing the risk of skin atrophy that is associated with chronic corticosteroid use [21, 22]. However, calcipotriene is a relatively unstable molecule that is inactivated by acidic substances, and as such, it is not compatible with some topical therapies used in psoriasis treatment such as salicylic acid. It is also known to be degraded to some extent in the presence of hydrocortisone valerate and ammonium lactate.

Efficacy

In randomized controlled trials, calcipotriene was found to be at least as effective as calcitriol, potent topical corticosteroids, hydrocortisone 0.5%, and coal tar [23]. Calcipotriene cream is less efficacious than ointment with efficacy comparable to betamethasone valerate and coal tar derivatives. However, many patients prefer to use the cream formulation on the body, and there is some evidence that patients are more likely to adhere to use of calcipotriene twice daily if they alternate between cream in the morning and ointment in the evening [24]. Monotherapy with calcipotriene foam is efficacious and is the preferred vehicle of calcipotriene in scalp psoriasis, with 40.9% of patients achieving clear or almost clear scalp after 8 weeks [25].

Side Effects

Skin irritation is the most common side effect of vitamin D analogs. This usually presents as lesional or perilesional burning, stinging, erythema, or scaling. Hypercalcemia is the only serious concern with the use of topical vitamin D preparations; however, this risk is minimized when using less than the recommended weekly maximum of 100 g of calcipotriene [26].

Combination Preparations with Corticosteroids

While mixing vitamin D analogs and corticosteroids is not always possible (due to the degradation of calcipotriene by some steroids as mentioned above), there are currently three stable combination preparations available in the United States: calcipotriene and betamethasone dipropionate ointment and suspension (Taclonex®) and calcipotriene and betamethasone dipropionate foam (Enstilar®).

The ointment, suspension, and foam preparations all contain calcipotriene 0.005% (equivalent to 50 µg/g) and betamethasone dipropionate 0.064% (equivalent to betamethasone 0.5 mg/g) and are indicated for the treatment of psoriasis in adults for up to four consecutive weeks [27]. When applied twice daily for 4 weeks, the combination ointment led to a greater mean Psoriasis Area and Severity Index (PASI) reduction (74.4%) than the individual components applied twice daily (betamethasone dipropionate 61.3% and calcipotriene ointment 55.3%) [28]. Once daily application of the combination ointment, which has been shown to lead to greater patient compliance than twice daily application, produced mean PASI reduction of 69–71% over 4 weeks [28, 29, 30].

The once daily application of the combination foam significantly reduced the mean modified PASI (mPASI) scores compared to once daily application of either individual component of calcipotriene or betamethasone foam alone (71% mean reduction versus 42% and 55%, respectively). Once daily application of the combination foam also achieved significantly greater PASI-75 response (≥75% improvement from the baseline PASI score) than either calcipotriene or betamethasone alone (49% versus 18% and 34%, respectively) [31]. The combination foam is efficacious not only on the body but also on the scalp. Compared to a gel formulation used for 8 weeks, the foam formulation of calcipotriol and betamethasone was more efficacious after just 4 weeks of treatment with a PASI-75 response rate of 52% versus 35% and a PASI-90 response rate of 22.2% versus 10.7% [32]. Furthermore, a greater proportion of patients using the foam reported that it was easier to apply and preferred it to their previous topical regimens. Once daily use of the foam formulation was more effective than the calcipotriol/betamethasone combination ointment in terms of treatment success rate and mPASI improvement (54.6% versus 43.0%). However, the PASI-75 and PASI-50 response rates were not statistically different between the foam versus ointment [33].

Based on above, the combination of a vitamin D analog and betamethasone dipropionate applied either once or twice daily in either ointment or foam vehicle appears to have superior efficacy compared to either component of the combinations applied as monotherapy.

Tazarotene

Tazarotene (Tazorac®) is a topical retinoid that was approved for treatment of psoriasis in 1997. It is available as a 0.1 and 0.05% gel and cream. While approved for use as a single agent, patients can often experience minimal effectiveness and significant local skin irritation that limits its use. The combination of this agent with other therapies (e.g., topical corticosteroids) has been used to minimize irritation and to increase efficacy, which has allowed tazarotene to become part of a long-term combination maintenance regimen. Tazarotene has also been used with ultraviolet (UV) B therapy for more rapid improvement, increased efficacy, and lower cumulative UV dosage exposure.

Mechanism of Action and Pharmacology

Tazarotene is a vitamin A-derived acetylene retinoid that selectively binds to the retinoic acid receptors (RARs) β and γ [34]. The active metabolite, tazarotenic acid, binds to RARs that leads to alteration of gene expression. The precise mechanism of action in psoriasis is unclear but may be related to both anti-inflammatory and antiproliferative actions (e.g., inhibition of transglutaminase expression and keratin 16 expression) [35].

A study by Hecker et al. demonstrated that tazarotene exhibits minimal degradation in vitro (<10%) when combined with a variety of topical corticosteroids and with calcipotriene [22]. It also did not appear to affect the stability of other compounds. A similar in vivo study analyzing tazarotene with these topical products in combination is needed.

Efficacy

Tazarotene gel at both 0.1 and 0.05% concentrations applied once daily has been shown to be similar in efficacy to fluocinonide 0.05% cream [36]. In one study, tazarotene 0.1% gel applied as a single agent once daily resulted in 70% of patients reaching the clinical endpoint of treatment success (≥75% improvement from baseline), with 41% maintaining significant improvement 12 weeks after stopping the drug [34]. When combining tazarotene with intermediate and superpotent topical corticosteroids, more rapid improvement, improved efficacy, and decreased irritation have been reported [37–39]. Combination of tazarotene and corticosteroids may also prevent atrophy [40, 41]. When combining tazarotene with calcipotriene, Bowman et al. showed comparable efficacy to clobetasol dipropionate 0.05% ointment [42]. Tazarotene has also been successfully combined with broadband and narrowband UVB for more rapid and effective clearing of psoriasis compared to either treatment alone [43–45].

Application

As monotherapy, tazarotene should be applied directly on the thick and scaly psoriatic lesions and the surrounding unaffected skin should be avoided. Application of tazarotene to sensitive areas such as the face and the neck may easily cause irritation. Genital areas should be avoided for the same reason. If significant irritation occurs, decreasing the frequency of application, starting at the lower 0.05% concentration and increasing the concentration as tolerated, switching formulations (e.g., gel to cream), or utilizing the "short-contact" method may be of benefit (Table 2.3) [46].

Side Effects

Application of tazarotene may lead to teratogenic systemic concentrations if applied to more than

Table 2.3 Tazarotene short-contact therapy

Apply tazarotene to plaques for a short time (5–20 min)
Wash medication off with water after prescribed time period
Gradually increase application time by 1–5 min as tolerated

20% of the total body surface area [47]. Therefore, women of childbearing potential must be cautioned of the risk before starting treatment. Adequate birth control measures must be utilized while on therapy.

Adverse local effects include a burning and stinging sensation, as well as peeling, erythema, and localized edema of the skin. This sensitivity occurs more commonly with the 0.1% concentration compared to 0.05% [46]. Burns and photosensitivity are of concern in those receiving UVB phototherapy and taking photosensitizing medications, respectively [50]. These patients should be cautioned to minimize sunlight exposure and to use sunscreens and protective clothing.

Calcineurin Inhibitors (Tacrolimus and Pimecrolimus)

Topical calcineurin inhibitors, tacrolimus 0.1% (Protopic®) and pimecrolimus 1% (Elidel®), have been shown to be effective in the treatment of psoriasis [48–51]. However, they are not officially FDA approved for the treatment of psoriasis and are commonly used off-label. Their use can be of benefit particularly in areas where topical corticosteroids should ideally be avoided (e.g., facial and intertriginous areas). Tacrolimus and pimecrolimus are available as topical therapy in ointment and cream formulations, respectively.

Mechanism of Action and Pharmacology

The mechanism of action of calcineurin inhibitors involves the reduction of T-cell proliferation through inhibition of calcineurin, a calcium- and calmodulin-dependent phosphatase enzyme [51, 52, 53]. This process inhibits the translocation of a family of transcription factors called nuclear factor of activated T cells (NFAT), leading to reduced transcriptional activation of cytokine genes, including IL-2, IL-3, IL-4, TNF-α, and IFN-γ.

Efficacy

Topical tacrolimus and pimecrolimus are generally well-tolerated when used to treat facial and intertriginous psoriasis and allow avoidance of chronic topical steroid use in these sensitive areas. However, it appears to be less effective in other areas, which may be due to differences in absorption.

In a clinical trial with tacrolimus 0.1% ointment, twice daily application to facial and intertriginous psoriasis lesions resulted in more patients achieving clear or almost clear psoriasis compared to placebo (65% versus 32%) [54]. Furthermore, the addition of 6% salicylic acid to tacrolimus 0.1% ointment has been shown to produce greater improvement of plaques than tacrolimus alone [55].

In a clinical trial with pimecrolimus 1% cream, twice daily application resulted in more patients achieving clear or almost clear inverse psoriasis compared with placebo (71% versus 21%) [56]. However, compared to topical corticosteroids, pimecrolimus appears to be less effective [57].

Application

A thin layer of tacrolimus 0.1% ointment or pimecrolimus 1% cream can be applied to the psoriatic lesions twice daily. Patients should be instructed to rub the ointment/cream gently and completely to the affected area. Burning and stinging is most common in the first few days of application but generally improve as the lesions improve. Application should continue as long as signs and symptoms persist and discontinued if resolution occurs.

Side Effects

Tacrolimus ointment and pimecrolimus cream are commonly associated with burning and stinging, particularly tacrolimus. There is also a black box warning regarding the possible link between topical calcineurin inhibitors and cases of lymphoma and skin cancer [58]. No definite causal relationship has been established, and subsequent studies have not found an increased incidence of lymphoma [59, 60].

Anthralin (Dithranol)

Topical anthralin (also known as dithranol) has been used effectively in the treatment of psoriasis since the early twentieth century. Anthralin is a synthesized version of the natural product chrysarobin, which comes from the South American araroba tree. Due to problem of staining and irritancy, anthralin has not been widely used as a first-line agent in treating psoriasis. Rather, it has been most commonly used in treating localized psoriasis plaques resistant to other therapies. It is approved for the treatment of chronic plaque-type psoriasis in the United States and is available as 1% and 1.2% creams and as a 1% shampoo.

Mechanism of Action and Pharmacology

Anthralin inhibits monocyte proinflammatory activity and induces extracellular generation of reactive oxygen species [61]. It also has an anti-Langerhans cell effects [62]. However, the precise mechanism of action of anthralin in psoriasis is not completely known. Its actions include the inhibition of DNA synthesis and a decrease in the mitotic rate of epidermal cells in psoriasis [63]. Anthralin also suppress the IFN-γ-induced upregulation of cytokeratin 17, which may be implicated in the pathogenesis of psoriasis [64].

Efficacy

Anthralin is typically used for short durations. Approximately 30% of psoriasis patients achieve clearance after an average of 5 weeks [65–67]. The efficacy of anthralin is increased when used in combination with other therapies.

Application

The adverse effects of anthralin, the permanent red-brown staining of clothing, and the temporary staining of the skin have limited the use of anthralin in the United States. As a result, the "short-contact anthralin therapy (SCAT) is often used in the outpatient setting where 1% or 1.2% anthralin is applied for 5–10 min per day." Subsequently, the application time is titrated up to 20–30 min as tolerated.

Side Effects

Skin irritation is a common side effect of anthralin and includes contact dermatitis, erythema, edema, and temporary staining of the hair, nails, and skin.

Salicylic Acid

Salicylic acid is a keratolytic agent that has been commonly used for the treatment of mild-to-moderate psoriasis for years. Its mechanism of action in psoriasis involves desquamation of hyperkeratotic epithelium via dissolution of the intercellular cement which causes thinning and scaling of the plaques [68]. Its use is limited as monotherapy since it only removes scales in the treatment of psoriasis. More commonly, salicylic acid is used as an adjunct to other topical medications. Although not commercially available as a compound with other types of topical agents, salicylic acid has been shown to increase the penetration and efficacy of topical corticosteroids, and the combination is overall more effective than either agent alone [69]. Salicylic acid can be used for the treatment of psoriasis as a 6% gel or shampoo and works well in combination with other psoriasis therapies including topical corticosteroids and coal tar. Of note, salicylic acid inactivates calcipotriol upon contact and blocks UVB; thus, it should not be used with calcipotriol or prior to UVB phototherapy [70]. Side effects of salicylic acid, such as tinnitus and fatigue, can occur if applied to >20% of the body surface area [76]. While rare, cases of hypoglycemia in diabetic patients have also been reported following the application of salicylic acid over a large surface area [76].

Coal Tar

Coal tar is the ancient modality of treating psoriasis, although its popularity has decreased since the development of newer and less messy topical treatment options. While long-existed as a treatment option for psoriasis, its mechanism of action is uncertain due to the countless ingredients in coal tar. However, clinically, it provides antipruritic, anti-inflammatory, and anti-psoriatic effects [71]. Coal tar can be found in several preparations, including ointment, lotion, cream, shampoo, gel, solutions, and soaps in multiple concentrations. Crude coal tar used in Goeckerman therapy includes 2, 5, and 10% concentrations. The Goeckerman therapy was first developed in 1925 and involves the application of crude coal tar to the entire body, including unaffected areas, for several hours a day along with UVB therapy.

Lactic Acid

Lactic acid is a less commonly used keratolytic agent for the treatment of psoriasis. This is an effective and useful second-line keratolytic agent when salicylic acid is not an option. It is commonly used in diabetic patients when salicylate toxicity is a concern. It has been shown that hairless mice exhibit increased desquamation of normal skin when this agent is applied [72].

References

1. Pearce DJ, Stealey KH, Balkrishnan R, ABJ F, Feldman SR. Psoriasis treatment in the United States at the end of the 20th century. Int J Dermatol. 2006;45(4):370–4.
2. Leung DY, Bloom JW. Update on glucocorticoid action and resistance. J Allergy Clin Immunol. 2003;111:3–22.

3. Kragballe K. Topical corticosteroids: mechanisms of action. Acta Derm Venereol Suppl (Stockh). 1989;151:7–10.

4. van de Kerkhof PCM, Vissers WHPM. The topical treatment of psoriasis. Skin Pharmacol Appl Ski Physiol. 2003;16(2):69–83.

5. Almawi WY, Saouda MS, Stevens AC, Lipman ML, Barth CM, Strom TB. Partial mediation of glucocorticoid antiproliferative effects by lipocortins. J Immunol. 1996;157(12):5231–9.

6. Cornell RC, Stoughton RB. Correlation of the vasoconstriction assay and clinical activity in psoriasis. Arch Dermatol. 1985;121(1):63–7.

7. Krueger GG, O'Reilly MA, Weidner M, Dromgoole SH, Killey FP. Comparative efficacy of once-daily flurandrenolide tape versus twice-daily diflorasone diacetate ointment in the treatment of psoriasis. J Am Acad Dermatol. 1998;38(2 Pt 1):186–90.

8. Katz HI, Gross E, Buxman M, Prawer SE, Schwartzel EH, Gibson JR. A double-blind, vehicle-controlled paired comparison of halobetasol propionate cream on patients with plaque psoriasis. J Am Acad Dermatol. 1991;25(6 Pt 2):1175–8.

9. Blum G, Yawalkar S. A comparative, multicenter, double blind trial of 0.05% halobetasol propionate ointment and 0.1% betamethasone valerate ointment in the treatment of patients with chronic, localized plaque psoriasis. J Am Acad Dermatol. 1991;25(6 Pt 2):1153–6.

10. Goldberg B, Hartdegen R, Presbury D, Smith EH, Yawalkar S. A double-blind, multicenter comparison of 0.05% halobetasol propionate ointment and 0.05% clobetasol propionate ointment in patients with chronic, localized plaque psoriasis. J Am Acad Dermatol. 1991;25(6 Pt 2):1145–8.

11. Katz HI, Hien NT, Prawer SE, Mastbaum LI, Mooney JJ, Samson CR. Superpotent topical steroid treatment of psoriasis vulgaris--clinical efficacy and adrenal function. J Am Acad Dermatol. 1987;16(4):804–11.

12. Bruce S, Epinette WW, Funicella T, Ison A, Jones EL, Loss RJ, et al. Comparative study of calcipotriene (MC 903) ointment and fluocinonide ointment in the treatment of psoriasis. J Am Acad Dermatol. 1994;31(5 Pt 1):755–9.

13. Molin L, Cutler TP, Helander I, Nyfors B, Downes N. Comparative efficacy of calcipotriol (MC903) cream and betamethasone 17-valerate cream in the treatment of chronic plaque psoriasis. A randomized, double-blind, parallel group multicentre study. Calcipotriol study group. Br J Dermatol. 1997;136(1):89–93.

14. Tristani-Firouzi P, Krueger GG. Efficacy and safety of treatment modalities for psoriasis. Cutis. 1998;61(2 Suppl):11–21.

15. Diprolene® lotion (augmented betamethasone dipropionate 0.05%) product information. Kenilworth, NJ:Schering Corp; 1999.

16. Fowler JF Jr, Hebert AA. Sugarman J.DFD-01, a novel medium potency betamethasone dipropionate 0.05% emollient spray, demonstrates similar efficacy to augmented betamethasone dipropionate 0.05% lotion for the treatment of moderate plaque psoriasis. J Drugs Dermatol. 2016;15(2):154–62.

17. Menter A, Korman NJ, Elmets CA, Feldman SR, Gelfand JM, Gordon KB, et al. Guidelines of care for the management of psoriasis and psoriatic arthritis. Section 3. Guidelines of care for the management and treatment of psoriasis with topical therapies. J Am Acad Dermatol. 2009;60(4):643–59.

18. Rizova E, Corroller M. Topical calcitriol--studies on local tolerance and systemic safety. Br J Dermatol. 2001;144(Suppl 58):3–10.

19. Kragballe K. Treatment of psoriasis with calcipotriol and other vitamin D analogues. J Am Acad Dermatol. 1992;27(6 Pt 1):1001–8.

20. Barna M, Bos JD, Kapsenberg ML, Snijdewint FG. Effect of calcitriol on the production of T-cell-derived cytokines in psoriasis. Br J Dermatol. 1997;136(4):536–41.

21. Patel B, Siskin S, Krazmien R, Lebwohl M. Compatibility of calcipotriene with other topical medications. J Am Acad Dermatol. 1998;38(6 Pt 1):1010–1.

22. Hecker D, Worsley J, Yueh G, Lebwohl M. In vitro compatibility of tazarotene with other topical treatments of psoriasis. J Am Acad Dermatol. 2000;42(6):1008–11.

23. Ashcroft DM, Po AL, Williams HC, Griffiths CE. Systematic review of comparative efficacy and tolerability of calcipotriol in treating chronic plaque psoriasis. BMJ. 2000;320(7240):963–7.

24. van de Kerkhof PC, Franssen M, de La Brassine M, Kuipers M. Calcipotriol cream in the morning and ointment in the evening: a novel regimen to improve compliance. J Dermatolog Treat. 2001;12(2):75–9.

25. Feldman SR, Mills M, Brundage T, Eastman WJ. A multicenter, randomized, double-blind study of the efficacy and safety of calcipotriene foam, 0.005%, vs vehicle foam in the treatment of plaque-type psoriasis of the scalp. J Drugs Dermatol. 2013;12(3):300–6.

26. Mortensen L, et al. Treatment of psoriasis vulgaris with topical calcipotriol has no short-term effect on calcium or bone metabolism. A randomized, double-blind, placebo-controlled study. Acta Derm Venereol. 1993;73(4):300–4.

27. Traulsen J. Bioavailability of betamethasone dipropionate when combined with calcipotriol. Int J Dermatol. 2004;43(8):611–7.

28. Douglas WS, Poulin Y, Decroix J, Ortonne JP, Mrowietz U, Gulliver W, et al. A new calcipotriol/betamethasone formulation with rapid onset of action was superior to monotherapy with betamethasone dipropionate or calcipotriol in psoriasis vulgaris. Acta Derm Venereol. 2002;82(2):131–5.

29. Kaufmann R, Bibby AJ, Bissonnette R, Cambazard F, Chu AC, Decroix J, et al. A new calcipotriol/betamethasone dipropionate formulation (Daivobet) is an effective once-daily treatment for psoriasis vulgaris. Dermatology. 2002;205(4):389–93.

30. Guenther L, Van de Kerkhof PCM, Snellman E, Kragballe K, Chu AC, Tegner E, et al. Efficacy and

safety of a new combination of calcipotriol and betamethasone dipropionate (once or twice daily) compared to calcipotriol (twice daily) in the treatment of psoriasis vulgaris: a randomized, double-blind, vehicle-controlled clinical trial. Br J Dermatol. 2002;147(2):316–23.

31. Lebwohl M, Tyring S, Bukhalo M, Alonso-Llamazares J, Olesen M, Lowson D, et al. Fixed combination aerosol foam Calcipotriene 0.005% (Cal) plus betamethasone Dipropionate 0.064% (BD) is more efficacious than Cal or BD aerosol foam alone for psoriasis vulgaris: a randomized, double-blind, multicenter, three-arm, phase 2 study. J Clin Aesthet Dermatol. 2016;9(2):34–41.

32. Paul C, Stein Gold L, Cambazard F, Kalb RE, Lowson D, Bang B, et al. Calcipotriol plus betamethasone dipropionate aerosol foam provides superior efficacy vs. gel in patients with psoriasis vulgaris: randomized, controlled. J Eur Acad Dermatol Venereol. 2017;31(1):119–26.

33. Koo J, Tyring S, Werschler WP, Bruce S, Olesen M, Villumsen J, et al. Superior efficacy of calcipotriene and betamethasone dipropionate aerosol foam versus ointment in patients with psoriasis vulgaris--a randomized phase II study. J Dermatolog Treat. 2016;27(2):120–7.

34. Krueger GG, Drake LA, Elias PM, Lowe NJ, Guzzo C, Weinstein GD, et al. The safety and efficacy of tazarotene gel, a topical acetylenic retinoid, in the treatment of psoriasis. Arch Dermatol. 1998;134(1):57–60.

35. Duvic M, Asano AT, Hager C, Mays S. The pathogenesis of psoriasis and the mechanism of action of tazarotene. J Am Acad Dermatol. 1998;39(4 Pt 2):S129–33.

36. Lebwohl M, Ast E, Callen JP, Cullen SI, Hong SR, Kulp-Shorten CL, et al. Once-daily tazarotene gel versus twice-daily fluocinonide cream in the treatment of plaque psoriasis. J Am Acad Dermatol. 1998;38(5 Pt 1):705–11.

37. Koo JY, Martin D. Investigator-masked comparison of tazarotene gel q.D. Plus mometasone furoate cream q.D. vs. mometasone furoate cream b.I.D. In the treatment of plaque psoriasis. Int J Dermatol. 2001;40(3):210–2.

38. Lebwohl M, Poulin Y. Tazarotene in combination with topical corticosteroids. J Am Acad Dermatol. 1998;39(4 Pt 2):S139–43.

39. Lesnik RH, Mezick JA, Capetola R, Kligman LH. Topical all-trans-retinoic acid prevents corticosteroid-induced skin atrophy without abrogating the anti-inflammatory effect. J Am Acad Dermatol. 1989;21(2 Pt 1):186–90.

40. Smith EL, Walworth NC, Holick MF. Effect of 1 alpha,25-dihydroxyvitamin D3 on the morphologic and biochemical differentiation of cultured human epidermal keratinocytes grown in serum-free conditions. J Invest Dermatol. 1986;86(6):709–14.

41. Lebwohl M, Lombardi K, Tan MH. Duration of improvement in psoriasis after treatment with tazarotene 0.1% gel plus clobetasol propionate 0.05% ointment: comparison of maintenance treatments. Int J Dermatol. 2001;40(1):64–6.

42. Bowman PH, Maloney JE, Koo JYM. Combination of calcipotriene (Dovonex) ointment and tazarotene (Tazorac) gel versus clobetasol ointment in the treatment of plaque psoriasis: a pilot study. J Am Acad Dermatol. 2002;46(6):907–13.

43. Lowe NJ. Optimizing therapy: tazarotene in combination with phototherapy. Br J Dermatol. 1999;140(Suppl 54):8–11.

44. Koo JY, Lowe NJ, Lew-Kaya DA, Vasilopoulos AI, Lue JC, Sefton J, et al. Tazarotene plus UVB phototherapy in the treatment of psoriasis. J Am Acad Dermatol. 2000;43(5 Pt 1):821–8.

45. Behrens S, Grundmann-Kollmann M, Schiener R, Peter RU, Kerscher M. Combination phototherapy of psoriasis with narrow-band UVB irradiation and topical tazarotene gel. J Am Acad Dermatol. 2000;42(3):493–5.

46. Veraldi S, Caputo R, Pacifico A, Peris K, Soda R, Chimenti S. Short contact therapy with tazarotene in psoriasis vulgaris. Dermatology. 2006;212(3):235–7.

47. Tazorac® gel product information. Irvine: Allergan Plc; 1997.

48. Freeman AK, Linowski GJ, Brady C, Lind L, Vanveldhuisen P, Singer G, et al. Tacrolimus ointment for the treatment of psoriasis on the face and intertriginous areas. J Am Acad Dermatol. 2003;48(4):564–8.

49. Wilsmann-Theis D, Hagemann T, Dederer H, Wenzel J, Bieber T, Novak N. Successful treatment of acrodermatitis continua suppurativa with topical tacrolimus 0.1% ointment. Br J Dermatol. 2004;150(6):1194–7.

50. Mrowietz U, Wustlich S, Hoexter G, Graeber M, Brautigam M, Luger T. An experimental ointment formulation of pimecrolimus is effective in psoriasis without occlusion. Acta Derm Venereol. 2003;83(5):351–3.

51. Yamamoto T, Nishioka K. Topical tacrolimus: an effective therapy for facial psoriasis. Eur J Dermatol. 2003;13(5):471–3.

52. Wiederrecht G, Lam E, Hung S, Martin M, Sigal N. The mechanism of action of FK-506 and cyclosporin a. Ann N Y Acad Sci. 1993;696:9–19.

53. Klintmalm GB. FK 506: an update. Clin Transpl. 1994;8(2 Pt 2):207–10.

54. Lebwohl M, Freeman AK, Chapman MS, Feldman SR, Hartle JE, Henning A. Tacrolimus ointment is effective for facial and intertriginous psoriasis. J Am Acad Dermatol. 2004;51(5):723–30.

55. Carroll CL, Clarke J, Camacho F, Balkrishnan R, Feldman SR. Topical tacrolimus ointment combined with 6% salicylic acid gel for plaque psoriasis treatment. Arch Dermatol. 2005;141(1):43–6.

56. Gribetz C, Ling M, Lebwohl M, Pariser D, Draelos Z, Gottlieb AB, et al. Pimecrolimus cream 1% in the treatment of intertriginous psoriasis: a double-blind, randomized study. J Am Acad Dermatol. 2004;51(5):731–8.

57. Kreuter A, Sommer A, Hyun J, Brautigam M, Brockmeyer NH, Altmeyer P, et al. 1% pimecrolimus, 0.005% calcipotriol, and 0.1% betamethasone in the treatment of intertriginous psoriasis: a double-blind, randomized controlled study. Arch Dermatol. 2006;142(9):1138–43.

58. Center for Drug Evaluation and Research. Postmarket Drug Safety Information for Patients and Providers—Public Health Advisory for Elidel and Protopic (3/10/2005). U Public Health Advisory for Elidel and Protopic. Center for Drug Evaluation and Research, 10 Mar. 2015. Web. 18 May 2017. https://www.fda.gov/Drugs/DrugSafety/PostmarketDrugSafetyInformationforPatientsandProviders/ucm153956.htm

59. Siegfried EC, Jaworski JC, Hebert AA. Topical calcineurin inhibitors and lymphoma risk: evidence update with implications for daily practice. Am J Clin Dermatol. 2013;14(3):163–78.

60. Tennis P, Gelfand JM, Rothman KJ. Evaluation of cancer risk related to atopic dermatitis and use of topical calcineurin inhibitors. Br J Dermatol. 2011;165(3):465–73.

61. Schmidt KN, Podda M, Packer L, Baeuerle PA. Antipsoriatic drug anthralin activates transcription factor NF-kappa B in murine keratinocytes. J Immunol. 1996;156(11):4514–9.

62. Morhenn VB, Orenberg EK, Kaplan J, Pfendt E, Terrell C, Engleman EG. Inhibition of a Langerhans cell-mediated immune response by treatment modalities useful in psoriasis. J Invest Dermatol. 1983;81(1):23–7.

63. Klem EB. Effects of antipsoriasis drugs and metabolic inhibitors on the growth of epidermal cells in culture. J Invest Dermatol. 1978;70(1):27–32.

64. Bonnekoh B, Bockelmann R, Ambach A, Gollnick H. Dithranol and dimethylfumarate suppress the interferon-gamma-induced up-regulation of cytokeratin 17 as a putative psoriasis autoantigen in vitro. Skin Pharmacol Appl Ski Physiol. 2001;14(4):217–25.

65. Schaefer H, Farber EM, Goldberg L, Schalla W. Limited application period for dithranol in psoriasis. Preliminary report on penetration and clinical efficacy. Br J Dermatol. 1980;102(5):571–3.

66. Goransson A. Comparison of dithranol and butantrone in short contact therapy of psoriasis. Acta Derm Venereol. 1987;67(2):149–53.

67. Statham BN, Ryatt KS, Rowell NR. Short-contact dithranol therapy—a comparison with the Ingram regime. Br J Dermatol. 1984;110(6):703–8.

68. Lebwohl M. The role of salicylic acid in the treatment of psoriasis. Int J Dermatol. 1999;38(1):16–24.

69. Koo J, Cuffie CA, Tanner DJ, Bressinck R, Cornell RC, DeVillez RL, et al. Mometasone furoate 0.1% salicylic acid 5% ointment versus mometasone furoate 0.1% ointment in the treatment of moderate-to-severe psoriasis: a multicenter study. Clin Ther. 1998;20(2):283–91.

70. Koo JY, Lebwohl MG, Lee CS, editors. Mild-to-Moderate psoriasis. New York: CRC Press; 2006.

71. Arnold WP. Tar. Clin Dermatol. 1997;15(5):739–44.

72. Kim TH, Choi EH, Kang YC, Lee SH, Ahn SK. The effects of topical alpha-hydroxy acids on the normal skin barrier of hairless mice. Br J Dermatol. 2001;144(2):267–73.

Phototherapy and Photochemotherapy

3

James L. Griffith, Allison J. Zarbo, and Henry W. Lim

Introduction

Since the start of its use over 3000 years ago, ultraviolet (UV)-based therapy has remained a cornerstone in the management of cutaneous conditions. It first attained this status when ancient Hindu and Egyptian healers discovered the synergistic effects of ambient sunlight and psoralen-containing plants in the repigmentation of vitiligo [1]. Over the subsequent centuries, this photochemotherapy began to be used in other conditions and continents. However, significant advances in the field of photomedicine did not occur until the early twentieth century with the advent of artificial UV lamps.

Shortly after Niels Finsen introduced artificial UV radiation (UVR) to the management of cutaneous disease, the field of photomedicine began to rapidly advance. In 1925, Goeckerman revolutionized the treatment of psoriasis by incorporating crude coal tar with UV light therapy [2]; this was later modified by Ingram with the substitution of anthralin (dithranol) for coal tar [3, 4]. With the subsequent development of the broadband UVB (BB-UVB) light source, BB-UVB phototherapy became an important treatment modality for psoriasis. As the light sources continued to improve, refinements in photosensitizers also occurred. Fahmy et al. isolated crystalline methoxsalen, 8-methoxsalen (8-MOP) and 5-methoxsalen (5-MOP), from the plant *Ammi majus Linnaeus* [5, 6]. This advancement was later utilized by Parish et al., who reported the successful treatment of psoriasis with oral 8-MOP and a newly developed, high-intensity UVA lamp in 1974 [7, 8]. This marked the development of what would later be termed psoralen plus ultraviolet A (PUVA) photochemotherapy. In 1982, the US Food and Drug Administration (FDA) approved the use of PUVA in the management of cutaneous psoriasis. With PUVA exhibiting superior efficacy over BB-UVB, more efficacious forms of UVB, including narrowband UVB (NB-UVB) and excimer laser, were developed as treatment options for psoriasis in 1988 and 1997, respectively [9–11]. More recently, two visible light therapies, pulsed dye laser and photodynamic therapy, have also been utilized in the management of psoriasis with varying degrees of efficacy [12, 13].

This chapter will include a brief review of the basic principles behind photomedicine before presenting a more thorough discussion of PUVA, NB-UVB, targeted UV phototherapies, pulsed dye laser, photodynamic therapy, and future directions of phototherapy in the management of psoriasis. For the purposes of this discussion, devices irradiating a significant portion of one's body surface area (BSA), such as a standing light box, will be considered conventional phototherapy

J. L. Griffith · A. J. Zarbo · H. W. Lim (✉)
Department of Dermatology, Henry Ford Hospital, Detroit, MI, USA
e-mail: azarbo2@hfhs.org; HLIM1@hfhs.org

© Springer International Publishing AG, part of Springer Nature 2018
T. Bhutani et al. (eds.), *Evidence-Based Psoriasis*, Updates in Clinical Dermatology,
https://doi.org/10.1007/978-3-319-90107-7_3

devices, while those that limit irradiation to a localized anatomical area or psoriatic lesion will be termed targeted phototherapy.

Basic Principles of Photomedicine and Photochemistry

Phototherapy is the therapeutic use of nonionizing electromagnetic radiation to induce a biologic response in irradiated tissue. Therapies are classified by the spectrum of their electromagnetic radiation (Table 3.1). Wavelengths within each spectrum display distinct, major photobiologic responses; however, overlaps do occur. For example, UVB is more effective than UVA in producing erythema, deoxyribonucleic acid (DNA) photodamage, and urocanic acid photoisomerization. UVA is more effective in producing immediate pigment darkening and delayed tanning; however, it also contributes to photocarcinogenesis [14–21]. If a photosensitizing chemical, such as psoralen, is added to modulate the photobiologic reaction, the therapy is termed photochemotherapy. When aminolevulinic acid (ALA) is used as part of the treatment, the term photodynamic therapy is preferred to reflect the essential requirement of oxygen in the process. Absorption of photons by the target molecule (i.e., chromophore) can result in the production of heat, emission of fluorescence, or change in the target molecule's chemical structure. The degree of these reactions depends upon several variables, including the wavelength(s) of radiation,

total energy delivered, and rate at which this energy is delivered.

Each wavelength has its own unique probability of being absorbed by molecules within the tissue. Molecules capable of absorbing photons from nonionizing radiation are known as chromophores. Most chromophores absorb photons across a wavelength range but retain one wavelength where the photons are most efficiently absorbed, known as the absorption maxima. For example, NADH can absorb UVB and UVA wavelengths, but displays an absorption maxima of 340 nm; protoporphyrin IX absorbs photons along a broad range of the visible light (VL) spectrum, but it absorbs most intensely at 405 nm with smaller peaks at 510, 545, 580, and 630 nm [22]. VL is also absorbed by riboflavin, hemoglobin, and bilirubin, while melanin absorbs UVB, UVA, and VL without displaying an absorption maxima. It should be noted that the absorption maxima does not necessarily equate to the specific chromophore's associated action spectrum, which is the spectrum that induces a biologic response; this difference is due to the effect of other chromophores within the tissue. For example, although purine and pyrimidine bases in DNA and RNA have an in vitro absorption maxima of 260 nm, the in vivo peak is approximately 300 nm because of the optical screening properties of other chromophores in the epidermis [17].

The degree of erythema and other photobiologic responses is usually proportional to the dose (fluence) and rate of energy delivered (power). While this generalization appears to remain true for UV radiation, recent evidence indicates that some wavelengths may incur greater photobiologic responses at lower powers; this understanding is the basis for low-level laser therapies. Similarly, visible light, which was once thought to be biologically inert, can induce greater levels of immediate and persistent pigment darkening than UV radiation. Visible light's therapeutic utility in the management of psoriasis is discussed later in this chapter [23–27].

While lamps in UV medical devices generally emit a narrow or broad spectrum of wavelengths peaking around a specific wavelength, xenon chloride excimer laser devices emit only

Table 3.1 Spectrums of radiation and their corresponding wavelengths

Spectrum of radiation	Abbreviation	Wavelength (nm)
Broadband ultraviolet B	BB-UVB	290–320
Narrowband ultraviolet B	NB-UVB	311–312
Ultraviolet A	UVA	320–400
Ultraviolet A-1	UVA1	340–400
Ultraviolet A-2	UVA2	320–340
Visible light	VL	400–760
Infrared	IR	760–1000

the 308-nm wavelength. Monochromatic excimer lights (MEL), also known as excimer lamps, emit an incoherent, nearly monochromatic spectrum (308 ± 2 nm). Excimer laser derives its name from the unstable "excited dimers" (excimer) of xenon and chloride gas [28]. When combined with a high-energy electric current, these dimers dissociate to their ground state and emit 308-nm coherent, monochromatic wavelengths in short pulses [28]. It is theorized that these 308-nm photons affect tissue by breaking the chemical bonds in molecules, which leads to the decomposition of organic matter [28]. This process is known as cold ablation. Therefore, when these photons penetrate keratinocytes, T-lymphocytes, Langerhans cells, fibroblasts, and other cells, the chromophore for the 308-nm photons (cellular DNA) absorbs this UVB radiation fracturing the DNA. Ultimately, this DNA damage leads to results in increased apoptosis and decreased proliferation of T-lymphocytes [29].

Ultraviolet Radiation (UVR)

Mechanism of Action in Psoriasis

Our understanding of the role of UV radiation in the management of cutaneous psoriasis has shifted from the inhibition of cellular turnover toward a focus on its immunosuppressive effects. While UV radiation induces a normalization of p53, cyclin D1, and antiproliferative proteins, the direct change in the cytokine profile of psoriatic plaques appears to be the key driver behind the therapeutic effects of UV-based therapy [30]. Both NB-UVB and PUVA shift the cytokine profile of localized psoriatic plaques and that of serum from a pro-inflammatory, T helper (Th) 1/Th 17 environment to a suppressive Th 2 phenotype with increased regulatory T cells [30, 31]. This altered cytokine profile, in turn, downregulates the immunologically driven hyperproliferation of keratinocytes. Additionally, UV radiation activates apoptotic cascades leading to the depletion of T cells, epidermal keratinocytes, and Langerhans cells [30, 31]. Thus, by reducing

antigen-presenting cells, effector T cells, keratinocyte hyperproliferation, and Th 1/17 phenotypes, phototherapy induces a series of multifaceted changes leading to an efficacious and prolonged therapeutic response.

The photobiologic effects of UV radiation can also be enhanced with topical or systemic psoralens. These naturally occurring tricyclic furocoumarins possess potent photosensitizing properties capable of cross-linking two strands of DNA. It does this through a bimolecular photoreaction between psoralen and pyrimidine nucleotides. Upon excitation by UVA radiation, psoralen, which intercalates between DNA nucleotides, reacts with thymine and cytosine to form monoadducts and cyclobutyl ring structures. Additional UV radiation can excite two cyclobutyl rings to react and cross-link two separate stands of DNA [32]. As the peak action spectrum for psoralen-induced erythema is approximately 335 nm, its primary action spectrum is UVA. Although plant-derived psoralens are still utilized by some practitioners of photomedicine, such as Ayurvedic doctors, synthetic forms of these plant-derived psoralens are more commonly used in Western medicine. Synthetic forms of methoxsalen include 8-methoxypsoralen (8-MOP), 5-methoxypsoralen (5-MOP), and trimethylpsoralen. 8-MOP is used worldwide, while 5-MOP is only available in Europe. Trimethylpsoralen is primarily used for bath-PUVA in Scandinavia.

UVR: Indications and Contraindications

After topical treatments, phototherapy is commonly recommended as the next therapeutic option for moderate-to-severe psoriasis before initiating oral, injectable, or intravenous systemic therapies [11, 33]; this is due to its high response rate, relative low cost, and minimal generalized immunosuppression compared to other systemic therapies [33]. UV therapy should be considered in patients with (a) moderate-to-severe psoriasis (BSA > 3–5%, Psoriasis Area and Severity Index [PASI] > 7–12) resistant to topical therapy, (b) severe psoriasis affecting limited areas (BSA < 5%, such as the scalp, palms, and soles) but causing disability and a poor quality of life, and (c) uncontrolled guttate psoriasis [11, 33, 34]. Phototherapy can be useful in cases of erythrodermic psoriasis, but requires cautious initial dosing and escalations to avoid exacerbating this condition. Topical corticosteroid wraps can be used to calm the inflammation before initiating phototherapy to avoid worsening the erythroderma. Application of topical corticosteroids after each phototherapy session may also help reduce the risk of exacerbation. Depending upon the extent of body surface area involvement (BSA) and lesions location, conventional NB- or BB-UVB phototherapy, targeted phototherapy, or oral, bath, or hand-foot PUVA photochemotherapy can be considered. Targeted phototherapy is an excellent choice for those with limited cutaneous involvement (BSA < 10%) or lesions involving difficult to irradiate locations, such as the scalp and genitals. Current targeted UVB modalities consist of excimer laser, MEL, and localized NB-UVB (i.e., handheld UVB devices or UVB scalp combs). Excimer laser and localized NB-UVB light sources are available in the United States, while MEL is not. For those with recalcitrant psoriasis on the palms and soles, excimer laser or topical or soak PUVA may be appropriate considerations.

If a patient is unable to regularly attend twice to thrice weekly office-based phototherapy, home phototherapy may be an appropriate therapeutic consideration in motivated, compliant patients. Additional considerations and practical issues regarding the use of home phototherapy are presented later in this chapter.

The National Institute for Clinical Health and Excellence (NICE) and the European S3 guidelines recommend a trial of NB-UVB prior to PUVA due to the increased skin cancer risk of PUVA and possible compounded risk with prior, future, or comcomitant use of systemic medications (e.g., cyclosporine) [33, 34]. PUVA should not be used in patients who are pregnant or nursing. Given the associated increased risk of skin cancer, particularly with PUVA therapy, careful consideration is recom-

mended before prescribing UV-based therapy to patients with a history of melanoma or nonmelanoma skin cancers, atypical or dysplastic nevi, organ transplantation (who are currently on immunosuppressive medications), arsenic exposure (e.g., Fowler's solution), ionizing radiation therapy, high cumulative number of PUVA treatments (>150–250), photosensitivity, epilepsy, or poor compliance [11, 33, 34]. While long-term concomitant use of cyclosporine and PUVA is associated with increased risks of squamous cell carcinoma, limited data is available on the risk with short-term administration [11, 34]. Therefore, concurrent treatment with cyclosporine and UVR is a relative, but not an absolute, contraindication. Furthermore, any physical or emotional inability to tolerate the prolonged heat and standing in a closed space may hinder the safe administration of phototherapy; this may be particularly true for pediatric or elderly populations.

Absolute contraindications for UVB and PUVA include photodermatoses or photoaggravated dermatoses (e.g., systemic lupus erythematosus) with action spectrum either in the UVB or UVA range, respectively. However, it should be noted that NB-UVB and PUVA are regularly used in the management of polymorphous light eruption. UVB and PUVA should not be administered in patients with diseases associated with increased skin cancer formation (e.g., xeroderma pigmentosum, Cockayne and Bloom syndrome) [11, 33, 34]. Additional PUVA-specific contraindications include its administration in patients with porphyrias (this is an absolute contraindication; the action spectrum in porphyrias is in the Soret band, which is immediately adjacent to the emission spectrum of UVA lamps), significant hepatic or renal impairment (relative contraindication for oral PUVA), and medically necessary photosensitizing medications (this is a relative contraindication; the action spectrum of practically all photosensitizing medications is limited to the UVA spectrum) [11, 17, 34, 35]. NB-UVB lamps, excimer laser, and MEL used in targeted phototherapy all emit negligible to no amounts of UVA; they can safely be administered in patients on photosensitizing medications.

Ultraviolet B (UVB): BB-UVB, NB-UVB, Goeckerman, and Targeted UVB Phototherapy

UVB: Efficacy

BB-UVB

BB-UVB therapy (emission, 270–390 nm with a peak at 313 nm) was one of the first treatment modalities for psoriasis. Its initial efficacy significantly improved with the addition of crude coal tar, anthralin (dithranol), and transparent emollients [2–4]. Although some transparent topical medications may limit or prevent the transmission of UVB, the addition of mineral oil, transparent cream, or white petroleum can minimize the reflection of UVB photons by psoriatic scales and therefore enhance the penetration of UVB, resulting in shorter treatment times and lower cumulative doses of UVB [36, 37]. The incorporation of these transparent topicals allowed the transition of BB-UVB from a tar-based inpatient or day-hospital treatment known as Goeckerman therapy to the outpatient setting [38, 39]. Improvement from BB-UVB can be noted after 4 weeks of daily therapy or 20–25 treatments, but remission persists in only 5% of patients after 1 year [11]. This remission can be prolonged with the addition of maintenance therapy [40–42]. Currently, BB-UVB's role in the management of psoriasis has been largely usurped by NB-UVB due to the better efficacy of the latter [43–46].

NB-UVB

NB-UVB has been shown to be more effective than BB-UVB in the management of psoriasis [45]. The clearance rate of psoriasis with NB-UVB (peak emission, 311–312 nm) occurs in approximately 70% of patients [47]. Initial improvement may be seen within the first 2 weeks. Based upon one study by Fowler et al., approximately 50% of patients who do not attain a PASI 50 by week 4 of NB-UVB will also fail to attain a PASI 75 by the completion of one course (about 18–24 sessions) of NB-UVB [48]. In contrast, 92% and 47% of those meeting this goal at week 4 will attain PASI 75 and PASI 90, respec-

tively, by the end of the treatment course [48]. NB-UVB has a relatively high 1-year remission rate of 38% [11]. This rate can be enhanced with maintenance therapy [39].

Goeckerman Therapy

Goeckerman therapy consists of the use of crude coal tar in combination with UVB. Because of the messiness of the tar preparation, this is usually done in a day-hospital setting. Despite the limited number of centers practicing this therapy, Goeckerman is a very effective treatment option for inducing clearance and a prolonged remission in patients with psoriasis. Menter et al. noted that 100% of their 300 patients achieved 75% improvement within 3 months of starting Goeckerman therapy [49]. Similar results have been echoed in publications from the University of California, San Francisco, and Mayo Clinic [50, 51]. These two US centers also noted its utility for cases recalcitrant to at least one biologic agent [52, 53]. In addition, Goeckerman therapy provided a prolonged remission (greater than 1 year) in the majority of patients undergoing treatment [49, 54–56]. The use of home phototherapy as maintenance treatment may further prolong remission to 2 years [54]. Alternatively, another round of Goeckerman therapy may be utilized upon recurrence, often with fewer treatments being needed [57]. When compared to NB-UVB, a small retrospective study with 65 patients demonstrated Goeckerman therapy to outperform NB-UVB with and without acitretin [58]. Therefore, even though a few centers continue to practice this therapy, Goeckerman remains one of the most efficacious, light-based treatment options for psoriasis [59].

Targeted UVB

Targeted phototherapy devices offer an effective therapeutic modality for the treatment of psoriasis with limited BSA (<10%) and involvement of anatomical areas with limited UV exposure with conventional phototherapy, such as the scalp, palms, and soles. Excimer laser is the most efficacious form of targeted UVB phototherapy, followed by excimer light, and localized NB-UVB, with a 75% improvement reported in 70%, 59%, and 49% of patients, respectively [12]. Targeted phototherapy with excimer laser is also amenable to body site-specific dosing as individual psoriatic lesions can be irradiated. Excimer laser requires fewer treatment sessions (less than 12) and lower cumulative UVB dose than conventional NB-UVB to achieve clearance [60, 61]. Thus, there is less concern for carcinogenicity and photoaging with targeted phototherapy [62, 63].

UVB: Dose and Administration

UVB phototherapy is indicated for generalized psoriasis and its variants, such as guttate psoriasis, which are unresponsive to topical therapy [11]. Patients should have a baseline full-body skin examination prior to starting phototherapy. Regular full-body skin examinations should also occur with phototherapy to monitor for response to treatment, development of photodermatoses (most commonly polymorphous light eruption), photoaging, and cutaneous malignancies [11]. Basic phototherapy education should be provided to all patients, including the necessity of goggles and, in male patients, shielding of genitalia. If BB-UVB is to be administered, a careful review of all medications must occur at baseline and with each treatment to minimize the risk of phototoxic reactions because BB-UVB light sources do emit a small amount of UVA.

BB-UVB and NB-UVB

BB-UVB and NB-UVB may be dosed according to skin phototype (SPT) or minimal erythema dose (MED) [11, 34, 64]. Guidelines for dosing per SPT differ among different organizations, with SPT I-VI addressed by the American Academy of Dermatology (AAD) and SPT I-IV by the European S3 guidelines [11, 34]. Initial dosing for both BB-UVB and NB-UVB are lower in the AAD guidelines for both SPT and MED regimens [11, 34]. Subsequent treatments should increase either by a set amount, with a maximum dose of NB-UVB specified according to SPT or by a percentile of the previous dose [11] (Table 3.2 [11, 34, 65, 66]). The European S3 guidelines recommend the dose to be increased based upon cutaneous findings from the last treat-

ment [34]. The AAD recommends capping the dose between 2000 and 5000 mJ/cm^2 based upon skin phototype [11]. However, the authors will often limit the dose administered to the face to 1000 mJ/cm^2 and place a soft cap of 3000 mJ/cm^2 for the body regardless of skin phototype; in our practice, it is uncommon that this soft cap needs to be limited or increased for skin phototypes I–VI.

A 2012 meta-analysis of five studies evaluating the role of various dose-increment strategies in the clearance rate of psoriasis found no significant differences between the ultimate efficacies of various initial dosing and dose escalation strategies [47]. However, there appears to be a potential difference in the initial speed of improvement with a more aggressive protocol of dose increments resulting in a more rapid response. The AAD has issued recommendations on dose de-escalation when phototherapy sessions are missed (Table 3.3 [11]).

Each course of treatment involves 15–30 sessions administered at a frequency of 2–5 sessions per week [11, 34]. While improvement can often be appreciated within 2–3 weeks for NB-UVB and 4 weeks for BB-UVB [11], the onset of this improvement can be hastened by more frequent treatments (e.g., five sessions per week). As maximum erythema occurs approximately 24 hours after NB-UVB irradiation, daily treatment is safe but may not be practical for most patients. Therefore, twice to thrice weekly phototherapy is more commonly practiced.

In the authors' experience, it is prudent to decrease the next treatment dose by 20% when new lamps are installed and the unit is recalibrated. If one lamp needs to be replaced, all lamps in the device should also be replaced to limit variations in radiation.

Home NB-UVB devices are effective and safe methods for extending this standard therapeutic option to those unable to attend regular in-office phototherapy. As additional considerations and patient instructions are required to safely prescribe home phototherapy, intricacies of patient selection, safety, and dosing are reviewed later in this chapter under the section entitled "UVB: Home Phototherapy."

Table 3.2 Initial and escalating dosages for NB-UVB

	Approach strategy	SPT	AAD initial dose (mJ/cm²)	European S3 initial dose (mJ/cm²)	AAD dose escalations [max dose] (mJ/cm²)	European S3 dose escalations
NB-UVB	SPT	I	130	200	15 [2000]	bBased upon the degree of erythema
		II	220	300	25 [2000]	
		III	260	500	40 [3000]	
		IV	330	600	45 [3000]	
		V	350	–	60 [5000]	
		VI	400	–	65 [5000]	
	MED	–	50%	70%	aBased upon treatment number	

SPT skin phototype
MED minimal erythema dose
aAAD dose escalation for NB-UVB according to treatment number:
Tx 1-20: 10% of initial MED
Tx 21+: Per ordering physician
bEuropean S3 dose escalation by the degree of erythema for NB-UVB
No erythema: increase by 30%
Minimal erythema: increase by 20% (15% after two treatments)
Persistent asymptomatic erythema: no increase
Painful erythema: break in therapy until symptoms fade, and then resume at 50% last dose with subsequent increases limited to 10%
Adapted from: Pathirana et al., Vassantachart et al., Herzinger et al., and Menter et al.

Table 3.3 Dose adjustment for missed treatment sessions

	Days since last treatment (days)	Dose adjustment
NB-UVB and BB-UVB	<4	Continue original dose protocol
	4–7	Hold at last treatment dose
	8–14	Decrease the dose by 25%
	15–21	Decrease the dose by 50%
	>21	Restart at initial dosing

Adapted from Menter et al.

Goeckerman Therapy

Gupta et al. provide an excellent description of the step-by-step approach to Goeckerman therapy, which will be briefly summarized here [57]. Goeckerman therapy consists of treatment with NB-UVB, which is used more commonly than BB-UVB for psoriasis, followed by at least 4 h of occlusion with a 2–10% crude coal tar in Aquaphor or 20% liquid carbonis detergens in Nutraderm for the body and scalp, respectively. Thick psoriatic lesions are treated with a compounded 2–10% salicylic acid and 10% crude coal tar. This process is repeated at least three times a week for at least the first month before tapering down to twice weekly and once weekly treatments. A more intensive 6-day per-week outpatient regimen has also been reported [54]. If the patient is erythrodermic, a "cooldown" procedure can be performed with topical corticosteroid occlusion before the treatment begins. A typical course of Goeckerman therapy requires 20–30 sessions before clearance is achieved; if further improvement is needed, treatment can be extended. Patients failing to improve with Goeckerman therapy should be reevaluated and the diagnosis confirmed with a skin biopsy to rule out other disorders.

Targeted Phototherapy

For excimer laser and MEL, the starting dose is usually based on SPT with consideration of plaque thickness [12]; other starting doses, which have been reported, include a minimal erythema dose (MED)-based protocol , a fixed-dose protocol, and an anatomically based dosing protocol [67–69]. The combined approach of SPT and plaque thickness is recommended by the AAD [11]. Initial and escalating dosages for excimer laser and light can

Table 3.4 Initial and escalating dosages for excimer laser and light

	Approach strategy	SPT	Plaque thickness	AAD initial dose (mJ/cm²)	AAD dose escalations
Excimer	SPT and plaque thickness	I	None	–	[a]Based upon the degree of erythema
		II	Mild	300	
		III	Moderate	500	
			Severe	700	
		IV	None	–	[a]Based upon the degree of erythema
		V	Mild	400	
		VI	Moderate	600	
			Severe	900	
	Approach strategy	–	–	European S3 initial dose	European S3 dose escalation
	MED	–	–	2–4× MED	[b]Based upon the degree of erythema

[a]*AAD dose escalation by degree of erythema for Excimer laser and light*
No erythema: increase by 25%
Slight erythema: increase by 15%
Mild to moderate erythema, tenderness, or significant improvement with plaque thinning, reduced scaliness, or pigmentation occurred: maintain or reduce dose by 15%
Moderate to severe erythema ± blistering: reduce by 25% avoiding the blistered area until it resolves
[b]*European S3 dose escalation by the degree of erythema for excimer*
Persistent asymptomatic erythema: increase by 1–2× MED
Painful erythema: break in therapy until symptoms fade, and then repeat with the last dose
Adapted from: Pathirana et al. and XTRAC Treatment Guidelines [34, 70]

be found in Table 3.4 [34, 70]. The treatment protocol for localized NB-UVB, such as a handheld UVB device, is similar to that of total body NB-UVB.

UVB: Adverse Effects

BB-UVB and NB-UVB have similar acute and chronic effects on the skin. Symptoms of acute exposure include sunburn (erythema, itching, burning, and stinging), tanning, vitamin D production, and the uncommon reactivation of herpes simplex virus, while those of chronic exposure are photoaging (wrinkling, lentigines, and telangiectasias) and theoretical risk of skin cancer. Although there is concern for photocarcinogenesis, no study to date has demonstrated an increased risk of skin cancer in psoriasis patients without a prior exposure to PUVA, a known risk factor for non-melanoma skin cancer (NMSC) formation [50, 71, 72]. Males are recommended to adhere to genital shielding as long-term exposure (>300 treatments) could potentially increase the risk of genital tumors [73, 74]. Shielding the face or limiting its dose, if treatment of this area is required, is considered prudent practice.

NB-UVB and BB-UVB display a few differences of their adverse effect profiles. BB-UVB is more erythemogenic than NB-UVB, therefore requiring approximately a 5–10 times lower dose of radiation to produce the same biologic effect (e.g., erythema). In murine models, carcinogenicity per MED of irradiation has been estimated to be 2–3 times greater with NB-UVB than with BB-UVB [75, 76]. However, due to the higher efficacy of NB-UVB, for a given treatment course, the total MED dose-equivalent of NB-UVB is less than that of BB-UVB, indicating that NB-UVB may not have a higher long-term risk of carcinogenesis [77]. To date, there has been no significant association of UVB phototherapy with basal cell carcinoma, squamous cell carcinoma, or melanoma [72].

Adverse effects from Goeckerman phototherapy typically consist of irritant dermatitis, mild local burning, and phototoxic reactions due to the use of tar [54, 57]. Folliculitis has also been reported [57]. Although there is a potential carcinogenic risk associated with crude coal tar, clinical studies have not identified an increased risk of the development of skin cancer with crude coal tar therapy compared to topical corticosteroids in psoriasis or atopic dermatitis patient cohorts [57].

UVB: Combination Therapies

Topical Therapies

Emollients increase the therapeutic efficacy of UVB phototherapy by enhancing the optical properties of psoriasis [78, 79]. Topical tazarotene enhances therapeutic efficacy, reduces the number of treatment sessions, and lowers the cumulative UVB exposure [77]; however, caution must be used as it enhances susceptibility to UV-induced erythema. Goeckerman therapy with topical crude coal tar and Ingram therapy with topical anthralin (dithranol) are efficacious but not commonly employed due to their time-consuming nature, messy formulations, and requirement for inpatient or day-hospital treatment with uncertain reimbursements [2, 4, 80, 81]. Short-contact anthralin does not sufficiently improve efficacy when combined with UVB [82, 83]. The role of topical corticosteroids in combination therapy with UVB is not recommended due to the lack of added efficacy and higher relapse rates despite initial early trials suggesting a beneficial role [84–87]. There is conflicting evidence regarding the role of vitamin D analogues, such as calcipotriol, with both BB-UVB and NB-UVB. Beneficial effects have been demonstrated with this combination therapy including reduction in relapse rate and reduced UVB exposure [88, 89]. However, a meta-analysis did not find this beneficial effect [90]. Unlike emollients, which are applied prior to phototherapy, vitamin D analogues can be degraded with UV exposure, necessitating application to occur after phototherapy [91, 92].

Systemic Therapies

Combining phototherapy with systemic therapies often provides additive or synergistic improvements but may also generate new therapeutic considerations. For example, methotrexate plus NB-UVB phototherapy produces heightened therapeutic efficacy [93]. If flaring occurs, the dose or frequency of NB-UVB can be increased, or the rate of the methotrexate dose taper can be reduced [94]. Cyclosporine reduces the cumulative UVB dose needed, and it improves clearance rates without the increased risk of an acute flare [95]. Despite this desirable outcome, the combination of cyclosporine and UVB should be used with caution as it can potentially increase the risk of NMSC development. It should also be noted that data on the risk of short-term cyclosporine with UVB phototherapy has not been published. In practice, this combination can be considered in severe, recalcitrant cases, as long as the combination is not used for longer than 2–3 months.

Acitretin is efficacious with concomitant BB-UVB, NB-UVB, Goeckerman phototherapy, and home phototherapy [57, 96–98]. It reduces the cumulative UVB and retinoid dosages in addition to accelerating the response to phototherapy [99–101]. In patients already undergoing phototherapy, the UVB dose should be reduced by approximately 20% upon initiating acitretin therapy. This is due to thinning of the epidermis as a result of the administration of acitretin, hence enhancing the penetration of UVB. However, ideally, acitretin should be started 2 weeks prior to beginning phototherapy. Standard dosing for acitretin is 25 mg per day for those weighing ≥ 70 kg or 10 mg per day for patients weighing <70 kg.

With the increasing development of biologics, there is need for large-scale studies and long-term data with three study arms: combination therapy, monotherapy with a biologic, and monotherapy with UVB. These data are currently lacking. However, alefacept and etanercept in combination with UVB have proven to be more effective than biologic monotherapy in most studies [102–104]; alefacept has been withdrawn from the US market due to adverse post-marketing safety data.

Phototherapy

PUVA in combination with UVB therapy has demonstrated more rapid clearing compared to either as monotherapy [105]; however, the long-term side effects are unknown; hence this combination is not typically used.

UVB: Special Patient Populations

Pregnancy

NB-UVB is the first-line therapy for patients with plaque or guttate psoriasis who are inadequately controlled with topical therapy [106–108]. UVB phototherapy is safe for use in pregnant patients, and expert opinion has also deemed it safe in nursing mothers [11, 109]. While there are no studies evaluating the use of the excimer laser and MEL in pregnant and nursing patients, they may be used safely, as the targeted nature of the therapy is unlikely to produce teratogenic effects [11]. There are no known teratogenic effects for BB-UVB or NB-UVB, but pregnant patients should be informed of the possible increased incidence of melasma [11, 109].

Data on UV-induced degradation of folate are still somewhat controversial. However, folate is known to have a crucial role in fetal neural tube development, which takes place in the first 4 weeks of gestation before women may know that they are pregnant. As such, it is now recommended that all women of childbearing age, whether or not they are receiving phototherapy, should take 0.8–1 mg of folate supplement daily [110, 111].

Pediatrics

NB-UVB and excimer phototherapy are the appropriate treatment options in the pediatric population when topical therapies have failed. Both types of UVB demonstrate efficacious responses without serious side effects in this population [112–114]. The most common side effect reported is erythema with an increased incidence of UVB-induced blisters in lesional skin with the excimer laser. Other reported adverse effects in the pediatric population include anxiety, two cases of herpes simplex virus reactivation, and one episode of varicella zoster treated with oral acyclovir [113].

Administering phototherapy in the pediatric population requires unique considerations. In addition to careful selection of those with appropriate demeanors to safely administer phototherapy, allowing the child to explore the phototherapy booth and become familiar with the environment before the first treatment may help reduce anxiety regarding this procedure. Additionally, decorating the area with child-friendly decorations, such as stickers or children's drawings, playing music during treatment, positioning a photo-protected parent in or near the booth with the door ajar, or incorporating a break during long-treatment sessions may help relieve a child's anxiety [112, 115–117]. To accommodate a school schedule, phototherapy may be arranged in the early morning or late afternoon [115].

UVB: Home Phototherapy

Home phototherapy with NB-UVB has equal efficacy and safety compared to outpatient NB-UVB in complaint, motivated, and educated patients when practiced under the supervision of experienced healthcare practitioners. A large randomized controlled trial involving 195 patients with psoriasis found no significant differences in the efficacy of home phototherapy to outpatient phototherapy. PASI scores decreased by 74% and 70% in home and outpatient treatment cohorts, respectively. Similar improvements in quality of life were also observed [118]. Home phototherapy is also associated with greater patient satisfaction, lower direct and indirect treatment burdens (e.g., medical costs and secondary costs of travel and loss of income), and superior patient access [118–120]. Home phototherapy is a cost-effective treatment for psoriasis and is less expensive than biologic therapies [121–124]. Ideally, patients should first demonstrate a clinical response to and familiarize themselves with in-office phototherapy before choosing to proceed with home phototherapy.

Common reasons to consider home phototherapy include but are not limited to distance from a local phototherapy unit, inability to access the unit due to limited transportation, inability to afford transportation costs for the entire treatment course, inability to regularly attend sessions due to work commitments, operational hours of the phototherapy unit, or responsibilities in the care of dependent children, elderly, or disabled family members [123]. Furthermore, if the patient is unable to attend periodic in-office appointments or does not have reliable access for contacting one's office, home phototherapy may not be appropriate. Inappropriate candidates for home phototherapy include the patients who are unable to attend office visits due to noncompliance, unwillingness, or inability to agree to supervision of home phototherapy service, inability to safely perform home phototherapy, or inability to tolerate the heat or standing required for treatment due to one's physical or mental state.

Dosing protocols for home NB-UVB phototherapy vary. Like office-administered NB-UVB, initial dosing may be based upon MED, SPT, or a fixed dose. While MED-based therapy may optimize the starting dose, SPT-based dosing is more convenient and commonly practiced; as previously discussed, office-based studies revealed no significant differences between MED and SPT approaches. Instructions on phototherapy safety and administration must be thoroughly reviewed prior to prescribing home phototherapy. These instructions include, but are not limited to, discussing protective eyewear, appropriate distance to stand from the lamps, and how to escalate or de-escalate treatment based upon clinical erythema, subjective burning sensations, and missed treatments. Since it is often difficult for patients to endure prolonged heat and standing, the authors limit the irradiation time for conventional home phototherapy devices to a maximum of 10 min of irradiation per side of the body.

Many types of phototherapy units are available on the market for home phototherapy. Often, depending upon the patient's preference and insurance coverage, the authors prescribe conventional NB-UVB devices with 6 foot panels with or without reflective wings or doors, which provide greater irradiation to the sides of the body. Patients are instructed to administer phototherapy 3 or 6 days per week. Most commonly, the patient is asked to expose the anterior and posterior body surfaces every other day, with increasing doses as tolerated with each treatment. In patients with significant involvement on the lateral trunk or extremities, a 6-day-a-week treatment may be used. This is accomplished by exposing the anterior and posterior body on day 1 and the left and right side of body on day 2, with the dose kept constant from

day 1. The dose is increased on day 3 (front-back) and day 4 (left-right sides). As with office-administered devices, it is prudent to decrease the dose by 20% when new lightbulbs are installed. All lamps should be replaced at the same time to provide even irradiation from the device.

It should be noted that the newer home phototherapy unit comes with a laminated table of irradiation times and doses. Therefore, the physician can have a clear idea on the dose that the patient is receiving. In addition, all units now have a computerized treatment number cutoff; once the maximum number of prescribed treatments is reached, the patient must contact the office of the dermatologist to obtain a new authorization code for additional treatment sessions.

Psoralen and UVA (PUVA)

PUVA: Efficacy

Systemic PUVA

PUVA is an effective therapeutic option for generalized psoriasis that is resistant to topical medications or NB-UVB therapy in adults [125, 126]. According to a meta-analysis, approximately 80% of patients on PUVA photochemotherapy achieve clearance of their lesions compared to 70% of those receiving NB-UVB [47]. This clearance with PUVA was on average 2.7 times more likely than NB-UVB to persist 6 months after the discontinuation of therapy. The average number of PUVA sessions needed for clearance in this analysis was 17, but a confidence interval could not be ascertained due to a lack of clearance data in almost half of these studies. Still, this finding supports the recommendation to define one PUVA treatment course as 20–30 sessions [127, 128]. Additional courses may be prescribed if needed.

It should be noted that one prospective study, which evaluated the efficacy of PUVA compared to NB-UVB, found that both forms of UV-based therapy were significantly less effective in clearing psoriatic lesions in patients with skin phototypes V and VI compared to those with lighter skin phototypes [129].

Topical, Soak, or Bath PUVA

Topical or soak PUVA is primarily utilized in the management of psoriasis of the palms and soles, and bath PUVA is used for generalized psoriasis in adults and children. These methods reduce systemic psoralen exposure compared to oral PUVA [130–133]. Bath PUVA is uncommon in the United States due to the prohibitive cost of operating bath PUVA units [11].

The recent meta-analysis by Almutawa et al. revealed that approximately 75% of patients achieve at least a 75% improvement in psoriatic lesions with topical PUVA therapy [12]. No statistically significant differences were identified between topical PUVA and targeted UV therapy, but none of the three comparative randomized controlled trials included in this meta-analysis utilized a xenon chloride laser. The typical treatment course for topical PUVA entails 30–40 sessions with improvement often evident within 30 sessions. Remission can last anywhere from 3 to 12 months; maintenance therapy is optional.

PUVA: Dosing and Administration

Systemic PUVA

Prior to starting oral (systemic) PUVA, patients should undergo a full-body skin screening, eye examination, and additional workup, if indicated, including ANA, anti-Ro/La antibodies, and liver enzyme profiles [11]. Throughout the course of therapy, regular full-body skin examinations and annual ophthalmologic examinations should be performed.

The dosage for oral 8-MOP and 5-MOP is weight-based at 0.4–0.6 mg/kg (maximum 70 mg) and 1.0–1.2 mg/kg, respectively. Although the time to peak serum levels may vary among individuals, patients are advised to ingest the methoxsalen 1 h before exposure to UVA. Ideally, food should be avoided 1 h before and after the methoxsalen dose to limit impaired absorption. A light meal, particularly one containing milk, may help alleviate nausea, a common side effect of methoxsalen. In such cases, it is important that patients standardize the type, amount, and timing of the food ingested to limit variations in psoralen absorption. Dividing the dose into two administrations taken twenty minutes apart can also help reduce one's nausea.

A typical course of systemic PUVA therapy consists of 20–30 treatments. The initial and final fluence of UVA, along with interval escalations during therapy, is based upon Fitzpatrick skin type. The recommended treatment frequency is two to three times per week with at least 48 h between sessions to permit assessment of UVA-induced erythema. The degree of erythema determines the next dose administered (Table 3.5 [34, 65, 66]). Once clearance has been achieved, the frequency of treatment can be tapered to every 1–2 weeks. Applying a thin layer of a clear emollient or mineral oil will improve the penetration of ultraviolet radiation, particularly in areas with thick adherent scale.

Topical, Soak, and Bath PUVA

In the United States, topical PUVA is delivered most commonly by diluting a 1% 8-MOP solution to 0.1% in either an ointment or lotion base for topical application onto lesional skin. UVA irradiation is administered 20–30 min later [11]. Care should be taken that topical 8-MOP is applied to the same area at each session to prevent an inadvertent, severe phototoxic reaction as the UVA dose is increased. The medication should be thoroughly washed off following irradiation. No baseline or routine monitoring is necessary [11].

For hand or foot soak PUVA, 10 mg of methoxsalen is dissolved in two quarts of warm water. For bath PUVA, 50 mg of methoxsalen is dissolved in a bathtub with 100 L of warm water. The patient then soaks the affected areas (hands, feet, or the entire body from the neck down) for approximately 30 min and then dries off completely without showering prior to receiving light exposure.

PUVA: Adverse Effects

Systemic PUVA

Oral 8-MOP can cause nausea and vomiting and, less commonly, dizziness and headache. PUVA can cause erythema peaking at 48–96 h post-therapy, xerosis, irregular pigmentation, and tanning (onset

Table 3.5 Initial and escalating dosages for PUVA

	Approach strategy	SPT	AAD initial dose (J/cm²)	European S3 initial dose (J/cm²)	AAD dose escalations [max dose] (J/cm²)	European S3 dose escalations
PUVA	SPT (oral)	I	0.5	0.3	0.5 [8]	[a]Based upon the degree of erythema
		II	1.0	0.5	0.5 [8]	
		III	1.5	0.8	1.0 [10]	
		IV	2.0	1.0	1.0 [10]	
		V	2.5	–	1.5 [20]	
		VI	3.0	–	1.5 [20]	
	MPD (oral)	–	–	75%	–	[a]Based upon the degree of erythema
	SPT (bath)	I		0.2		[a]Based upon the degree of erythema
		II		0.3		
		III		0.4		
		IV		0.6		
		V		–		
		VI		–		
	MPD (bath)	–	–	30%	–	[a]Based upon the degree of erythema

SPT skin phototype, *MPD* minimal phototoxic dose
[a]*European S3 dose escalation by the degree of erythema for PUVA*
No erythema: increase by 20–30% (no more than 2×/week)
Minimal erythema: no further increase
Persistent asymptomatic erythema: no increase
Painful erythema: break in therapy until symptoms fade, and then resume at 50% last dose with subsequent increases limited to 10%
Adapted from Pathirana et al., Vassantachart et al., and Herzinger et al.

Fig. 3.1 PUVA-induced distal onycholysis

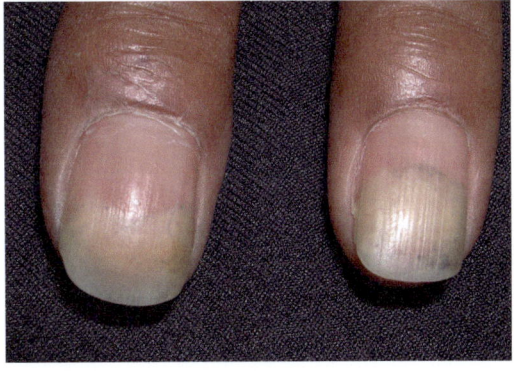

1 week after PUVA initiation); in some, pruritus may occur. Erythema can be managed by adjusting the dose of UVA or, if necessary, the dose of 8-MOP. Pruritus can be managed by using emollients and antipruritics. Nausea can often be improved using the previously discussed strategies. Other side effects include blisters, photo-onycholysis (Fig 3.1), melanonychia (especially in dark-skinned individuals) (Fig 3.2), and hepatotoxicity.

Chronic effects of PUVA include photocarcinogenesis, especially squamous cell carcinomas (SCC) of the body and male genitalia and basal cell carcinomas [74, 134–136]. The risk of melanoma remains unclear, with conflicting data between United States and European studies [137–142]. SCC is the most common NMSC associated with PUVA occurring primarily in Caucasians with skin phototypes I–III who

Fig. 3.2 PUVA-induced transverse melanonychia

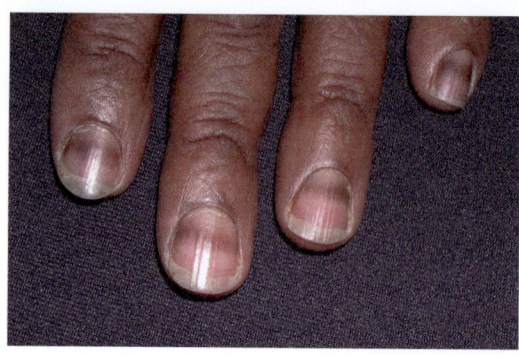

received over 200–400 treatments [143]. This increased risk of NMSC has not been reported in non-Caucasian populations or those treated with bath-PUVA therapy [144]. Long-term coadministration of PUVA with cyclosporine is associated with a significantly greater risk of developing SCC than either therapy alone [145].

In addition, photoaging with elastosis and poikiloderma and PUVA lentigines are more common in skin types I–III and are associated with higher cumulative UVA doses. Hypertrichosis is another uncommon reported side effect. In animal models, PUVA has been associated with cataract formation. Therefore, the current recommendations include wearing protective goggles during treatment and sunglasses when outdoors for 8–12 h after ingestion of oral psoralen. It should be noted that, in humans, studies have not demonstrated an increased risk of cataract formation with oral PUVA, which could be due to adherence to eye protection or lack of other risk factors [11, 146].

Drug interactions with PUVA may occur. These include carbamazepine-, phenytoin-, or phenobarbital-induced reduction of 8-MOP levels, increased serum levels of caffeine or theophylline with 8-MOP, and an increased risk of phototoxicity when taken with other photosensitizers, such as NSAIDs, sulfonamides, diuretics (furosemide, chlorothiazide), sulfonylurea drugs, antifungals, neuroleptics, tetracyclines, and fluoroquinolones; UVA is the action spectrum for these phototoxic medications [143]. In patients who are already on PUVA, additional administration of systemic retinoids would necessitate a

reduction in the UVA dose by 20–30% to prevent a phototoxic reaction due to retinoid-induced thinning of the epidermis.

Topical PUVA

Acute toxicity includes erythema, blistering, and hyperpigmentation. While there is a potential increased risk of skin cancer formation, no association with topical PUVA therapy has been reported [144, 147, 148].

PUVA: Combination Therapy

Combination therapies are an appealing alternative to PUVA monotherapy, with the goal of reducing PUVA dosage to decrease side effects [149].

Topical Therapies

Topical calcipotriol is a useful adjunct to PUVA therapy for decreasing the duration of PUVA therapy and improving clinical response if applied after irradiation [150–152]. Tazarotene also may improve the efficacy of PUVA. However, more research is needed to verify these anecdotal reports [153, 154]. The role of topical corticosteroids remains unclear. While topical corticosteroids have been shown to hasten clearance of psoriatic lesions, there is conflicting evidence about its effect on the duration of remission [155, 156].

Systemic Therapies

Oral retinoids, when used in conjunction with PUVA, are more effective than PUVA or retinoid monotherapy [157–159]. The concomitant use of these treatments decreases both the number of

PUVA sessions and the total UVA dose [159, 160]. In addition, acitretin in combination with PUVA decreases the incidence of SCC [161]. This decrease is likely due to the known suppressive effect of acitretin on the formation of NMSC [162–165]. Methotrexate and PUVA therapy are more effective together than as monotherapies [166, 167]; however, the long-term safety profile of this combination is unclear [168]. Cyclosporine, on the other hand, should be avoided when possible, due to the increased risk of SCC [145]. No increased risk of malignancy has been reported from concomitant biologic and PUVA therapies, but no systematic studies have been performed utilizing this dual therapy.

Phototherapy

Combinations of PUVA with BB-UVB, NB-UVB, and excimer laser have demonstrated efficacy but are seldom used in current practice due to concerns regarding the long-term side effects of such combinations [60, 105, 169, 170].

Special Patient Populations

Pregnancy

Systemic PUVA
Systemic PUVA is a category C therapy. The AAD recommends against its use in pregnant patients and recommends cautious use in those breastfeeding [11]. Nursing mothers should wait at least 24 h after ingesting psoralen before breastfeeding. The European S3 guidelines list pregnancy and breastfeeding as contraindications for PUVA therapy [34]. In practice, due to the availability of many other therapeutic options, it is prudent and appropriate to avoid PUVA in these groups of patients.

Topical PUVA
Because of the short duration of contact and the short treatment course, topical PUVA is likely safe for use in pregnancy. However, there is no data on this topic; in view of other available treatment modalities, including targeted phototherapy, alternative treatments should be used in pregnancy or in nursing mothers. Of note, pso-

ralen has not been demonstrated in the blood of patients using topical PUVA [171]. However, bath PUVA or other topical preparations could potentially involve enough BSA to induce a measurable quantity in the blood from cutaneous absorption [172].

Pediatrics

Systemic PUVA
Caution is advised in pediatric patients <18 years of age due to the long-term risk of photocarcinogenicity [11, 173].

Topical PUVA
Topical PUVA is safe in the pediatric population if the patient is able to follow directions. Bath PUVA is not approved by the FDA for use in children; however, this approach would be preferred over oral PUVA due to lower systemic absorption [11, 174].

Visible Light Radiation (VLR)

VLR: Indications and Contraindications

The use of VL as monotherapy in the management of psoriasis has been investigated. While VL has less carcinogenic potential compared to the already low-risk option of NB-UVB and excimer phototherapies, no VL treatment option has consistently demonstrated superior efficacy compared to UVB in the management of psoriasis.

Photodynamic Therapy (PDT)

Historically, PDT has demonstrated poor therapeutic utility in the management of psoriasis. Studies investigating topical ALA-PDT have consistently revealed a low degree of efficacy and intolerable pain in up to one-third of patients [12]. In addition, PDT performed on ALA-soaked immune cells harvested by apheresis, a process known as extracorporeal PDT, failed to consistently demonstrate efficacious outcomes for psoriasis when used as monotherapy [175–179]. Thus, after reviewing the evidence for extracorporeal PDT in the management of psoriasis, the British Photodermatology Group and the UK Skin Lymphoma Group stated that there was poor evidence to support its use in the management of cutaneous psoriasis or psoriatic arthritis [180]. Similarly, a systematic review and meta-analysis evaluating the evidence for topical PDT agreed with the British Association of Dermatologists guidelines on the limited therapeutic role of ALA-PDT for psoriasis [12].

Future Frontiers of Phototherapy in Psoriasis

Blue Light Therapy and Psoriasis

Over the past 10 years, scientific investigations have revealed that blue light is not in the inert spectrum as previously thought. Investigations on pigmentation demonstrated blue light to have a greater impact on the induction of immediate and persistent pigment darkening than UVA [23]. With regard to psoriasis, the most relevant spectra were proposed to be at 420 and 453 nm [181]. Unlike UVR, blue light is not absorbed by DNA nor leads to cell death below fluences of 500 J/cm^2 [27]. Instead, blue light's chromophores are flavins, cryptochromes, and porphyrins [181]. These chromophores are thought to mediate the effects of blue light irradiation primarily through the release of nitric oxide and reactive oxygen species. These downstream effects lead to a reduction in keratinocyte proliferation and dendritic cell activation while inducing differentiation of keratinocytes [181]. Additional effects of blue light that are not fully understood include T-cell-induced apoptosis, altered immune response, and decreased inflammation after treatment. Like other photobiologic responses, these effects appear to be wavelength and fluence dependent.

Clinical investigations with blue light radiation have generally supported its role in the management of mild to moderate, localized psoriatic lesions. Of the four clinical investigations on blue light in psoriasis, only the initial investigation by Maari et al. revealed no statistical difference following treatment [182]. The subsequent three trials and a computational model demonstrated blue light to be a potentially beneficial therapy for psoriasis [24–26]. Interestingly, the computational model predicts blue light to transiently improve psoriatic lesions with limited utility for producing a prolonged remission [182]. Unlike UVR, blue light does not induce apoptosis of keratinocytes [27]. Therefore, the population of hyperproliferating keratinocytes experiences only a transient decrease in their proliferating capacity during blue light therapy, lacking the long remissions brought about with PUVA, Goeckerman, and NB-UVB therapies. This steady decline in posttreatment remission was also noted clinically by Weinstabl et al. [24].

Nail Psoriasis

Nail psoriasis is a common and notoriously difficult to treat cutaneous manifestation of psoriasis without the use of systemic medications. In recent years, laser and light-based therapies have become increasingly investigated in the management of nail psoriasis. Initially, most of the investigations were limited to UVR. Although a human cadaveric study suggested that a limited amount of UVA and nearly no UVB penetrates through the nail plate, in vivo clinical studies have reported some beneficial effects from oral PUVA, solar PUVA, NB-UVB, excimer light, and excimer laser [13]. More recently, pulsed dye laser (PDL, 595 nm) has gained traction in the literature as an effective therapeutic modality for psoriatic nail dystrophy [183–185]. In fact, a 42-patient, left-to-right comparison study of PDL versus excimer laser observed a significantly greater improvement in the PDL cohort [183]. Onycholysis and subungual hyperkeratosis are the most likely manifestations to respond to PDL treatment. Nail pitting often remains recalcitrant to treatment. The addition of methyl aminolevulinic acid, a known photosensitizer, or a change in pulse duration does not improve the response to PDL [185, 186]. Long-pulse PDL is associated with a higher frequency of transient petechial hyperpigmentation and significant pain. Intense pulsed light with a 550-nm filter has also been reported to improve nail dystrophy from nail bed and nail matrix disease [187]. Nail matrix disease, particularly nail pitting, is less responsive to IPL treatment. Future refinements in the delivery of laser and light therapy may offer an effective therapeutic modality for the management of recalcitrant nail psoriasis.

Summary

Phototherapy and photochemotherapy remain some of the most cost-effective and safe therapeutic strategies for the management of cutaneous psoriasis. For these reasons, NB-UVB has been endorsed by the AAD and S3 European guidelines as a first-line UV-based therapy for this disorder. It can safely be administered to pregnant women and most pediatric patients. PUVA and Goeckerman therapy are both efficacious therapeutic options for recalcitrant psoriatic lesions but pose greater carcinogenic risks and difficulty in administration, respectively, than NB-UVB. These, in turn, limit their clinical use and availability. As not all patients can comply with twice or thrice weekly office-based phototherapy, home NB-UVB phototherapy is also an excellent therapeutic option for the appropriate patient. Like the new VL devices in the field of acne, UV-free, VL devices have emerged as another potential tool in the management of psoriasis. Future randomized controlled trials are needed to determine the true efficacy and longevity of remission for such devices compared to existing technologies such as NB-UVB.

References

1. Fitzpatrick TB, Pathak MA. Historical aspects of methoxsalen and other furocoumarins. J Invest Dermatol. 1959;32(2, Part 2):229–31.
2. Goeckerman WH. Treatment of psoriasis. Northwest Med. 1925;24:229–31.
3. Ingram JT. The approach to psoriasis. Br Med J. 1953;2(4836):591–4.
4. Ingram JT. The significance and management of psoriasis. Br Med J. 1954;2(4892):823–8.
5. Fahmy IR, Abu-Shady H, Schönberg A, Sina A. A crystalline principle from Ammi majus L. Nature. 1947;160:468–9.
6. Fahmy IR, Abu-Shady H. Ammi majus Linn: pharmacognostical study and isolation of a crystalline constituent, ammoidin. Q J Pharm Pharmacol. 1947;20:281–91.
7. Parrish JA, Fitzpatrick TB, Tanenbaum L, Pathak MA. Photochemotherapy of psoriasis with oral methoxsalen and longwave ultraviolet light. N Engl J Med. 1974;291(23):1207–11.
8. Roelandts R. History of human photobiology. In: Lim HW, Hönigsmann H, Hawk JLM, editors. Photodermatology. New York: Informa Healthcare USA, Inc.; 2007. p. 1–14.
9. van Weelden H, De La Faille HB, Young E, van der Leun JC. A new development in UVB phototherapy of psoriasis. Br J Dermatol. 1988;119(1):11–9.
10. Green C, Ferguson J, Lakshmipathi T, Johnson BE. 311 nm UVB phototherapy—an effective treatment for psoriasis. Br J Dermatol. 1988;119(6):691–6.
11. Menter A, Korman NJ, Elmets CA, Feldman SR, Gelfand JM, Gordon KB, et al. Guidelines of care for the management of psoriasis and psoriatic arthritis: Section 5. Guidelines of care for the treatment of psoriasis with phototherapy and photochemotherapy. J Am Acad Dermatol. 2010;62(1):114–35.
12. Almutawa F, Thalib L, Hekman D, Sun Q, Hamzavi I, Lim HW. Efficacy of localized phototherapy and photodynamic therapy for psoriasis: a systematic review and meta-analysis. Photodermatol Photoimmunol Photomed. 2015;31(1):5–14.
13. Maranda EL, Nguyen AH, Lim VM, Hafeez F, Jimenez JJ. Laser and light therapies for the treatment of nail psoriasis. J Eur Acad Dermatol Venereol. 2016;30(8):1278–84.
14. Anders A, Altheide HJ, Knalmann M, Tronnier H. Action spectrum for erythema in humans investigated with dye lasers. Photochem Photobiol. 1995;61(2):200–5.
15. Diffey BL. Observed and predicted minimal erythema doses: a comparative study. Photochem Photobiol. 1994;60(4):380–2.
16. CIE Standard. Erythema reference action spectrum and standard erythema dose. CIE S 007/E-1998.1998; Vienna: Commission Internationale de l'Eclairage.
17. Young AR, Chadwick CA, Harrison GI, Nikaido O, Ramsden J, Potten CS. The similarity of action spectra for thymine dimers in human epidermis and erythema suggests that DNA is the chromophore for erythema. J Invest Dermatol. 1998;111(6):982–8.
18. McLoone P, Simics E, Barton A, Norval M, Gibbs NK. An action spectrum for the production of cis-urocanic acid in human skin in vivo. J Invest Dermatol. 2005;124(5):1071–4.
19. de Gruijl FR. Action spectrum for photocarcinogenesis. Recent Results Cancer Res. 1995;139:21–30.

20. CIE 132/2; TC 6-32 report: action spectrum for photocarcinogenesis (non-melanoma skin cancers). Commission Internationale de l'Eclairage; 2000; Vienna.

21. Irwin C, Barnes A, Veres D, Kaidbey K. An ultraviolet radiation action spectrum for immediate pigment darkening. Photochem Photobiol. 1993;57(3):504–7.

22. Calzavara-Pinton PG, Venturini M, Sala R. Photodynamic therapy: update 2006. Part 1: Photochemistry and photobiology. J Eur Acad Dermatol Venereol. 2007;21(3):293–302.

23. Mahmoud BH, Ruvolo E, Hexsel CL, Liu Y, Owen MR, Kollias N, et al. Impact of long-wavelength UVA and visible light on melanocompetent skin. J Invest Dermatol. 2010;130(8):2092–7.

24. Weinstabl A, Hoff-Lesch S, Merk HF, von Felbert V. Prospective randomized study on the efficacy of blue light in the treatment of psoriasis vulgaris. Dermatology. 2011;223(3):251–9.

25. Pfaff S, Liebmann J, Born M, Merk HF, von Felbert V. Prospective randomized long-term study on the efficacy and safety of UV-free blue light for treating mild psoriasis vulgaris. Dermatology. 2015;231(1):24–34.

26. Kleinpenning MM, Otero ME, van Erp PE, Gerritsen MJ, van de Kerkhof PC. Efficacy of blue light vs. red light in the treatment of psoriasis: a double-blind, randomized comparative study. J Eur Acad Dermatol Venereol. 2012;26(2):219–25.

27. Awakowicz P, Bibinov N, Born M, Busse B, Gesche R, Helmke A, et al. Biological stimulation of the human skin applying health promoting light and plasma sources. Contrib Plasma Physics. 2009;49:641–7.

28. Spencer JM, Hadi SM. The excimer lasers. J Drugs Dermatol. 2004;3(5):522–5.

29. Bulat V, Situm M, Dediol I, Ljubicic I, Bradic L. The mechanisms of action of phototherapy in the treatment of the most common dermatoses. Coll Antropol. 2011;35(Suppl 2):147–51.

30. Wong T, Hsu L, Liao W. Phototherapy in psoriasis: a review of mechanisms of action. J Cutan Med Surg. 2013;17(1):6–12.

31. Tartar D, Bhutani T, Huynh M, Berger T, Koo J. Update on the immunological mechanism of action behind phototherapy. J Drugs Dermatol. 2014;13(5):564–8.

32. Diffey BL, Kochevar IE. Basic principles of photobiology. In: Lim HW, Hönigsmann H, Hawk JLM, editors. Photodermatology. New York: Informa Healthcare USA, Inc.; 2007. p. 15–28.

33. NCGC. Psoriasis: assessment and management of psoriasis. National Institute for Health and Clinical Excellence (NICE): Guidance. London: Royal College of Physicians; 2012.

34. Pathirana D, Ormerod AD, Saiag P, Smith C, Spuls PI, Nast A, et al. European S3-guidelines on the systemic treatment of psoriasis vulgaris. J Eur Acad Dermatol Venereol. 2009;23(Suppl 2):1–70.

35. Kerstein RL, Lister T, Cole R. Laser therapy and photosensitive medication: a review of the evidence. Lasers Med Sci. 2014;29(9):1449–52.

36. Berne B, Blom I, Spangberg S. Enhanced response of psoriasis to UVB therapy after pretreatment with a lubricating base. A single-blind controlled study. Acta Derm Venereol. 1990;70(6):474–7.

37. Fetil E, Akarsu S, Ilknur T, Kusku E, Gunes AT. Effects of some emollients on the transmission of ultraviolet. Photodermatol Photoimmunol Photomed. 2006;22(3):137–40.

38. LeVine MJ, Parrish JA. Outpatient phototherapy of psoriasis. Arch Dermatol. 1980;116(5):552–4.

39. Larkö O, Swanbeck G. Home solarium treatment of psoriasis. Br J Dermatol. 1979;101(1):13–6.

40. Boer J, Schothorst AA, Suurmond D. UV-B phototherapy of psoriasis. Dermatologica. 1980;161(4):250–8.

41. Stern RS, Armstrong RB, Anderson TF, Bickers DR, Lowe NJ, Harber L, et al. Effect of continued ultraviolet B phototherapy on the duration of remission of psoriasis: a randomized study. J Am Acad Dermatol. 1986;15(3):546–52.

42. Boztepe G, Karaduman A, Sahin S, Hayran M, Kolemen F. The effect of maintenance narrow-band ultraviolet B therapy on the duration of remission for psoriasis: a prospective randomized clinical trial. Int J Dermatol. 2006;45(3):245–50.

43. Karvonen J, Kokkonen EL, Ruotsalainen E. 311 nm UVB lamps in the treatment of psoriasis with the Ingram regimen. Acta Derm Venereol. 1989;69(1):82–5.

44. Larkö O. Treatment of psoriasis with a new UVB-lamp. Acta Derm Venereol. 1989;69(4):357–9.

45. Coven TR, Burack LH, Gilleaudeau R, Keogh M, Ozawa M, Krueger JG. Narrowband UV-B produces superior clinical and histopathological resolution of moderate-to-severe psoriasis in patients compared with broadband UV-B. Arch Dermatol. 1997;133(12):1514–22.

46. Walters IB, Burack LH, Coven TR, Gilleaudeau P, Krueger JG. Suberythemogenic narrow-band UVB is markedly more effective than conventional UVB in treatment of psoriasis vulgaris. J Am Acad Dermatol. 1999;40(6 Pt 1):893–900.

47. Archier E, Devaux S, Castela E, Gallini A, Aubin F, Le Maitre M, et al. Efficacy of psoralen UV-A therapy vs. narrowband UV-B therapy in chronic plaque psoriasis: a systematic literature review. J Eur Acad Dermatol Venereol. 2012;26(Suppl 3):11–21.

48. Fowler J, Weatherhead S. Can the Psoriasis Area and Severity Index score measured 4 weeks into a course of narrowband ultraviolet B phototherapy be used to predict final Psoriasis Area and Severity Index response? Br J Dermatol. 2016;175(Suppl 1):102–3.

49. Menter A, Cram DL. The Goeckerman regimen in two psoriasis day care centers. J Am Acad Dermatol. 1983;9(1):59–65.

50. Lee E, Koo J, Berger T. UVB phototherapy and skin cancer risk: a review of the literature. Int J Dermatol. 2005;44(5):355–60.

51. Perry HO, Soderstrom CW, Schulze RW. The Goeckerman treatment of psoriasis. Arch Dermatol. 1968;98(2):178–82.

52. Fitzmaurice S, Bhutani T, Koo J. Goeckerman regimen for management of psoriasis refractory to biologic therapy: the University of California San Francisco experience. J Am Acad Dermatol. 2013;69(4):648–9.

53. Serrao R, Davis MD. Goeckerman treatment for remission of psoriasis refractory to biologic therapy. J Am Acad Dermatol. 2009;60(2):348–9.

54. de Miguel R, el-Azhary R. Efficacy, safety, and cost of Goeckerman therapy compared with biologics in the treatment of moderate to severe psoriasis. Int J Dermatol. 2009;48(6):653–8.

55. Cort DH, Schleider NR, Moskowitz RS, Horwitz SN, Frost P. Retrospective analysis of a modified Goeckerman regimen for the treatment of psoriasis. Cutis. 1980;25(2):201–3. 6-9

56. DesGroseilliers JP, Cullen AE, Rouleau GA. Ambulatory Goeckerman treatment of psoriasis: experience with 200 patients. Can Med Assoc J. 1981;124(8):1018–20.

57. Gupta R, Debbaneh M, Butler D, Huynh M, Levin E, Leon A, et al. The Goeckerman regimen for the treatment of moderate to severe psoriasis. J Vis Exp. 2013;11(77):e50509.

58. Çaliskan E, Tunca M, Açikgöz G, Arca E, Yürekli A, Akar A. Narrow band ultraviolet-B versus Goeckerman therapy for psoriasis with and without acritretin: a retrospective study. Indian J Dermatol Venereol Leprol. 2015;81(6):584–7.

59. Feldman SR. Where has Goeckerman treatment gone? J Dermatol Treat. 2005;16(2):73–4.

60. Trott J, Gerber W, Hammes S, Ockenfels HM. The effectiveness of PUVA treatment in severe psoriasis is significantly increased by additional UV 308-nm excimer laser sessions. Eur J Dermatol. 2008;18(1):55–60.

61. Feldman SR, Mellen BG, Housman TS, Fitzpatrick RE, Geronemus RG, Friedman PM, et al. Efficacy of the 308-nm excimer laser for treatment of psoriasis: results of a multicenter study. J Am Acad Dermatol. 2002;46(6):900–6.

62. Bónis B, Kemény L, Dobozy A, Bor Z, Szabó G, Ignácz F. 308 nm UVB excimer laser for psoriasis. Lancet (London, England). 1997;350(9090):1522.

63. Mudigonda T, Dabade TS, Feldman SR. A review of targeted ultraviolet B phototherapy for psoriasis. J Am Acad Dermatol. 2012;66(4):664–72.

64. Wolff K, Gschnait F, Honigsmann H, Konrad K, Parrish JA, Fitzpatrick TB. Phototesting and dosimetry for photochemotherapy. Br J Dermatol. 1977;96(1):1–10.

65. Vassantachart JM, Soleymani T, Wu JJ. Comparison of phototherapy guidelines for psoriasis: a critical appraisal and comprehensive review. J Drugs Dermatol. 2016;15(8):995–1000.

66. Herzinger T, Berneburg M, Ghoreschi K, Gollnick H, Hölzle E, Hönigsmann H, et al. S1-Guidelines on UV phototherapy and photochemotherapy. J Dtsch Dermatol Ges. 2016;14(8):853–76.

67. Asawanonda P, Anderson RR, Chang Y, Taylor CR. 308-nm excimer laser for the treatment of psoriasis: a dose-response study. Arch Dermatol. 2000;136(5):619–24.

68. Trehan M, Taylor CR. High-dose 308-nm excimer laser for the treatment of psoriasis. J Am Acad Dermatol. 2002;46(5):732–7.

69. PHAROS EX-308 Operations Guide. Carlsbad: Ra Medical Systems.

70. XTRAC treatment guidelines card. 12-95359-01. Rev. E. Carlsbad: PhotoMedex; 2009.

71. Stern RS, Laird N. The carcinogenic risk of treatments for severe psoriasis. Photochemotherapy Follow-up Study. Cancer. 1994;73(11):2759–64.

72. Hearn RM, Kerr AC, Rahim KF, Ferguson J, Dawe RS. Incidence of skin cancers in 3867 patients treated with narrow-band ultraviolet B phototherapy. Br J Dermatol. 2008;159(4):931–5.

73. Studniberg HM, Weller P. PUVA, UVB, psoriasis, and nonmelanoma skin cancer. J Am Acad Dermatol. 1993;29(6):1013–22.

74. Stern RS. Genital tumors among men with psoriasis exposed to psoralens and ultraviolet A radiation (PUVA) and ultraviolet B radiation. The Photochemotherapy Follow-up Study. N Engl J Med. 1990;322(16):1093–7.

75. Flindt-Hansen H, McFadden N, Eeg-Larsen T, Thune P. Effect of a new narrow-band UVB lamp on photocarcinogenesis in mice. Acta Derm Venereol. 1991;71(3):245–8.

76. Gibbs NK, Traynor NJ, MacKie RM, Campbell I, Johnson BE, Ferguson J. The phototumorigenic potential of broad-band (270-350 nm) and narrow-band (311-313 nm) phototherapy sources cannot be predicted by their edematogenic potential in hairless mouse skin. J Invest Dermatol. 1995;104(3):359–63.

77. Man I, Crombie IK, Dawe RS, Ibbotson SH, Ferguson J. The photocarcinogenic risk of narrow-band UVB (TL-01) phototherapy: early follow-up data. Br J Dermatol. 2005;152(4):755–7.

78. Schleider NR, Moskowitz RS, Cort DH, Horwitz SN, Frost P. Effects of emollients on ultraviolet-radiation-induced erythema of the skin. Arch Dermatol. 1979;115(10):1188–91.

79. Lebwohl M, Martinez J, Weber P, DeLuca R. Effects of topical preparations on the erythemogenicity of UVB: implications for psoriasis phototherapy. J Am Acad Dermatol. 1995;32(3):469–71.

80. Lowe NJ, Wortzman MS, Breeding J, Koudsi H, Taylor L. Coal tar phototherapy for psoriasis reevaluated: erythemogenic versus suberythemogenic ultraviolet with a tar extract in oil and crude coal tar. J Am Acad Dermatol. 1983;8(6):781–9.

81. Pittelkow MR, Perry HO, Muller SA, Maughan WZ, O'Brien PC. Skin cancer in patients with psoriasis treated with coal tar. A 25-year follow-up study. Arch Dermatol. 1981;117(8):465–8.

82. Boer J, Smeenk G. Effect of short-contact anthralin therapy on ultraviolet B irradiation of psoriasis. J Am Acad Dermatol. 1986;15(2 Pt 1):198–204.

83. Lebwohl M, Berman B, France DS. Addition of short-contact anthralin therapy to an ultraviolet B phototherapy regimen: assessment of efficacy. J Am Acad Dermatol. 1985;13(5 Pt 1):780–4.

84. Meola T Jr, Soter NA, Lim HW. Are topical corticosteroids useful adjunctive therapy for the treatment of psoriasis with ultraviolet radiation? A review of the literature. Arch Dermatol. 1991;127(11):1708–13.

85. Petrozzi JW. Topical steroids and UV radiation in psoriasis. Arch Dermatol. 1983;119(3):207–10.

86. Larkö O, Swanbeck G, Svartholm H. The effect on psoriasis of clobetasol propionate used alone or in combination with UVB. Acta Derm Venereol. 1984;64(2):151–4.

87. Dover JS, McEvoy MT, Rosen CF, Arndt KA, Stern RS. Are topical corticosteroids useful in phototherapy for psoriasis? J Am Acad Dermatol. 1989;20(5 Pt 1):748–54.

88. Molin L. Topical calcipotriol combined with phototherapy for psoriasis. The results of two randomized trials and a review of the literature. Calcipotriol-UVB Study Group. Dermatology. 1999;198(4):375–81.

89. Ramsay CA, Schwartz BE, Lowson D, Papp K, Bolduc A, Gilbert M. Calcipotriol cream combined with twice weekly broad-band UVB phototherapy: a safe, effective and UVB-sparing antipsoriatic combination treatment. The Canadian Calcipotriol and UVB Study Group. Dermatology. 2000;200(1):17–24.

90. Ashcroft DM, Li Wan Po A, Williams HC, Griffiths CE. Combination regimens of topical calcipotriene in chronic plaque psoriasis: systematic review of efficacy and tolerability. Arch Dermatol. 2000;136(12):1536–43.

91. Lebwohl M, Hecker D, Martinez J, Sapadin A, Patel B. Interactions between calcipotriene and ultraviolet light. J Am Acad Dermatol. 1997;37(1):93–5.

92. Lebwohl M, Quijije J, Gilliard J, Rollin T, Watts O. Topical calcitriol is degraded by ultraviolet light. J Invest Dermatol. 2003;121(3):594–5.

93. Asawanonda P, Nateetongrungsak Y. Methotrexate plus narrowband UVB phototherapy versus narrowband UVB phototherapy alone in the treatment of plaque-type psoriasis: a randomized, placebo-controlled study. J Am Acad Dermatol. 2006;54(6):1013–8.

94. Paul BS, Momtaz K, Stern RS, Arndt KA, Parrish JA. Combined methotrexate—ultraviolet B therapy in the treatment of psoriasis. J Am Acad Dermatol. 1982;7(6):758–62.

95. Calzavara-Pinton P, Leone G, Venturini M, Sala R, Colombo D, La Parola IL, et al. A comparative non randomized study of narrow-band (NB) (312 +/- 2 nm) UVB phototherapy versus sequential therapy with oral administration of low-dose Cyclosporin A and NB-UVB phototherapy in patients with severe psoriasis vulgaris. Eur J Dermatol. 2005;15(6):470–3.

96. Kampitak T, Asawanonda P. The efficacy of combination treatment with narrowband UVB (TL-01) and acitretin vs narrowband UVB alone in plaque-type psoriasis: a retrospective study. J Med Assoc Thai. 2006;89(Suppl 3):S20–4.

97. Yelverton CB, Yentzer BA, Clark A, Pearce DJ, Balkrishnan R, Camacho FT, et al. Home narrowband UV-B phototherapy in combination with low-dose acitretin in patients with moderate to severe psoriasis. Arch Dermatol. 2008;144(9):1224–5.

98. Yentzer BA, Yelverton CB, Pearce DJ, Camacho FT, Makhzoumi Z, Clark A, et al. Adherence to acitretin and home narrowband ultraviolet B phototherapy in patients with psoriasis. J Am Acad Dermatol. 2008;59(4):577–81.

99. Lowe NJ, Prystowsky JH, Bourget T, Edelstein J, Nychay S, Armstrong R. Acitretin plus UVB therapy for psoriasis. Comparisons with placebo plus UVB and acitretin alone. J Am Acad Dermatol. 1991;24(4):591–4.

100. Ruzicka T, Sommerburg C, Braun-Falco O, Koster W, Lengen W, Lensing W, et al. Efficiency of acitretin in combination with UV-B in the treatment of severe psoriasis. Arch Dermatol. 1990;126(4):482–6.

101. Ozdemir M, Engin B, Baysal I, Mevlitoglu I. A randomized comparison of acitretin-narrow-band TL-01 phototherapy and acitretin-psoralen plus ultraviolet A for psoriasis. Acta Derm Venereol. 2008;88(6):589–93.

102. Ortonne JP, Khemis A, Koo JY, Choi J. An open-label study of alefacept plus ultraviolet B light as combination therapy for chronic plaque psoriasis. J Eur Acad Dermatol Venereol. 2005;19(5):556–63.

103. Legat FJ, Hofer A, Wackernagel A, Salmhofer W, Quehenberger F, Kerl H, et al. Narrowband UV-B phototherapy, alefacept, and clearance of psoriasis. Arch Dermatol. 2007;143(8):1016–22.

104. Kircik L, Bagel J, Korman N, Menter A, Elmets CA, Koo J, et al. Utilization of narrow-band ultraviolet light B therapy and etanercept for the treatment of psoriasis (UNITE): efficacy, safety, and patient-reported outcomes. J Drugs Dermatol. 2008;7(3):245–53.

105. Momtaz TK, Parrish JA. Combination of psoralens and ultraviolet A and ultraviolet B in the treatment of psoriasis vulgaris: a bilateral comparison study. J Am Acad Dermatol. 1984;10(3):481–6.

106. Wainwright NJ, Dawe RS, Ferguson J. Narrowband ultraviolet B (TL-01) phototherapy for psoriasis: which incremental regimen? Br J Dermatol. 1998;139(3):410–4.

107. Vun YY, Jones B, Al-Mudhaffer M, Egan C. Generalized pustular psoriasis of pregnancy treated with narrowband UVB and topical steroids. J Am Acad Dermatol. 2006;54(2 Suppl):S28–30.

108. Spuls PI, Bossuyt PM, van Everdingen JJ, Witkamp L, Bos JD. The development of practice guidelines for the treatment of severe plaque form psoriasis. Arch Dermatol. 1998;134(12):1591–6.

109. Tauscher AE, Fleischer AB Jr, Phelps KC, Feldman SR. Psoriasis and pregnancy. J Cutan Med Surg. 2002;6(6):561–70.

110. Bibbins-Domingo K, Grossman DC, Curry SJ, Davidson KW, Epling JWJ, García FA, et al. Folic acid supplementation for the prevention of neural tube defects: US Preventive Services Task Force Recommendation Statement. JAMA. 2017;317(2):183–9.

111. Zhang M, Goyert G, Lim HW. Folate and phototherapy: what should we inform our patients? J Am Acad Dermatol. 2017;77(5):958–64.

112. Tay YK, Morelli JG, Weston WL. Experience with UVB phototherapy in children. Pediatr Dermatol. 1996;13(5):406–9.

113. Jury CS, McHenry P, Burden AD, Lever R, Bilsland D. Narrowband ultraviolet B (UVB) phototherapy in children. Clin Exp Dermatol. 2006;31(2):196–9.

114. Pahlajani N, Katz BJ, Lozano AM, Murphy F, Gottlieb A. Comparison of the efficacy and safety of the 308 nm excimer laser for the treatment of localized psoriasis in adults and in children: a pilot study. Pediatr Dermatol. 2005;22(2):161–5.

115. Song E, Reja D, Silverberg N, Rothe MJ. Phototherapy: kids are not just little people. Clin Dermatol. 2015;33(6):672–80.

116. Holme SA, Anstey AV. Phototherapy and PUVA photochemotherapy in children. Photodermatol Photoimmunol Photomed. 2004;20(2):69–75.

117. Collins P, Ferguson J. Narrowband (TL-01) UVB air-conditioned phototherapy for atopic eczema in children. Br J Dermatol. 1995;133(4):653–5.

118. Koek MB, Buskens E, van Weelden H, Steegmans PH, Bruijnzeel-Koomen CA, Sigurdsson V. Home versus outpatient ultraviolet B phototherapy for mild to severe psoriasis: pragmatic multicentre randomised controlled non-inferiority trial (PLUTO study). BMJ. 2009;b1542:338.

119. Rajpara AN, O'Neill JL, Nolan BV, Yentzer BA, Feldman SR. Review of home phototherapy. Dermatol Online J. 2010;16(12):2.

120. Lapolla W, Yentzer BA, Bagel J, Halvorson CR, Feldman SR. A review of phototherapy protocols for psoriasis treatment. J Am Acad Dermatol. 2011;64(5):936–49.

121. Yelverton CB, Kulkarni AS, Balkrishnan R, Feldman SR. Home ultraviolet B phototherapy: a cost-effective option for severe psoriasis. Manag Care Interface. 2006;19(1):33–6. 9

122. Koek MB, Sigurdsson V, van Weelden H, Steegmans PH, Bruijnzeel-Koomen CA, Buskens E. Cost effectiveness of home ultraviolet B phototherapy for psoriasis: economic evaluation of a randomized controlled trial (PLUTO study). BMJ. 2010;340:c1490.

123. Hung R, Ungureanu S, Edwards C, Gambles B, Anstey AV. Home phototherapy for psoriasis: a review and update. Clin Exp Dermatol. 2015;40(8):827–2; quiz 32–3

124. Psoriasis: the assessment and managing of psoriasis. Cost report. Implementing NICE guidance. January 1, 2017. https://www.nice.org.uk/guidance/cg153/resources/costing-report-188311357

125. Henseler T, Wolff K, Honigsmann H, Christophers E. Oral 8-methoxypsoralen photochemotherapy of psoriasis. The European PUVA study: a cooperative study among 18 European centres. Lancet. 1981;1(8225):853–7.

126. Melski JW, Tanenbaum L, Parrish JA, Fitzpatrick TB, Bleich HL. Oral methoxsalen photochemotherapy for the treatment of psoriasis: a cooperative clinical trial. J Invest Dermatol. 1977;68(6):328–35.

127. Spuls PI, Witkamp L, Bossuyt PM, Bos JD. A systematic review of five systemic treatments for severe psoriasis. Br J Dermatol. 1997;137(6):943–9.

128. Griffiths CE, Clark CM, Chalmers RJ, Li Wan Po A, Williams HC. A systematic review of treatments for severe psoriasis. Health Technol Assess. 2000;4(40):1–125.

129. Yones SS, Palmer RA, Garibaldinos TT, Hawk JL. Randomized double-blind trial of the treatment of chronic plaque psoriasis: efficacy of psoralen-UV-A therapy vs narrowband UV-B therapy. Arch Dermatol. 2006;142(7):836–42.

130. Cooper EJ, Herd RM, Priestley GC, Hunter JA. A comparison of bathwater and oral delivery of 8-methoxypsoralen in PUVA therapy for plaque psoriasis. Clin Exp Dermatol. 2000;25(2):111–4.

131. Collins P, Rogers S. Bath-water compared with oral delivery of 8-methoxypsoralen PUVA therapy for chronic plaque psoriasis. Br J Dermatol. 1992;127(4):392–5.

132. Lowe NJ, Weingarten D, Bourget T, Moy LS. PUVA therapy for psoriasis: comparison of oral and bath-water delivery of 8-methoxypsoralen. J Am Acad Dermatol. 1986;14(5 Pt 1):754–60.

133. Turjanmaa K, Salo H, Reunala T. Comparison of trioxsalen bath and oral methoxsalen PUVA in psoriasis. Acta Derm Venereol. 1985;65(1):86–8.

134. Stern RS, Thibodeau LA, Kleinerman RA, Parrish JA, Fitzpatrick TB. Risk of cutaneous carcinoma in patients treated with oral methoxsalen photochemotherapy for psoriasis. N Engl J Med. 1979;300(15):809–13.

135. Stern RS, Laird N, Melski J, Parrish JA, Fitzpatrick TB, Bleich HL. Cutaneous squamous-cell carcinoma in patients treated with PUVA. N Engl J Med. 1984;310(18):1156–61.

136. Nijsten TE, Stern RS. The increased risk of skin cancer is persistent after discontinuation of psoralen+ultraviolet A: a cohort study. J Invest Dermatol. 2003;121(2):252–8.

137. Morison WL, Baughman RD, Day RM, Forbes PD, Hoenigsmann H, Krueger GG, et al. Consensus workshop on the toxic effects of long-term PUVA therapy. Arch Dermatol. 1998;134(5):595–8.

138. Lindelöf B. Risk of melanoma with psoralen/ultraviolet A therapy for psoriasis. Do the known risks now outweigh the benefits? Drug Saf. 1999;20(4):289–97.

139. Stern RS, Nichols KT, Vakeva LH. Malignant melanoma in patients treated for psoriasis with methoxsalen (psoralen) and ultraviolet A radiation (PUVA). The PUVA Follow-Up Study. N Engl J Med. 1997;336(15):1041–5.

140. Forman AB, Roenigk HH Jr, Caro WA, Magid ML. Long-term follow-up of skin cancer in the PUVA-48 cooperative study. Arch Dermatol. 1989;125(4):515–9.

141. Chuang TY, Heinrich LA, Schultz MD, Reizner GT, Kumm RC, Cripps DJ. PUVA and skin cancer. A historical cohort study on 492 patients. J Am Acad Dermatol. 1992;26(2 Pt 1):173–7.

142. Wolff K. Should PUVA be abandoned? N Engl J Med. 1997;336(15):1090–1.

143. Stern RS, Kleinerman RA, Parrish JA, Fitzpatrick TB, Bleich HL. Phototoxic reactions to photoactive drugs in patients treated with PUVA. Arch Dermatol. 1980;116(11):1269–71.

144. Murase JE, Lee EE, Koo J. Effect of ethnicity on the risk of developing nonmelanoma skin cancer following long-term PUVA therapy. Int J Dermatol. 2005;44(12):1016–21.

145. Marcil I, Stern RS. Squamous-cell cancer of the skin in patients given PUVA and cyclosporin: nested cohort crossover study. Lancet. 2001;358(9287):1042–5.

146. Malanos D, Stern RS. Psoralen plus ultraviolet A does not increase the risk of cataracts: a 25-year prospective study. J Am Acad Dermatol. 2007;57(2):231–7.

147. Hannuksela-Svahn A, Sigurgeirsson B, Pukkala E, Lindelof B, Berne B, Hannuksela M, et al. Trioxsalen bath PUVA did not increase the risk of squamous cell skin carcinoma and cutaneous malignant melanoma in a joint analysis of 944 Swedish and Finnish patients with psoriasis. Br J Dermatol. 1999;141(3):497–501.

148. Hannuksela A, Pukkala E, Hannuksela M, Karvonen J. Cancer incidence among Finnish patients with psoriasis treated with trioxsalen bath PUVA. J Am Acad Dermatol. 1996;35(5 Pt 1):685–9.

149. Menter MA, See JA, Amend WJ, Ellis CN, Krueger GG, Lebwohl M, et al. Proceedings of the psoriasis combination and rotation therapy conference. Deer Valley, Utah, Oct. 7–9, 1994. J Am Acad Dermatol. 1996;34(2 Pt 1):315–21.

150. Torras H, Aliaga A, Lopez-Estebaranz JL, Hernandez I, Gardeazabal J, Quintanilla E, et al. A combination therapy of calcipotriol cream and PUVA reduces the UVA dose and improves the response of psoriasis vulgaris. J Dermatolog Treat. 2004;15(2):98–103.

151. Youn JI, Park BS, Park SB, Kim SD, Suh DH. Comparison of calcipotriol and PUVA with conventional PUVA in the treatment of psoriasis. J Dermatol Treat. 2000;11:125–30.

152. Frappaz A, Thivolet J. Calcipotriol in combination with PUVA: a randomized double blind placebo study in severe psoriasis. Eur J Dermatol. 1993;3:351–4.

153. Tzaneva S, Honigsmann H, Tanew A, Seeber A. A comparison of psoralen plus ultraviolet A (PUVA) monotherapy, tacalcitol plus PUVA and tazarotene plus PUVA in patients with chronic plaque-type psoriasis. Br J Dermatol. 2002;147(4):748–53.

154. Behrens S, Grundmann-Kollmann M, Peter RU, Kerscher M. Combination treatment of psoriasis with photochemotherapy and tazarotene gel, a receptor-selective topical retinoid. Br J Dermatol. 1999;141(1):177.

155. Schmoll M, Henseler T, Christophers E. Evaluation of PUVA, topical corticosteroids and the combination of both in the treatment of psoriasis. Br J Dermatol. 1978;99(6):693–702.

156. Morison WL, Parrish JA, Fitzpatrick TB. Controlled study of PUVA and adjunctive topical therapy in the management of psoriasis. Br J Dermatol. 1978;98(2):125–32.

157. Lauharanta J, Geiger JM. A double-blind comparison of acitretin and etretinate in combination with bath PUVA in the treatment of extensive psoriasis. Br J Dermatol. 1989;121(1):107–12.

158. Saurat JH, Geiger JM, Amblard P, Beani JC, Boulanger A, Claudy A, et al. Randomized double-blind multicenter study comparing acitretin-PUVA, etretinate-PUVA and placebo-PUVA in the treatment of severe psoriasis. Dermatologica. 1988;177(4):218–24.

159. Tanew A, Guggenbichler A, Honigsmann H, Geiger JM, Fritsch P. Photochemotherapy for severe psoriasis without or in combination with acitretin: a randomized, double-blind comparison study. J Am Acad Dermatol. 1991;25(4):682–4.

160. Lebwohl M. Acitretin in combination with UVB or PUVA. J Am Acad Dermatol. 1999;41(3 Pt 2):S22–4.

161. Nijsten TE, Stern RS. Oral retinoid use reduces cutaneous squamous cell carcinoma risk in patients with psoriasis treated with psoralen-UVA: a nested cohort study. J Am Acad Dermatol. 2003;49(4):644–50.

162. Bavinck JN, Tieben LM, Van der Woude FJ, Tegzess AM, Hermans J, ter Schegget J, et al. Prevention of skin cancer and reduction of keratotic skin lesions during acitretin therapy in renal transplant recipients: a double-blind, placebo-controlled study. J Clin Oncol. 1995;13(8):1933–8.

163. McKenna DB, Murphy GM. Skin cancer chemoprophylaxis in renal transplant recipients: 5 years of experience using low-dose acitretin. Br J Dermatol. 1999;140(4):656–60.

164. McNamara IR, Muir J, Galbraith AJ. Acitretin for prophylaxis of cutaneous malignancies after cardiac transplantation. J Heart Lung Transplant. 2002;21(11):1201–5.

165. Yuan ZF, Davis A, Macdonald K, Bailey RR. Use of acitretin for the skin complications in renal transplant recipients. N Z Med J. 1995;108(1002):255–6.

166. Morison WL, Momtaz K, Parrish JA, Fitzpatrick TB. Combined methotrexate-PUVA therapy in the treatment of psoriasis. J Am Acad Dermatol. 1982;6(1):46–51.

167. Shehzad T, Dar NR, Zakria M. Efficacy of concomitant use of PUVA and methotrexate in disease clearance time in plaque type psoriasis. J Pak Med Assoc. 2004;54(9):453–5.

168. MacKie RM, Fitzsimons CP. Risk of carcinogenicity in patients with psoriasis treated with methotrexate or PUVA singly or in combination. J Am Acad Dermatol. 1983;9(3):467–9.

169. Calzavara-Pinton P. Narrow band UVB (311 nm) phototherapy and PUVA photochemotherapy: a combination. J Am Acad Dermatol. 1998;38(5 Pt 1):687–90.

170. Grundmann-Kollmann M, Ludwig R, Zollner TM, Ochsendorf F, Thaci D, Boehncke WH, et al. Narrowband UVB and cream psoralen-UVA combination therapy for plaque-type psoriasis. J Am Acad Dermatol. 2004;50(5):734–9.

171. Pham CT, Koo JY. Plasma levels of 8-methoxypsoralen after topical paint PUVA. J Am Acad Dermatol. 1993;28(3):460–6.

172. Neild VS, Scott LV. Plasma levels of 8-methoxypsoralen in psoriatic patients receiving topical 8-methoxypsoralen. Br J Dermatol. 1982;106(2):199–203.

173. Stern RS, Nichols KT. Therapy with orally administered methoxsalen and ultraviolet A radiation during childhood increases the risk of basal cell carcinoma. The PUVA Follow-up Study. J Pediatr. 1996;129(6):915–7.

174. Pasić A, Ceović R, Lipozencić J, Husar K, Susić SM, Skerlev M, et al. Phototherapy in pediatric patients. Pediatr Dermatol. 2003;20(1):71–7.

175. Vonderheid EC, Bigler RD, Rogers RD, Rogers TJ, Kadin ME, Griffin TD. Effect of extracorporeal photopheresis on selected immunologic parameters in psoriasis vulgaris. Yale J Biol Med. 1989;62(6):653–64.

176. Wilfert H, Hönigsmann H, Steiner G, Smolen J, Wolff K. Treatment of psoriatic arthritis by extracorporeal photochemotherapy. Br J Dermatol. 1990;122(2):225–32.

177. Vonderheid EC, Kang CA, Kadin M, Bigler RD, Griffin TD, Rogers TJ. Extracorporeal photopheresis in psoriasis vulgaris: clinical and immunologic observations. J Am Acad Dermatol. 1990;23(4 Pt 1):703–12.

178. de Misa RF, Azaña JM, Harto A, Boizeda P, Moreno R, Ledo A. Psoriatic arthritis: one year of treatment with extracorporeal photochemotherapy. J Am Acad Dermatol. 1994;30(6):1037–8.

179. Vahlquist C, Larsson M, Ernerudh J, Berlin G, Skogh T, Vahlquist A. Treatment of psoriatic arthritis with extracorporeal photochemotherapy and conventional psoralen-ultraviolet A irradiation. Arthritis Rheum. 1996;39(9):1519–23.

180. McKenna KE, Whittaker S, Rhodes LE, Taylor P, Lloyd JJ, Ibbotson S, et al. Evidence-based practice of photopheresis 1987–2001: a report of a workshop of the British Photodermatology Group and the U. K. Skin Lymphoma Group. Br J Dermatol. 2006;154(1):7–20.

181. Garza FZC, Liebmann J, Born M, Hilbers PA, van Riel NA. A dynamic model for prediction of psoriasis management by blue light irradiation. Front Physiol. 2017;26(8):28.

182. Maari C, Viau G, Bissonnette R. Repeated exposure to blue light does not improve psoriasis. J Am Acad Dermatol. 2003;49(1):55–8.

183. Al-Mutairi N, Noor T, Al-Haddad A. Single blinded left-to-right comparison study of excimer laser versus pulsed dye laser for the treatment of nail psoriasis. Dermatol Ther (Heidelb). 2014;4(2):197–205.

184. Huang YC, Chou CL, Chiang YY. Efficacy of pulsed dye laser plus topical tazarotene versus topical tazarotene alone in psoriatic nail disease: a single-blind, intrapatient left-to-right controlled study. Lasers Surg Med. 2012;45(2):102–7.

185. Treewittayapoom C, Singvahanont P, Chanprapaph K, Haneke E. The effect of different pulse durations in the treatment of nail psoriasis with 595-nm pulsed dye laser: a randomised, double-blind, intrapatient left-to-right study. J Am Acad Dermatol. 2012;66(5):807–12.

186. Fernández-Guarino M, Harto A, Sánchez-Ronco M, García-Morales I, Jaén P. Pulsed dye laser vs. photodynamic therapy in the treatment of refractory nail psoriasis: a comparative pilot study. J Eur Acad Dermatol Venereol. 2009;23(8):891–5.

187. Tawfik AA. Novel treatment of nail psoriasis using the intense pulsed light: a one-year follow-up study. Dermatol Surg. 2014;40(7):763–8.

Kristen M. Beck, Eric J. Yang, Ladi Afifian, Di Yan,
and Tina Bhutani

Methotrexate

Background

The antifolate agent aminopterin was first synthesized in 1947 to treat childhood leukemia [1] but was soon found to have efficacy in various nonneoplastic disease states. In 1951, aminopterin was shown to improve symptoms of psoriasis and psoriatic arthritis [2, 3]. This initial folate analog was subsequently modified to produce amethopterin, now termed methotrexate (MTX), a safer antifolate compound that continued to demonstrate efficacy in improving psoriasis symptoms [4–8]. By 1972, MTX was officially approved by the FDA for use in patients with severe, recalcitrant, disabling psoriasis [9] and has remained a mainstay of treatment for psoriatic disease for the last 50 years.

Mechanism of Action

MTX inhibits dihydrofolate reductase (DHFR), an enzyme that catalyzes the reduction of dihydrofolic acid to tetrahydrofolic acid, the active form of folate. Without tetrahydrofolic acid, thymidylate synthase is unable to methylate deoxyuridine monophosphate to produce thymidine, a nucleoside essential for DNA synthesis. Although the mechanism of action of MTX in psoriasis has not been fully elucidated, this process obstructs the S phase of the cell cycle, which inhibits epidermal cell hyperproliferation [10, 11], prevents the growth of activated lymphocytes [12], triggers T-cell apoptosis [13], and impedes neutrophil chemotaxis [14]. MTX also reduces levels of pro-inflammatory cytokines such as interleukin (IL)-6, IL-8, and IL-1 [15–17].

Pharmacokinetics

Oral doses of MTX are rapidly absorbed across the gut but demonstrate highly variable incomplete absorption [18]. Food intake does not affect MTX absorption in adults [19] but may reduce MTX bioavailability in children [20]. Once absorbed, the mean half-life of MTX in adults is 5–8 h [18]. MTX has a mean protein binding to serum albumin of 42–57% and is active when unbound [18]. Thus, drugs that decrease protein binding of MTX, such as salicylates,

K. M. Beck · L. Afifian · Di Yan
Department of Dermatology, UCSF Medical Center,
San Francisco, CA, USA
e-mail: Kristen.beck@ucsf.edu

T. Bhutani (✉) · E. J. Yang
Department of Dermatology, UCSF Psoriasis Center,
University of California San Francisco,
San Francisco, CA, USA
e-mail: tina.bhutani@ucsf.edu

© Springer International Publishing AG, part of Springer Nature 2018

T. Bhutani et al. (eds.), *Evidence-Based Psoriasis*, Updates in Clinical Dermatology,
https://doi.org/10.1007/978-3-319-90107-7_4

sulfonamides, and probenecid, can increase the risk of toxicity of this medication [21–23]. MTX is primarily excreted through renal clearance of the drug in its unchanged form, which is filtered through the glomeruli and also undergoes active tubular secretion [18, 24].

Indications

MTX is approved in dermatology for patients with severe, recalcitrant, disabling psoriasis that is not adequately responsive to other forms of therapy [25, 26]. MTX has also demonstrated efficacy in treating various forms of psoriasis, including plaque, guttate, pustular, and erythrodermic subtypes [9] and efficacy for patients with concurrent psoriatic arthritis as well.

Efficacy

The use of MTX for psoriasis predates the FDA requirement for randomized controlled trials in new drug applications. Although MTX has long been used as a treatment for psoriatic disease, to date there are only a few clinical studies to guide evidence-based use of MTX in psoriasis.

The first placebo-controlled clinical trial of oral MTX in psoriasis, CHAMPION, examined the efficacy MTX to adalimumab and placebo [27]. In this study, patients with moderate-to-severe plaque psoriasis were randomized to receive a starting oral dose of 7.5 mg of MTX that was increased to 25 mg weekly as needed (n = 110), adalimumab (n = 108), or placebo (n = 53). After 16 weeks, 36% of patients in the MTX group using a mean weekly dose of 19 ± 5 mg reached psoriasis area severity index (PASI) 75 response, significantly more than the placebo group (19%) but lower than the adalimumab group (79.6%). In trials that compared MTX to cyclosporine without a placebo arm, the PASI 75 response rate varied from 60% (maximum dose 22.5 mg/week MTX) [28] to 24% (maximum dose 15 mg/week MTX) at 16 weeks [29].

Combination Therapy

A variety of therapies, including other oral agents, phototherapy, and biologics may be used concurrently, in rotation, or sequentially with MTX. Combination therapy is often more effective than monotherapy and should be considered in patients for whom MTX alone is ineffective or in patients who desire a faster skin response or greater likelihood of skin clearance [30]. Synergistic effects of combining MTX with other treatment modalities may also result in clinical improvement at lower doses than those used in MTX monotherapy, which reduces of the risk of liver toxicity.

Several studies have shown that the effects of phototherapy in combination with MTX are synergistic [30], with faster clearance achieved with lower doses of MTX and ultraviolet B (UVB) or narrowband UVB (NBUVB) compared to monotherapy with either modality alone [31, 32]. Combination treatment of psoralen plus ultraviolet A (PUVA) and MTX may lead to faster skin clearance compared to MTX alone with fewer PUVA sessions compared to PUVA alone [33, 34]; however this advantage must be weighed against the risks of carcinogenesis, especially with regard to increased risk for squamous cell carcinoma [35, 36].

MTX and cyclosporine have been an especially successful treatment combination for psoriatic arthritis and generalized pustular psoriasis, as well as plaque psoriasis. Studies of MTX (7.5–15 mg/week) and cyclosporine (3 mg/kg/day) resulted in superior clearance with fewer side effects compared to either alone [37, 38]. These two drugs may also be used in rotation, alternating use of each for several months at full dose with a one-week washout period in between, so as to avoid nephrotoxicity and hepatotoxicity [30].

Although acitretin and hydroxyurea have been used in combination with MTX, this is generally not recommended. The primary concern of using acitretin and MTX together is the increased risk of hepatotoxicity. Hydroxyurea is generally contraindicated with MTX out of concern for bone marrow suppression. However, each of these has been used in combination with MTX success-fully without an increase in liver toxicity or wors-ening of blood counts, respectively [14, 39–42]. Careful laboratory monitoring is imperative if either of these combinations are prescribed.

MTX may be considered for use with biolog-ics. Most evidence is for either etanercept [43] or infliximab, since both of these are frequently used with MTX in rheumatoid arthritis [30, 44]. In one study, psoriasis patients who had not responded to MTX monotherapy showed signifi-cantly more improvement when etanercept was added to MTX compared to switch to etanercept monotherapy [45]. MTX is also often added to etanercept therapy to preserve the efficacy of the medication, an effect at least partially explained by its effects on neutralizing antibodies [46]. In a small study, psoriasis patients with treatment fail-ure on etanercept monotherapy had significant improvement when switched to a combination of etanercept with low-dose MTX therapy [47].

Adverse Effects and Monitoring

MTX is most commonly associated with hepato-toxic effects, ranging from elevated liver enzymes to hepatic steatosis, cirrhosis, and fibrosis [25, 26]. Patients with psoriatic disease are at increased risk of developing hepatotoxicity with MTX use compared to rheumatoid arthritis patients [48]. Risk factors for hepatotoxicity include a history or current excessive use of alco-hol, diabetes, hyperlipidemia, persistently abnor-mal liver tests, personal history of liver disease, family history of heritable liver disease, and past exposure to hepatotoxic compounds. The American Academy of Dermatology (AAD) and the National Psoriasis Foundation (NPF) recom-mend separate monitoring strategies for patients based on the presence or absence of risk factors for hepatotoxicity [9, 49]. To minimize the risk of hepatotoxicity, patients should be counseled to avoid or minimize alcohol intake while using MTX.

Myelosuppression is another potential serious adverse effect of MTX therapy. Risk factors for hematopoietic toxicity include advanced age,

renal insufficiency, hypoalbuminemia, and exces-sive alcohol consumption. A complete blood count should be monitored every 2–4 weeks for the first few months of therapy and then every 1–3 months thereafter. Folic or folinic acid may be added in 1–5 mg oral doses to protect against MTX toxicity [9, 49–51]. MTX should be tempo-rarily ceased or decreased if leukocyte or platelet counts become abnormally low. If toxicity is detected, folinic acid (leucovorin) should be administered without delay.

Potential short-term side effects of MTX include nausea, anorexia, headache, and fatigue [25, 26]. Other side effects associated with MTX include infections such as *Pneumocystis carinii* pneumonia, nocardiosis, cryptococcosis, and var-icella zoster. MTX pneumonitis is very rare in psoriasis patients but can be fatal and irrevers-ible, so age-appropriate vaccinations before com-mencing therapy are recommended. HIV testing and tuberculosis screening may be considered in patients with a history of risk factors for these infections [9].

Medications known to interact with MTX and possibly increase toxicity include nonsteroidal anti-inflammatories, antibiotics (trimethoprim/sulfamethoxazole, ciprofloxacin, minocycline, and penicillins), barbiturates, colchicine, dipyri-damole, sulfonylureas, furosemide, phenytoin, and thiazide diuretics [9].

Contraindications

Absolute contraindications to MTX include cir-rhosis and bone marrow abnormalities such as leukopenia, severe anemia, or thrombocytopenia [25, 26, 49]. MTX is pregnancy category X. The benefits and risks of MTX should be carefully weighed prior to initiating therapy in women of childbearing potential, due to the known terato-genic effects of this medication. Although MTX is not thought to have mutagenic effects, males are advised to wait 3 months after discontinuing MTX before attempting to conceive a child [49].

Relative contraindications to MTX use include renal impairment, liver dysfunction, active or recur-rent hepatitis, alcoholism, and immunosuppression.

Obesity, diabetes mellitus, and active severe infections such as HIV or tuberculosis are also relative contraindications.

Dosing

MTX is usually given as a single weekly dose [25, 26] but may be divided into three doses, each given 12 hours apart, which aims to decrease gastrointestinal side effects [49, 52]. The weekly dose typically ranges from 7.5 to 25 mg per week [52] and should not exceed 30 mg [53]. The AAD recommends an initial test dose of 2.5–5 mg prior to therapeutic dosing to evaluate for myelosuppression in susceptible patients [49]. Improvement is typically seen after 16 to 24 weeks. A minimum of 4–8 weeks is recommended before dose modification or cessation [52]. Once therapeutic results are achieved, MTX can be gradually titrated to the minimum dose necessary to achieve optimal control of symptoms. MTX may be used indefinitely at the lowest effective dose of the drug as long-term maintenance therapy [52].

Patients with impaired renal function, ascites, or pleural effusions require reduced dosing due to diminished MTX elimination [25, 26, 53]. MTX may also be used in children with recalcitrant, severe psoriasis for up to 6 months at 0.2–0.7 mg/kg weekly [54].

Acitretin

Background

Acitretin, the active metabolite of etretinate, is the most widely used systemic retinoid in the treatment of psoriasis. Etretinate was previously used for psoriasis since the 1970s but was removed from the market in 1997 due its teratogenicity and ability to be detected for years after cessation of the medication [55, 56]. Acitretin is 50 times less lipophilic, resulting in a much shorter half-life. Thus, acitretin has replaced etretinate for the treatment of psoriasis due to a more favorable pharmacokinetic profile.

Mechanism of Action

Acitretin is unique in comparison to other psoriasis treatments as it does not directly suppress immune system pathways. Retinoids activate receptors in the nucleus that mediate gene transcription, ultimately resulting in a broad range of downstream effects. Acitretin has been shown to decrease the quantity of Th1 and Th17 cells, resulting in reduced expression of pro-inflammatory cytokines implicated in the pathogenesis of psoriasis, such as IFN-γ and IL-17 [57]. Additionally, retinoids play a critical role in promoting keratinocyte differentiation and maturation, ultimately resulting in decreased skin cell turnover and decreased epidermal hyperplasia [58, 59].

Pharmacokinetics

Due to the lipophilic nature of retinoids, bioavailability of acitretin is enhanced by food, particularly fatty meals [60]. Acitretin is considerably less lipophilic than etretinate, with a half-life of approximately 50–60 h and is undetectable in the serum 1 month after stopping medication [58, 61]. Retinoids are metabolized in the liver via oxidation and chain shortening, processes which are induced by retinoic acid and possibly cytochrome P450 3A4 inducers [62, 63]. The resulting metabolites are then primarily excreted in the urine and feces. Notably, transesterification of acitretin into etretinate can occur with concurrent ethanol ingestion [64]. Due to the lipophilicity of etretinate, it may stay in the body for up to 3 years and contribute to increased risk of toxicity and teratogenicity [58]. Thus, patients are advised to refrain from alcohol intake during treatment.

Indications

Acitretin is used for moderate-to-severe psoriasis, with notable efficacy in pustular and erythrodermic subtypes. Since the mechanism of action of acitretin does directly not involve immunological pathways, acitretin is a particularly good choice in immunosuppressed individuals and those affected with chronic infections, such as viral hepatitis or HIV [65].

Efficacy

Acitretin monotherapy is particularly efficacious in pustular [66] and erythrodermic psoriasis [58, 67, 68]. A systematic review of 12 clinical trials found that among patients receiving acitretin, there was marked improvement in 100% of patients with pustular, 83% with erythrodermic, and 77% with other forms of psoriasis [69]. Several studies report improvement following retinoid use for pustular psoriasis [70–73]. Acitretin in HIV-associated psoriasis has also shown excellent results [65]. In comparison, studies of acitretin in chronic plaque psoriasis demonstrate relatively modest results. A study of 28 patients found high doses of acitretin (50 and 75 mg) for 8 weeks to significantly reduce PASI score versus placebo, while low doses (10 and 25 mg) did not; however, high doses were accompanied by an increase in adverse events [74]. However, other studies have reported improvement at lower doses. In a double-blind trial of 175 patients on 10, 25, or 50 mg/day of acitretin or 50 mg of etretinate for 8 weeks, PASI 50 was achieved in 50%, 41%, 54%, and 61% of patients, respectively [68]. One study looking at various dosing regimens in chronic plaque psoriasis patients found comparative efficacy among patients treated for 6 weeks with acitretin by either dose escalation (starting at 10 mg, increasing to 50 mg), constant dosing at 30 mg, or dose de-escalation (starting at 50 mg, tapering down to 10 mg) [75]. All three groups demonstrated more than 80% clinical improvement, while group 1 experienced the lowest drug toxicity rate [75]. Another study also demonstrated a higher safety profile with similarly low dose despite excellent efficacy [76].

Combination Therapy

Acitretin is a useful addition to other oral agents, phototherapy, and biologics, due to its non-immunomodulatory mechanism of action and anticarcinogenic qualities. Acitretin is synergist with phototherapy, allowing for lower doses of both to achieve therapeutic effect [36]. Re-PUVA refers to use of acitretin (typically 10–25 mg) in combination with PUVA, while Re-UVB refers to use with UVB. Acitretin is photosensitizing and results in clinical response at lower levels of UVA and UVB. Notably, acitretin is also the only psoriasis agent used in combination with phototherapy that is thought to be preventative against skin cancer, owing to its tumor-suppressing properties [77]. Use of acitretin in combination with MTX was discussed previously in this chapter. Sequential therapy of acitretin with cyclosporine has also been described [78].

Adverse Effects

Systemic retinoid use is associated with a variety of adverse effects that are primarily related to hypervitaminosis A. The risk is dose-dependent, particularly with doses greater than 25 mg [79]. Aside from the possible musculoskeletal effects, most of these adverse effects resolve or subside with drug tolerability, a reduced dosing regimen, or drug discontinuation.

Mucocutaneous adverse effects are expected to occur in nearly every patient. Cheilitis occurs in about 70–75% of patients, even on low doses [80]. However, incidence of xerosis and skin peeling is substantially increased at higher doses (high dose, 50% and 50–75%; low dose, 4% and 30%, respectively). Other mucocutaneous side effects include rhinitis, dry mouth, pruritus, photosensitivity, sticky skin, dermatitis, alopecia, paronychia, and nail deformities. Most of these are generally mild and reversible [81] and can be managed with bland emollients or mild topical steroids. A reduction in the retinoid dose can also be considered if these effects prove intolerable.

Acitretin is potentially hepatotoxic. About 15% of patients develop elevated serum liver enzymes, generally 2–8 weeks after initiating treatment [36, 82]. The risk increases with higher doses [83]. This increase in serum liver enzymes is usually transient and subsides with dose reduction; severe or persistent cases are rare, though alcoholics, diabetics, and obese patients are at increased risk. Patients are advised to refrain from alcohol intake while on acitretin.

Hyperlipidemia is observed in 25–40% of patients taking systemic retinoids, with hypertriglyceridemia more common than hypercholesterolemia [82, 84]. Obese patients, alcoholics, smokers, and diabetics are at especially high risk. Patients with familial hyperlipidemia or those who are taking medications such as beta-blockers, contraceptives, and thiazides are also at increased risk. Elevations can be managed with an initial trial of lifestyle modifications, but if this proves insufficient, use of anti-lipidemic drugs may be indicated [83].

Musculoskeletal side effects are less common, associated with cumulative long-term therapy, and generally irreversible. Specific associated musculoskeletal effects include premature fusion of epiphyses, diffuse idiopathic skeletal hyperostosis syndrome, calcification of ligaments, osteoporosis, as well as modeling abnormalities of long bones. Overall, conflicting reports within the literature have made it challenging to elucidate the true risk of skeletal toxicity with the use of systemic retinoids [85–91].

Major human fetal abnormalities are associated with retinoid use during pregnancy [81]. Other side effects include xerophthalmia, night blindness, nausea, and abdominal pain. Although acitretin is implicated in the development of pseudotumor cerebri, however, no evidence exists demonstrating a causal role [92]. Concomitant therapy with tetracyclines increases the risk and should be avoided [93–96]. Patients should be counseled on the signs and symptoms and the need for prompt ophthalmic evaluation if necessary.

Contraindications

There are very few absolute contraindications to the use of acitretin outside of hypersensitivity reactions. Relative contraindications to the use of retinoid therapy include women of childbearing age, liver and/or kidney dysfunction, and severe hyperlipidemia. Retinoid therapy should be used with caution in patients taking drugs with potential for drug interactions and/or hepatic toxicity as well as in patients with a history of alcohol abuse [49].

Acitretin is considered a pregnancy category X drug and highly teratogenic [89]. Women of childbearing potential should not take acitretin unless monitored with monthly pregnancy tests. Women of childbearing age should be counseled on contraception during and after use of acitretin for a minimum of 3 years after drug.

Monitoring

Laboratory assessments should include a complete blood cell count, liver function tests, basic metabolic panel, and lipid panel prior to initiation of therapy and with period reassessments no less than every 3 months while on treatment [49, 97].

Dosing

Usual dosing of acitretin ranges from 25 to 50 mg, every day or every other day. Typically initiation starts with a low dose (10–25 mg or less) and is titrated up, with dose adjustments no sooner than every 2–4 weeks, until psoriasis improvement or maximal tolerated side effects [98]. Therapeutic benefit is generally observed after 3–6 months, after which the dose can be tapered to a lower maintenance dose. Initial high doses may be necessary for acute flares of generalized pustular psoriasis or erythrodermic psoriasis.

Cyclosporine

Background

The immunomodulatory role of cyclosporine was originally demonstrated by its successful prevention of renal transplant rejection in 1978 [99]. The following year, it was incidentally observed that organ transplant patients receiving the medication experienced improvement in their psoriasis [100]. This resulted in a paradigm shift regarding the pathogenesis of psoriasis. Previously considered a disease of keratinocyte hyperproliferation, psoriasis was recognized for the first time as an immune-mediated disease. Eighteen years later, the FDA approved cyclosporine for treatment of psoriasis. Since then, cyclosporine has proven to be an excellent therapeutic option for psoriasis, especially in severe cases and flares requiring immediate control.

Mechanism of Action

Cyclosporine's various effects on immune function are well-characterized. Cyclosporine inhibits calcineurin, an enzyme important in mediating cytokine gene expression, primarily in T cells [101]. T-cell receptor activation leads to the activation of calcineurin, which subsequently activates nuclear factor of activated T cell (NFAT), a key transcription factor for the expression of many cytokines implicated in the psoriasis pathogenesis, such as interleukin-2 (IL-2), interferon gamma (IFN-γ), and tumor necrosis factor (TNF-α). Thus, cyclosporine inhibition of calcineurin prevents activation of NFAT and consequently expression of the NFAT-dependent cytokines. Cyclosporine's inhibition of IL-2 production results in substantial reductions of CD4 and CD8 T cells in the epidermis [102]. Decreased expression of genes within the Th1 and Th17 pathways in psoriatic skin with cyclosporine use likely also contribute to its efficacy in psoriasis [103]. Cyclosporine also downregulates intercellular adhesion molecule 1 (ICAM-1) expression on keratinocytes and endothelial cells, thus impairing leukocyte extravasation and inflammatory signaling [104, 105].

Pharmacokinetics

Due to the high lipophilicity of cyclosporine, its bioavailability is enhanced by food [106–108]. Thus patients should take cyclosporine at consistent times each day to ensure consistent levels

[109, 110]. Cyclosporine is metabolized in the liver by the CYP3A4 enzyme [111]. Patients with severe liver disease will have impaired breakdown of cyclosporine, and thus require careful monitoring and possible dosing adjustment [49]. This medication has a half-life of approximately 20 hours [109]. Cyclosporine metabolites are mainly eliminated via biliary excretion, with only 6% of the drug being excreted in the urine [109]. Of note, the two primary marketed formulations of cyclosporine, Sandimmune® and Neoral® (modified cyclosporine), are not bioequivalent and cannot be used interchangeably; the bioavailability of Sandimmune® is 76% that of Neoral® [112].

Indications

Cyclosporine is used for severe psoriasis. It is recommended as first-line treatment by the NPF and AAD for severe flares of erythrodermic and pustular psoriasis [49, 113, 114]. Cyclosporine is also particularly useful when a patient requests temporary but quick and complete clearance of their psoriasis—often in the context of major life events, such as weddings. Although cyclosporine is fast-acting and highly efficacious, its use is limited by its high toxicity profile. Importantly, patients must be counseled to expect only temporary use of cyclosporine since, despite its efficacy, long-term use carries serious risk of irreversible adverse effects.

Efficacy

The ability of cyclosporine to lead to rapid clearing of severe psoriasis is well-documented. A study of refractory erythrodermic psoriasis patients treated with cyclosporine 3–5 mg/kg/day led to full remission in 67% of patients and marked improvement in 27% [115]. Several studies of cyclosporine (2.5–5 mg/kg/day for 12–16 weeks) for severe, recalcitrant plaque psoriasis yielded rapid improvement in 80–90% of patients [116–118].

Subsequent studies have been performed to test the optimal dose of cyclosporine to achieve comparable efficacy while also reducing the toxicity profile. A 16-week double-blind placebo-controlled trial compared cyclosporine doses of 3, 5, or 7.5 mg/kg/day and found after 8 weeks of fixed-dose therapy that 35%, 65%, and 80% of patients achieved clearing or almost clearing of their psoriasis, respectively, and the 5 mg/kg/day group required the least amount of dosage changes [116]. In a study of "step-up therapy" (2.5 mg/kg/day with a standard increase in dose) versus "step-down therapy" (5 mg/kg/day with a gradual decrease), more patients in the step-down therapy group achieved PASI 75 in a shorter average timeframe, more rapidly [119].

A randomized, double-blind study comparing the efficacy of two formulations of cyclosporine, Sandimmune® and Neoral®, for severe, chronic plaque psoriasis found that while both had similar rate of adverse events, Neoral® required a ~10% lower dose and fewer dose adjustments [120]. Most patients require 3–4 mg/kg/day of Neoral® to achieve desired response and could be tapered down to 2.5–3.0 mg/kg/day for the maintenance period [121–123].

Adverse Events

Adverse effects of cyclosporine are dose-dependent and cumulative [49, 53, 124–128]. The two most clinically significant side effects are hypertension and nephrotoxicity. Although the exact mechanism for the new-onset or cyclosporine-induced hypertension is not clearly understood, an increase of 5 mmHg in mean arterial blood pressure has been observed when 3–5 mg/kg/day of cyclosporine is used [129]. Management options for new-onset hypertension include reducing the dose of cyclosporine or initiating antihypertensive medication [49, 53]. Nephrotoxicity is another serious concern in patients taking cyclosporine. Low-dose regimens can minimize the risk of nephrotoxicity and should be used whenever possible. Changes in serum creatinine may be observed as early as a few weeks after starting therapy and are gener-

ally reversible once the drug is discontinued [116, 130]. Hypomagnesemia may also occur, requiring replacement therapy. However, permanent renal dysfunction can develop after prolonged therapy at high doses (greater than or equal to 5 mg/kg/day). An increase in creatinine to 25–30% from baseline warrants a reduction in the cyclosporine dose [49, 53, 128].

Cyclosporine is also associated with an increased risk for certain cancers and infections. There may be a slight increase in non-melanoma skin cancers in patients with cyclosporine for psoriasis [131, 132] and increased in squamous cell carcinoma particularly in patients who received greater than 200 PUVA treatments prior to cyclosporine [131, 133]. Other reported side effects of cyclosporine include dyslipidemia, headaches, tremors, seizures, pseudotumor cerebri, gingival hyperplasia, and hypertrichosis [128, 134–139].

Contraindications

Absolute contraindications include hypersensitivity reactions to cyclosporine, abnormal renal function, uncontrolled hypertension, current malignancy, pregnancy, breastfeeding, history of >200 PUVA treatments, or concomitant use of any of the following: phototherapy, immunosuppression, coal tar therapy, or radiation therapy [49]. Relative contraindications include active infection, dyslipidemia, poorly controlled diabetes, elderly, morbid obesity, history of less than 200 cumulative PUVA treatments, and immunosuppression [49]. Cyclosporine use in any of these special populations requires close monitoring if it is initiated.

Cyclosporine is considered pregnancy category C. The AAD has not provided any specific guidelines for the use of cyclosporine in pregnancy but do recommend that nursing mothers avoid cyclosporine [49]. Cyclosporine capsules contain 12.7% alcohol, and both cyclosporine and alcohol enter breastmilk. Cyclosporine has been used in children and infants for several indications, including psoriasis, without any unexpected side effects [109].

Monitoring

The AAD recommends the following studies prior to initiation of cyclosporine: blood pressure, creatinine (obtain at least two measurements), basic metabolic panel (including BUN and electrolytes), complete blood count, magnesium, urinalysis, urine sediment, uric acid, lipid panel (including cholesterol and triglycerides), hepatic function (including enzymes and bilirubin), and a urine pregnancy test [49, 53]. Testing for tuberculosis should also be performed and all vaccinations current. Screening for HIV and Hepatitis B and C can be performed in high-risk patients. A thorough review of current medications to particularly assess for use of immunosuppressive agents, nephrotoxic agents, or other agents that may interfere with cyclosporine use should be performed. Review of concurrent medications or dietary regimens that inhibit or induce hepatic CYP3A4 activity is also necessary. Contraception should be encouraged for women of childbearing age.

Dosing

The usual dose of cyclosporine for psoriasis is 3–5 mg/kg per day, divided into two doses daily. The therapeutic benefit of doses higher than 5 mg/kg/day is offset by an increase in toxicity [140]. Most patients can be effectively maintained on 2.5–3.0 mg/kg/day [121–123]. AAD guidelines recommend initial doses of 2.5–3 mg/kg/day for 4–6 months, followed by gradual increases as needed. Once near-clearing is achieved, doses can be tapered 0.5–1.0 mg/kg/day at 2-week intervals or 1 mg/kg/day every week over 4 weeks to minimize chances of relapse [49, 53]. High initiation doses may be used for severe flares of erythrodermic or generalized pustular psoriasis. If rapid improvement is necessary, then generally, the maximum dose (5 mg/kg/day) is initiated followed by stepwise decreases (0.5–1.0 mg/kg per week) after adequate response.

Although the cyclosporine package insert recommends dosing is based on ideal body weight, the AAD recommends dosing obese patients at their actual body weight [49]. Cyclosporine withdrawal due to ineffectiveness is recommended following a 3-month trial period at the maximum dose of 5 mg/kg/day [49]. For intolerable side effects, the dosage can be decreased by 1 mg/kg/day and if side effects persist, then further reductions can be employed. Ultra-low doses (1.5 mg/kg/day) can be administered for patients who are unable to tolerate higher doses [141].

Duration of Use

In general, cyclosporine is used as intermittent short-term therapy, not long-term maintenance therapy [49, 53, 142, 143]. Once an adequate response is reached, cyclosporine can be tapered off to prevent relapses. After a brief rest period, treatment can be restarted and followed by subsequent intervals if clinically indicated. AAD guidelines limit the continuous maximum dose of 5 mg/kg/day use of cyclosporine to 1 year [125]; European guidelines allow up to 2 years [143]. Cyclosporine is also suitable as a bridge or sequential therapy. Sequential therapy of acitretin with cyclosporine is one example of this [78]; for example, patients typically start with 1 month of cyclosporine 5 mg/kg/day, then add acitretin 25 mg and increase as tolerated over the next months, and then slowly taper off cyclosporine and continue on maintenance acitretin [78]. However, in cases when cyclosporine is the only efficacious option available for severe, recalcitrant disease, long-term continuous therapy may be used with vigorous monitoring [130, 144–146]. In these cases the goal is not for remission, but rather acceptable improvement with the most minimal dose.

Apremilast

Background

Prior to use in psoriasis, small molecule inhibitors of phosphodiesterase 4 (PDE4) inhibitors were successfully used in other inflammatory diseases. Following the success of roflumilast in COPD, interest arose in PDE4 inhibitors as promising candidates for psoriatic disease. Apremilast is the first PDE4 inhibitor for psoriasis, approved for use in 2014. With its unique mechanism of action and ease of use, apremilast has already proven to be a valuable new addition to the armamentarium of psoriasis treatments. With more long-term data and clinical experience, a clearer picture of apremilast's niche among psoriasis therapeutics will emerge.

Mechanism of Action

Apremilast is a potent and selective small molecule inhibitor of PDE4, which mediates degradation of cyclic adenosine monophosphate (cAMP), an intracellular secondary messenger that promotes anti-inflammatory processes [147]. PDE4 inhibition increases cAMP accumulation, which activates protein kinase A (PKA) and other effector proteins that in turn activate transcription factors like cAMP-responsive element-binding protein (CREB) and activating transcription factor-1 (ATF-1), and inhibit nuclear factor kappa B (NF-κB) [147, 148]. These effects lead to decreased transcription of gene coding for cytokines and other inflammatory mediators and increased expression of anti-inflammatory genes [148]. PDE4 is overexpressed in psoriatic skin [149]. PDE4 inhibition in psoriasis reduces epidermal thickness, decreases dermal and epidermal T cells, and reduces Th1, Th2, and Th17 immune responses [150]. PDE4 inhibition blocks the production of pro-inflammatory cytokines implicated in the pathogenesis of psoriasis, including IFN-γ, TNF-α, IL-17, and IL-23 [151, 152], and increases levels of anti-inflammatory IL-10 [153, 154]. Since apremilast prevents T-cell activation and inflammatory cytokine production, it intervenes earlier in the inflammatory cascade than biologic antibodies that target TNF-alpha, IL-12/23, and IL-17A.

Pharmacokinetics

Apremilast reaches maximum plasma concentration in approximately 1.5–2.5 h and has a half-life of 5–7 h [155]. Oral administration has an absolute bioavailability of 73% [153] and is not altered by food consumption [155]. Apremilast metabolized predominantly by the isoenzyme CYP3A4 [156]. Concurrent use of CYP450 inducers and apremilast may reduce the efficacy of apremilast and should be avoided [155].

Indications

Apremilast is approved for the treatment of adult patients with moderate to severe plaque psoriasis who are candidates for systemic or phototherapy. Apremilast also has FDA approval for psoriatic arthritis.

Efficacy

Apremilast was approved for use in psoriasis based on one phase 2 and two phase 3 clinical trials ESTEEM1 and ESTEEM2 [157–159]. A phase 2b study of 352 patients with moderate to severe psoriasis demonstrate dose-dependent clinical response for apremilast, with PASI75 achieved by week 16 in 29% of those on 20 mg twice daily and 41% of those on 30 mg twice daily, compared to 6% on placebo [157]. ESTEEM 1 ($n = 844$) and ESTEEM 2 ($n = 413$) were randomized, placebo-controlled phase 3 trial that evaluated the safety and efficacy of apremilast in adults moderate to severe plaque psoriasis in three phases. In phase 1 of these studies, patients were randomly assigned to treatment with apremilast 30 mg twice daily or placebo. In both studies, subjects on apremilast arm had significantly higher PASI 75 response at week 16 compared to placebo (ESTEEM1: 33% vs. 5% [158]; ESTEEM 2: 29% vs. 6%) [159]. Nail, scalp, and palmoplantar psoriasis were all noted to have significant improvement, as well [159].

Combination Therapy

Due to the relatively recent approval of apremilast, clinical experience with combination therapy is limited. Results from a retrospective review suggest that apremilast may be a safe and effective addition to biologics, traditional systemic, and phototherapy [160]. In psoriatic arthritis, one study found concurrent use of apremilast and MTX is overall well-tolerated [161].

Adverse Effects

The most common adverse effects of apremilast are diarrhea, nausea, upper respiratory tract infection, headache, and weight loss. Most of these effects are mild in severity, occur within the first 2 weeks of treatment, and resolve without intervention [159, 162]. Diarrhea and nausea are most common, occurring in 15–20% of patients. Initiating a low dose and slowing ramping up to maintenance levels improves tolerability and reduces the risk of diarrhea. Although the mechanism by which apremilast causes diarrhea is yet unknown, it is thought that it may be due to interaction between the PDE4 isoforms and the cystic fibrosis transmembrane regulator (CFTR) in the gut, leading to inappropriate activation of CFTR and excessive fluid secretion [163].

Patients on apremilast may also experience weight loss and depression. In clinical trials, roughly 10% of patients lost 5–10% of their body weight [158, 159]. Weight loss did not lead to any medical complications and was not associated with nausea or diarrhea [159]. There is no evidence of cardiac, renal, or hepatic adverse effects. Apremilast is not associated with risk of malignancy, reactivation of occult infection, or opportunistic infections [164].

Monitoring

Unlike most other systemic therapies for psoriasis, apremilast does not require routine laboratory monitoring. Periodic monitoring of body weight is recommended [153, 155]. In the event of unexplained or clinically significant weight loss, cessation of apremilast may be considered. Patients and their caregivers should also be alert to any changes in mood, depression, or suicidal ideations during treatment [155].

Contraindications

Apremilast is contraindicated in those with a history of hypersensitivity to apremilast, or to any component of its formulation. While depression is not an absolute contraindication, apremilast is marketed with a warning label for the potential to increase the risk of depression [162].

Apremilast is designated as pregnancy category C [153]. Due to limited pre-market data in humans, the FDA has mandated a post-marketing, prospective, pregnancy registry to follow pregnant women who have been exposed to apremilast. Apremilast is not approved for use in children; however, use in 14-year-old boy with severe psoriasis at the usual adult dosage has been reported [165].

Dosing

The usual dose of apremilast is 30 mg twice daily. Initiation dosing follows a 5-day dose escalation regimen to minimize the risk of gastrointestinal side effects [153]. Day 1 of the initiation regimen starts with one dose of 10 mg. On day 2, the dose is doubled to two doses of 10 mg, one in the morning and one in the evening. On day 3, the evening dose is increased to 20 mg, and on day 4, the morning dose is increased to 20 mg. The evening dose is again increased on day 5–30 mg. On day 6, patients begin maintenance therapy at a dose of 30 mg twice daily. Patients with severe renal impairment should be given an alternative titration schedule using only the morning dose, followed by 30 mg once daily [155].

References

1. Farber S, Diamond LK. Temporary remissions in acute leukemia in children produced by folic acid antagonist, 4-aminopteroyl-glutamic acid. N Engl J Med. 1948;238(23):787–93.
2. Gubner R, August S, Ginsberg V. Therapeutic suppression of tissue reactivity. II. Effect of aminopterin in rheumatoid arthritis and psoriasis. Am J Med Sci. 1951;221(2):176–82.
3. Gubner R. Effect of aminopterin on epithelial tissues. AMA Arch Derm Syphilol. 1951;64(6):688–99.
4. Edmundson WF, Guy WB. Treatment of psoriasis with folic acid antagonists. AMA Arch Derm. 1958;78(2):200–3.
5. Roenigk HH Jr, Haserick JR, Curtis GH. MTX for psoriasis. A preliminary report. Cleve Clin Q. 1965;32(4):211–5.
6. Callaway JL, McAfee WC, Finlayson GR. Management of psoriasis using MTX orally in a single weekly dose. South Med J. 1966;59(4):424–6.
7. Strakosch EA. A study of the folic acid antagonists in the treatment of psoriasis (aminopterin vs. MTX vs. aminopterin and a corticosteroid). Dermatologica. 1963;126:259–67.
8. Rees RB, Bennett JH. MTX vs. aminopterin for psoriasis. Arch Dermatol. 1961;83:970–2.
9. Kalb RE, Strober B, Weinstein G, Lebwohl M. MTX and psoriasis: 2009 National Psoriasis Foundation Consensus Conference. J Am Acad Dermatol. 2009;60(5):824–37.
10. Taylor JR, Halprin KM, Levine V, Woodyard C. Effects of MTX in vitro on epidermal cell proliferation. Br J Dermatol. 1983;108(1):45–61.
11. Newburger AE, Weinstein GD, McCullough JL. Biological and biochemical actions of MTX in psoriasis. J Invest Dermatol. 1978;70(4):183–6.
12. Herman S, Zurgil N, Deutsch M. Low dose MTX induces apoptosis with reactive oxygen species involvement in T lymphocytic cell lines to a greater extent than in monocytic lines. Inflamm Res. 2005;54(7):273–80.
13. Genestier L, Paillot R, Fournel S, Ferraro C, Miossec P, Revillard JP. Immunosuppressive properties of MTX: apoptosis and clonal deletion of activated peripheral T cells. J Clin Invest. 1998;102(2):322–8.
14. Cream JJ, Pole DS. The effect of MTX and hydroxyurea on neutrophil chemotaxis. Br J Dermatol. 1980;102(5):557–63.
15. Seitz M, Dewald B, Ceska M, Gerber N, Baggiolini M. Interleukin-8 in inflammatory rheumatic diseases: synovial fluid levels, relation to rheumatoid factors, production by mononuclear cells, and effects of gold sodium thiomalate and MTX. Rheumatol Int. 1992;12(4):159–64.
16. Aggarwal A, Misra R. MTX inhibits interleukin-6 production in patients with juvenile rheumatoid arthritis. Rheumatol Int. 2003;23(3):134–7.
17. Nishina N, Kaneko Y, Kameda H, Kuwana M, Takeuchi T. Reduction of plasma IL-6 but not TNF-alpha by MTX in patients with early rheumatoid arthritis: a potential biomarker for radiographic progression. Clin Rheumatol. 2013;32(11):1661–6.
18. Bannwarth B, Pehourcq F, Schaeverbeke T, Dehais J. Clinical pharmacokinetics of low-dose pulse MTX in rheumatoid arthritis. Clin Pharmacokinet. 1996;30(3):194–210.
19. Hamilton RA, Kremer JM. The effects of food on MTX absorption. J Rheumatol. 1995;22(4):630–2.
20. Dupuis LL, Koren G, Silverman ED, Laxer RM. Influence of food on the bioavailability of oral MTX in children. J Rheumatol. 1995;22(8):1570–3.
21. Claudepierre P, Urien S, Chevalier X, Chassany O, Larget-Piet B, Tillement JP. MTX serum binding in rheumatoid arthritis. Int J Clin Pharmacol Ther. 1994;32(3):113–5.
22. Paxton JW. Interaction of probenecid with the protein binding of MTX. Pharmacology. 1984;28(2):86–9.
23. Hande K, Gober J, Fletcher R. Trimethoprim interferes with serum MTX assay by the competitive protein binding technique. Clin Chem. 1980;26(11):1617–9.
24. Widemann BC, Sung E, Anderson L, Salzer WL, Balis FM, Monitjo KS, et al. Pharmacokinetics and metabolism of the MTX metabolite 2,4-diamino-N(10)-methylpteroic acid. J Pharmacol Exp Ther. 2000;294(3):894–901.
25. MTX Injection, USP [package insert]. Lake Forest: Hospira, Inc.; 2011.
26. MTX Tablets USP, 2.5 mg [package insert]. RLI; 2015.
27. Saurat JH, Stingl G, Dubertret L, Papp K, Langley RG, Ortonne JP, et al. Efficacy and safety results from the randomized controlled comparative study of adalimumab vs. MTX vs. placebo in patients with psoriasis (CHAMPION). Br J Dermatol. 2008;158(3):558–66.
28. Heydendael VM, Spuls PI, Opmeer BC, de Borgie CA, Reitsma JB, Goldschmidt WF, et al. MTX versus cyclosporine in moderate-to-severe chronic plaque psoriasis. N Engl J Med. 2003;349(7):658–65.
29. Flytstrom I, Stenberg B, Svensson A, Bergbrant IM. MTX vs. ciclosporin in psoriasis: effectiveness, quality of life and safety. A randomized controlled trial. Br J Dermatol. 2008;158(1):116–21.
30. Lebwohl M, Menter A, Koo J, Feldman SR. Combination therapy to treat moderate to severe psoriasis. J Am Acad Dermatol. 2004;50(3):416–30.
31. Paul BS, Momtaz K, Stern RS, Arndt KA, Parrish JA. Combined MTX--ultraviolet B therapy in the treatment of psoriasis. J Am Acad Dermatol. 1982;7(6):758–62.
32. Mahajan R, Kaur I, Kanwar AJ. MTX/narrowband UVB phototherapy combination vs. narrowband UVB phototherapy in the treatment of chronic plaque-type psoriasis--a randomized single-blinded placebo-controlled study. J Eur Acad Dermatol Venereol. 2010;24(5):595–600.

33. Shehzad T, Dar NR, Zakria M. Efficacy of concomitant use of PUVA and MTX in disease clearance time in plaque type psoriasis. J Pak Med Assoc. 2004;54(9):453–5.

34. Laxmisha C, Vinod Kumar P, Thappa DM. Modified combined MTX PUVA therapy in the treatment of recalcitrant psoriasis: a preliminary report. Indian J Dermatol Venereol Leprol. 2006;72(2):153–5.

35. Morison WL, Momtaz K, Parrish JA, Fitzpatrick TB. Combined MTX-PUVA therapy in the treatment of psoriasis. J Am Acad Dermatol. 1982;6(1):46–51.

36. Lebwohl M, Ali S. Treatment of psoriasis. Part 2. Systemic therapies. J Am Acad Dermatol. 2001;45(5):649–61. quiz 62-4

37. Mazzanti G, Coloni L, De Sabbata G, Paladini G. MTX and cyclosporin combined therapy in severe psoriatic arthritis. A pilot study. Acta Derm Venereol Suppl (Stockh). 1994;186:116–7.

38. Clark CM, Kirby B, Morris AD, Davison S, Zaki I, Emerson R, et al. Combination treatment with MTX and cyclosporin for severe recalcitrant psoriasis. Br J Dermatol. 1999;141(2):279–82.

39. Rosenbaum MM, Roenigk HH Jr. Treatment of generalized pustular psoriasis with etretinate (Ro 10-9359) and MTX. J Am Acad Dermatol. 1984;10(2 Pt 2):357–61.

40. Vanderveen EE, Ellis CN, Campbell JP, Case PC, Voorhees JJ. MTX and etretinate as concurrent therapies in severe psoriasis. Arch Dermatol. 1982;118(9):660–2.

41. An J, Zhang D, Wu J, Li J, Teng X, Gao X, et al. The acitretin and MTX combination therapy for psoriasis vulgaris achieves higher effectiveness and less liver fibrosis. Pharmacol Res. 2017;121:158–68.

42. Sauer GC. Combined MTX and hydroxyurea therapy for psoriasis. Arch Dermatol. 1973;107(3):369–70.

43. Iyer S, Yamauchi P, Lowe NJ. Etanercept for severe psoriasis and psoriatic arthritis: observations on combination therapy. Br J Dermatol. 2002;146(1):118–21.

44. Armstrong AW, Bagel J, Van Voorhees AS, Robertson AD, Yamauchi PS. Combining biologic therapies with other systemic treatments in psoriasis: evidence-based, best-practice recommendations from the Medical Board of the National Psoriasis Foundation. JAMA Dermatol. 2015;151(4):432–8.

45. Zachariae C, Mork NJ, Reunala T, Lorentzen H, Falk E, Karvonen SL, et al. The combination of etanercept and MTX increases the effectiveness of treatment in active psoriasis despite inadequate effect of MTX therapy. Acta Derm Venereol. 2008;88(5):495–501.

46. Hsu L, Snodgrass BT, Armstrong AW. Antidrug antibodies in psoriasis: a systematic review. Br J Dermatol. 2014;170(2):261–73.

47. Sherman S, Hodak E, Pavlovsky L. Can etanercept treatment failure in moderate-to-severe psoriasis be overcome by addition of low-dose MTX? A single-center experience. J Dermatolog Treat. 2018:1–5. https://doi.org/10.1080/09546634.2018.1441491

48. Helliwell PS, Taylor WJ. Treatment of psoriatic arthritis and rheumatoid arthritis with disease modifying drugs—comparison of drugs and adverse reactions. J Rheumatol. 2008;35(3):472–6.

49. Menter A, Korman NJ, Elmets CA, Feldman SR, Gelfand JM, Gordon KB, et al. Guidelines of care for the management of psoriasis and psoriatic arthritis: section 4. Guidelines of care for the management and treatment of psoriasis with traditional systemic agents. J Am Acad Dermatol. 2009;61(3):451–85.

50. Gisondi P, Fantuzzi F, Malerba M, Girolomoni G. Folic acid in general medicine and dermatology. J Dermatolog Treat. 2007;18(3):138–46.

51. Strober BE, Menon K. Folate supplementation during MTX therapy for patients with psoriasis. J Am Acad Dermatol. 2005;53(4):652–9.

52. Czarnecka-Operacz M, Sadowska-Przytocka A. The possibilities and principles of MTX treatment of psoriasis—the updated knowledge. Postepy Dermatol Alergol. 2014;31(6):392–400.

53. Pathirana D, Ormerod AD, Saiag P, Smith C, Spuls PI, Nast A, et al. European S3-guidelines on the systemic treatment of psoriasis vulgaris. J Eur Acad Dermatol Venereol. 2009;23(Suppl 2):1–70.

54. Silverberg NB. Pediatric psoriasis: an update. Ther Clin Risk Manag. 2009;5:849–56.

55. Qureshi ZP, Seoane-Vazquez E, Rodriguez-Monguio R, Stevenson KB, Szeinbach SL. Market withdrawal of new molecular entities approved in the United States from 1980 to 2009. Pharmacoepidemiol Drug Saf. 2011;20(7):772–7.

56. O'Brien TJ. Etretin. A replacement for etretinate. Int J Dermatol. 1990;29(4):270–1.

57. Niu X, Cao W, Ma H, Feng J, Li X, Zhang X. Acitretin exerted a greater influence on T-helper (Th)1 and Th17 than on Th2 cells in treatment of psoriasis vulgaris. J Dermatol. 2012;39(11):916–21.

58. Pilkington T, Brogden RN. Acitretin : a review of its pharmacology and therapeutic use. Drugs. 1992;43(4):597–627.

59. Orfanos CE, Zouboulis CC, Almond-Roesler B, Geilen CC. Current use and future potential role of retinoids in dermatology. Drugs. 1997;53(3):358–88.

60. McNamara PJ, Jewell RC, Jensen BK, Brindley CJ. Food increases the bioavailability of acitretin. J Clin Pharmacol. 1988;28(11):1051–5.

61. Wiegand UW, Chou RC. Pharmacokinetics of acitretin and etretinate. J Am Acad Dermatol. 1998;39(2 Pt 3):S25–33.

62. Roberts AB. Microsomal oxidation of retinoic acid in hamster liver, intestine, and testis. Ann N Y Acad Sci. 1981;359:45–53.

63. Howell SR, Shirley MA, Ulm EH. Effects of retinoid treatment of rats on hepatic microsomal metabolism and cytochromes P450. Correlation between retinoic acid receptor/retinoid x receptor selectivity and effects on metabolic enzymes. Drug Metab Dispos. 1998;26(3):234–9.

64. Larsen FG, Jakobsen P, Knudsen J, Weismann K, Kragballe K, Nielsen-Kudsk F. Conversion of acitre-

tin to etretinate in psoriatic patients is influenced by ethanol. J Invest Dermatol. 1993;100(5):623–7.

65. Buccheri L, Katchen BR, Karter AJ, Cohen SR. Acitretin therapy is effective for psoriasis associated with human immunodeficiency virus infection. Arch Dermatol. 1997;133(6):711–5.

66. Schroder K, Zaun H, Holzmann H, Altmeyer P, el-Gammal S. Pustulosis palmo-plantaris. Clinical and histological changes during etretin (acitretin) therapy. Acta Derm Venereol Suppl (Stockh). 1989;146:111–6.

67. Kragballe K, Jansen CT, Geiger JM, Bjerke JR, Falk ES, Gip L, et al. A double-blind comparison of acitretin and etretinate in the treatment of severe psoriasis. Results of a Nordic multicentre study. Acta Derm Venereol. 1989;69(1):35–40.

68. Gollnick H, Bauer R, Brindley C, Orfanos CE, Plewig G, Wokalek H, et al. Acitretin versus etretinate in psoriasis. Clinical and pharmacokinetic results of a German multicenter study. J Am Acad Dermatol. 1988;19(3):458–68.

69. Geiger JM, Czarnetzki BM. Acitretin (Ro 10-1670, etretin): overall evaluation of clinical studies. Dermatologica. 1988;176(4):182–90.

70. Lassus A, Geiger JM, Nyblom M, Virrankoski T, Kaartamaa M, Ingervo L. Treatment of severe psoriasis with etretin (RO 10-1670). Br J Dermatol. 1987;117(3):333–41.

71. Wolska H, Jablonska S, Langner A, Fraczykowska M. Etretinate therapy in generalized pustular psoriasis (Zumbusch type). Immediate and long-term results. Dermatologica. 1985;171(5):297–304.

72. Ozawa A, Ohkido M, Haruki Y, Kobayashi H, Ohkawara A, Ohno Y, et al. Treatments of generalized pustular psoriasis: a multicenter study in Japan. J Dermatol. 1999;26(3):141–9.

73. Ettler K, Richards B. Acitretin therapy for palmoplantar pustulosis combined with UVA and topical 8-MOP. Int J Dermatol. 2001;40(8):541–2.

74. Goldfarb MT, Ellis CN, Gupta AK, Tincoff T, Hamilton TA, Voorhees JJ. Acitretin improves psoriasis in a dose-dependent fashion. J Am Acad Dermatol. 1988;18(4 Pt 1):655–62.

75. Berbis P, Geiger JM, Vaisse C, Rognin C, Privat Y. Benefit of progressively increasing doses during the initial treatment with acitretin in psoriasis. Dermatologica. 1989;178(2):88–92.

76. Dogra S, Jain A, Kanwar AJ. Efficacy and safety of acitretin in three fixed doses of 25, 35 and 50 mg in adult patients with severe plaque type psoriasis: a randomized, double blind, parallel group, dose ranging study. J Eur Acad Dermatol Venereol. 2013;27(3):e305–11.

77. Levine N. Role of retinoids in skin cancer treatment and prevention. J Am Acad Dermatol. 1998;39(2 Pt 3):S62–6.

78. Koo J. Systemic sequential therapy of psoriasis: a new paradigm for improved therapeutic results. J Am Acad Dermatol. 1999;41(3 Pt 2):S25–8.

79. SORIATANE (acitretin) [package insert]. Research Triangle Park: Stiefel Laboratories, Inc.; 2017.

80. Conley J, Nanton J, Dhawan S, Pearce DJ, Feldman SR. Novel combination regimens: biologics and acitretin for the treatment of psoriasis—a case series. J Dermatolog Treat. 2006;17(2):86–9.

81. Dogra S, Yadav S. Acitretin in psoriasis: an evolving scenario. Int J Dermatol. 2014;53(5):525–38.

82. Vahlquist C, Michaelsson G, Vahlquist A, Vessby B. A sequential comparison of etretinate (Tigason) and isotretinoin (Roaccutane) with special regard to their effects on serum lipoproteins. Br J Dermatol. 1985;112(1):69–76.

83. Otley CC, Stasko T, Tope WD, Lebwohl M. Chemoprevention of nonmelanoma skin cancer with systemic retinoids: practical dosing and management of adverse effects. Dermatol Surg. 2006;32(4):562–8.

84. Pearce DJ, Klinger S, Ziel KK, Murad EJ, Rowell R, Feldman SR. Low-dose acitretin is associated with fewer adverse events than high-dose acitretin in the treatment of psoriasis. Arch Dermatol. 2006;142(8):1000–4.

85. Prendiville J, Bingham EA, Burrows D. Premature epiphyseal closure—a complication of etretinate therapy in children. J Am Acad Dermatol. 1986;15(6):1259–62.

86. Halkier-Sorensen L, Laurberg G, Andresen J. Bone changes in children on long-term treatment with etretinate. J Am Acad Dermatol. 1987;16(5 Pt 1):999–1006.

87. Gilbert M, Ellis CN, Voorhees JJ. Lack of skeletal radiographic changes during short-term etretinate therapy for psoriasis. Dermatologica. 1986;172(3):160–3.

88. Van Dooren-Greebe RJ, Lemmens JA, De Boo T, Hangx NM, Kuijpers AL, Van de Kerkhof PC. Prolonged treatment with oral retinoids in adults: no influence on the frequency and severity of spinal abnormalities. Br J Dermatol. 1996;134(1):71–6.

89. Katz HI, Waalen J, Leach EE. Acitretin in psoriasis: an overview of adverse effects. J Am Acad Dermatol. 1999;41(3 Pt 2):S7–s12.

90. Lee E, Koo J. Single-center retrospective study of long-term use of low-dose acitretin (Soriatane) for psoriasis. J Dermatolog Treat. 2004;15(1):8–13.

91. Orfanos CE. Retinoids: the new status. Maintenance therapy, disorders of resorption in "non-responders", interactions and interferences with drugs, treatment of children and bone toxicity, acitetin and 13-cis-acitretin. Hautarzt. 1989;40(3):123–9.

92. Starling J 3rd, Koo J. Evidence based or theoretical concern? Pseudotumor cerebri and depression as acitretin side effects. J Drugs Dermatol. 2005;4(6):690–6.

93. Fraunfelder FW, Fraunfelder FT. Evidence for a probable causal relationship between tretinoin, acitretin, and etretinate and intracranial hypertension. J Neuroophthalmol. 2004;24(3):214–6.

94. Roytman M, Frumkin A, Bohn TG. Pseudotumor cerebri caused by isotretinoin. Cutis. 1988; 42(5):399–400.

95. Bigby M, Stern RS. Adverse reactions to isotretinoin. A report from the adverse drug reaction reporting system. J Am Acad Dermatol. 1988;18(3):543–52.

96. Lee AG. Pseudotumor cerebri after treatment with tetracycline and isotretinoin for acne. Cutis. 1995;55(3):165–8.

97. Ormerod AD, Campalani E, Goodfield MJ. British Association of Dermatologists guidelines on the efficacy and use of acitretin in dermatology. Br J Dermatol. 2010;162(5):952–63.

98. Ling MR. Acitretin: optimal dosing strategies. J Am Acad Dermatol. 1999;41(3 Pt 2):S13–7.

99. Calne RY, White DJ, Thiru S, Evans DB, McMaster P, Dunn DC, et al. Cyclosporin A in patients receiving renal allografts from cadaver donors. Lancet. 1978;2(8104–5):1323–7.

100. Mueller W, Herrmann B. Cyclosporin A for psoriasis. N Engl J Med. 1979;301(10):555.

101. Macian F. NFAT proteins: key regulators of T-cell development and function. Nat Rev Immunol. 2005;5(6):472–84.

102. Baker BS, Griffiths CE, Lambert S, Powles AV, Leonard JN, Valdimarsson H, et al. The effects of cyclosporin A on T lymphocyte and dendritic cell sub-populations in psoriasis. Br J Dermatol. 1987;116(4):503–10.

103. Haider AS, Lowes MA, Suarez-Farinas M, Zaba LC, Cardinale I, Khatcherian A, et al. Identification of cellular pathways of "type 1," Th17 T cells, and TNF- and inducible nitric oxide synthase-producing dendritic cells in autoimmune inflammation through pharmacogenomic study of cyclosporine A in psoriasis. J Immunol. 2008;180(3):1913–20.

104. Bharadwaj AS, Schewitz-Bowers LP, Wei L, Lee RW, Smith JR. Intercellular adhesion molecule 1 mediates migration of Th1 and Th17 cells across human retinal vascular endothelium. Invest Ophthalmol Vis Sci. 2013;54(10):6917–25.

105. Muller WA. How endothelial cells regulate transmigration of leukocytes in the inflammatory response. Am J Pathol. 2014;184(4):886–96.

106. Gupta SK, Manfro RC, Tomlanovich SJ, Gambertoglio JG, Garovoy MR, Benet LZ. Effect of food on the pharmacokinetics of cyclosporine in healthy subjects following oral and intravenous administration. J Clin Pharmacol. 1990;30(7):643–53.

107. Curtis JJ, Jones P, Barbeito R. Large within-day variation in cyclosporine absorption: circadian variation or food effect? Clin J Am Soc Nephrol. 2006;1(3):462–6.

108. Honcharik N. The effect of food on cyclosporine absorption. Clin Biochem. 1991;24(1):89–92.

109. NEORAL (cyclosporine) [package insert]. East Hanover: Novartis Pharmaceuticals Corporation; 2015.

110. SANDIMMUNE (cyclosporine) [package insert]. East Hanover: Novartis Pharmaceuticals Corporation; 2015.

111. Fahr A. Cyclosporin clinical pharmacokinetics. Clin Pharmacokinet. 1993;24(6):472–95.

112. Colombo D, Egan CG. Bioavailability of Sandimmun(R) versus Sandimmun Neoral(R): a meta-analysis of published studies. Int J Immunopathol Pharmacol. 2010;23(4):1177–83.

113. Rosenbach M, Hsu S, Korman NJ, Lebwohl MG, Young M, Bebo BF Jr, et al. Treatment of erythrodermic psoriasis: from the medical board of the National Psoriasis Foundation. J Am Acad Dermatol. 2010;62(4):655–62.

114. Robinson A, Van Voorhees AS, Hsu S, Korman NJ, Lebwohl MG, Bebo BF Jr, et al. Treatment of pustular psoriasis: from the Medical Board of the National Psoriasis Foundation. J Am Acad Dermatol. 2012;67(2):279–88.

115. Management of erythrodermic psoriasis with low-dose cyclosporin. Studio Italiano Multicentrico nella Psoriasi (SIMPSO). Dermatology. 1993;187 Suppl 1:30–7.

116. Ellis CN, Fradin MS, Messana JM, Brown MD, Siegel MT, Hartley AH, et al. Cyclosporine for plaque-type psoriasis. Results of a multidose, double-blind trial. N Engl J Med. 1991;324(5):277–84.

117. Berth-Jones J, Henderson CA, Munro CS, Rogers S, Chalmers RJ, Boffa MJ, et al. Treatment of psoriasis with intermittent short course cyclosporin (Neoral). A multicentre study. Br J Dermatol. 1997;136(4):527–30.

118. Ho VC, Griffiths CE, Berth-Jones J, Papp KA, Vanaclocha F, Dauden E, et al. Intermittent short courses of cyclosporine microemulsion for the long-term management of psoriasis: a 2-year cohort study. J Am Acad Dermatol. 2001;44(4):643–51.

119. Yoon HS, Youn JI. A comparison of two cyclosporine dosage regimens for the treatment of severe psoriasis. J Dermatolog Treat. 2007;18(5):286–90.

120. Koo J. A randomized, double-blind study comparing the efficacy, safety and optimal dose of two formulations of cyclosporin, Neoral and Sandimmun, in patients with severe psoriasis. OLP302 Study Group. Br J Dermatol. 1998;139(1):88–95.

121. Ellis CN, Fradin MS, Hamilton TA, Voorhees JJ. Duration of remission during maintenance cyclosporine therapy for psoriasis. Relationship to maintenance dose and degree of improvement during initial therapy. Arch Dermatol. 1995;131(7):791–5.

122. Mahrle G, Schulze HJ, Farber L, Weidinger G, Steigleder GK. Low-dose short-term cyclosporine versus etretinate in psoriasis: improvement of skin, nail, and joint involvement. J Am Acad Dermatol. 1995;32(1):78–88.

123. Shupack J, Abel E, Bauer E, Brown M, Drake L, Freinkel R, et al. Cyclosporine as maintenance therapy in patients with severe psoriasis. J Am Acad Dermatol. 1997;36(3 Pt 1):423–32.

124. Amor KT, Ryan C, Menter A. The use of cyclosporine in dermatology: part I. J Am Acad Dermatol. 2010;63(6):925–46; quiz 47–8

125. Lebwohl M, Ellis C, Gottlieb A, Koo J, Krueger G, Linden K, et al. Cyclosporine consensus conference: with emphasis on the treatment of psoriasis. J Am Acad Dermatol. 1998;39(3):464–75.

126. Rosmarin DM, Lebwohl M, Elewski BE, Gottlieb AB. Cyclosporine and psoriasis: 2008 National Psoriasis Foundation Consensus Conference. J Am Acad Dermatol. 2010;62(5):838–53.

127. Mihatsch MJ, Thiel G, Ryffel B. Renal side-effects of cyclosporin A with special reference to autoimmune diseases. Br J Dermatol. 1990;122(Suppl 36):101–15.

128. Ryan C, Amor KT, Menter A. The use of cyclosporine in dermatology: part II. J Am Acad Dermatol. 2010;63(6):949–72. quiz 73-4

129. Robert N, Wong GW, Wright JM. Effect of cyclosporine on blood pressure. Cochrane Database Syst Rev. 2010;(1):CD007893.

130. Powles AV, Hardman CM, Porter WM, Cook T, Hulme B, Fry L. Renal function after 10 years' treatment with cyclosporin for psoriasis. Br J Dermatol. 1998;138(3):443–9.

131. Paul CF, Ho VC, McGeown C, Christophers E, Schmidtmann B, Guillaume JC, et al. Risk of malignancies in psoriasis patients treated with cyclosporine: a 5 y cohort study. J Invest Dermatol. 2003;120(2):211–6.

132. Lain EL, Markus RF. Early and explosive development of nodular basal cell carcinoma and multiple keratoacanthomas in psoriasis patients treated with cyclosporine. J Drugs Dermatol. 2004;3(6):680–2.

133. Marcil I, Stern RS. Squamous-cell cancer of the skin in patients given PUVA and ciclosporin: nested cohort crossover study. Lancet. 2001;358(9287):1042–5.

134. Thompson CB, June CH, Sullivan KM, Thomas ED. Association between cyclosporin neurotoxicity and hypomagnesaemia. Lancet. 1984;2(8412):1116–20.

135. Lima MA, Maradei S, Maranhao Filho P. Cyclosporine-induced parkinsonism. J Neurol. 2009;256(4):674–5.

136. Cruz OA, Fogg SG, Roper-Hall G. Pseudotumor cerebri associated with cyclosporine use. Am J Ophthalmol. 1996;122(3):436–7.

137. Gonzalez Vicent M, Diaz MA, Madero L. "Pseudotumor cerebri" following allogeneic bone marrow transplantation (BMT). Ann Hematol. 2001;80(4):236–7.

138. Seymour RA, Jacobs DJ. Cyclosporin and the gingival tissues. J Clin Periodontol. 1992;19(1):1–11.

139. Doufexi A, Mina M, Ioannidou E. Gingival overgrowth in children: epidemiology, pathogenesis, and complications. A literature review. J Periodontol. 2005;76(1):3–10.

140. Fradin MS, Ellis CN, Voorhees JJ. Management of patients and side effects during cyclosporine therapy for cutaneous disorders. J Am Acad Dermatol. 1990;23(6 Pt 2):1265–73; discussion 73–5

141. Shintani Y, Kaneko N, Furuhashi T, Saito C, Morita A. Safety and efficacy of a fixed-dose cyclosporin microemulsion (100 mg) for the treatment of psoriasis. J Dermatol. 2011;38(10):966–72.

142. Papp K, Gulliver W, Lynde C, Poulin Y, Ashkenas J. Canadian guidelines for the management of plaque psoriasis: overview. J Cutan Med Surg. 2011;15(4):210–9.

143. National Clinical Guideline Centre. National Institute for Health and Clinical Excellence: Guidance. Psoriasis: assessment and Management of Psoriasis. London: Royal College of Physicians; 2012.

144. Lowe NJ, Wieder JM, Rosenbach A, Johnson K, Kunkel R, Bainbridge C, et al. Long-term low-dose cyclosporine therapy for severe psoriasis: effects on renal function and structure. J Am Acad Dermatol. 1996;35(5 Pt 1):710–9.

145. Grossman RM, Chevret S, Abi-Rached J, Blanchet F, Dubertret L. Long-term safety of cyclosporine in the treatment of psoriasis. Arch Dermatol. 1996;132(6):623–9.

146. Mrowietz U, Farber L, Henneicke-von Zepelin HH, Bachmann H, Welzel D, Christophers E. Long-term maintenance therapy with cyclosporine and posttreatment survey in severe psoriasis: results of a multicenter study. German Multicenter Study. J Am Acad Dermatol. 1995;33(3):470–5.

147. Houslay MD, Schafer P, Zhang KY. Keynote review: phosphodiesterase-4 as a therapeutic target. Drug Discov Today. 2005;10(22):1503–19.

148. Schafer P. Apremilast mechanism of action and application to psoriasis and psoriatic arthritis. Biochem Pharmacol. 2012;83(12):1583–90.

149. Schafer PH, Truzzi F, Parton A, Wu L, Kosek J, Zhang LH, et al. Phosphodiesterase 4 in inflammatory diseases: effects of apremilast in psoriatic blood and in dermal myofibroblasts through the PDE4/CD271 complex. Cell Signal. 2016;28(7):753–63.

150. Baumer W, Hoppmann J, Rundfeldt C, Kietzmann M. Highly selective phosphodiesterase 4 inhibitors for the treatment of allergic skin diseases and psoriasis. Inflamm Allergy Drug Targets. 2007;6(1):17–26.

151. Gottlieb AB, Strober B, Krueger JG, Rohane P, Zeldis JB, Hu CC, et al. An open-label, single-arm pilot study in patients with severe plaque-type psoriasis treated with an oral anti-inflammatory agent, apremilast. Curr Med Res Opin. 2008;24(5):1529–38.

152. Schafer PH, Parton A, Gandhi AK, Capone L, Adams M, Wu L, et al. Apremilast, a cAMP phosphodiesterase-4 inhibitor, demonstrates anti-inflammatory activity in vitro and in a model of psoriasis. Br J Pharmacol. 2010;159(4):842–55.

153. Zerilli T, Ocheretyaner E. Apremilast (Otezla): a new oral treatment for adults with psoriasis and psoriatic arthritis. P T. 2015;40(8):495–500.

154. Man HW, Schafer P, Wong LM, Patterson RT, Corral LG, Raymon H, et al. Discovery of (S)-N-[2-[1-(3-ethoxy-4-methoxyphenyl)-2-methanesulfonylethyl]-1,3-dioxo-2,3-dihydro-1H-isoindol-4-yl] acetamide (apremilast), a potent and orally active phosphodiesterase 4 and tumor necrosis factor-alpha inhibitor. J Med Chem. 2009;52(6):1522–4.

155. OTEZLA (apremilast) [package insert]. Summit: Celgene Corporation; 2017.

156. Cada DJ, Ingram K, Baker DE. Apremilast. Hosp Pharm. 2014;49(8):752–62.

157. Papp K, Cather JC, Rosoph L, Sofen H, Langley RG, Matheson RT, et al. Efficacy of apremilast in the treatment of moderate to severe psoriasis: a randomised controlled trial. Lancet. 2012;380(9843):738–46.

158. Papp K, Reich K, Leonardi CL, Kircik L, Chimenti S, Langley RG, et al. Apremilast, an oral phosphodiesterase 4 (PDE4) inhibitor, in patients with moderate to severe plaque psoriasis: results of a phase III, randomized, controlled trial (Efficacy and Safety Trial Evaluating the Effects of Apremilast in Psoriasis [ESTEEM] 1). J Am Acad Dermatol. 2015;73(1):37–49.

159. Paul C, Cather J, Gooderham M, Poulin Y, Mrowietz U, Ferrandiz C, et al. Efficacy and safety of apremilast, an oral phosphodiesterase 4 inhibitor, in patients with moderate-to-severe plaque psoriasis over 52 weeks: a phase III, randomized controlled trial (ESTEEM 2). Br J Dermatol. 2015;173(6):1387–99.

160. AbuHilal M, Walsh S, Shear N. Use of Apremilast in combination with other therapies for treatment of chronic plaque psoriasis: a retrospective study. J Cutan Med Surg. 2016;20(4):313–6.

161. Liu Y, Zhou S, Nissel J, Wu A, Lau H, Palmisano M. The pharmacokinetic effect of coadministration of apremilast and MTX in individuals with rheumatoid arthritis and psoriatic arthritis. Clin Pharmacol Drug Dev. 2014;3(6):456–65.

162. Keating GM. Apremilast: a review in psoriasis and psoriatic arthritis. Drugs. 2017;77(4):459–72.

163. Moon C, Zhang W, Sundaram N, Yarlagadda S, Reddy VS, Arora K, et al. Drug-induced secretory diarrhea: a role for CFTR. Pharmacol Res. 2015;102:107–12.

164. Crowley J, Thaci D, Joly P, Peris K, Papp KA, Goncalves J, et al. Long-term safety and tolerability of apremilast in patients with psoriasis: pooled safety analysis for >/=156 weeks from 2 phase 3, randomized, controlled trials (ESTEEM 1 and 2). J Am Acad Dermatol. 2017;77(2):310–7.e1.

165. Smith RL. Pediatric psoriasis treated with apremilast. JAAD Case Rep. 2016;2(1):89–91.

Biologics

5

Sahil Sekhon, Caleb Jeon, and Wilson Liao

Classes

TNF-α

Biologics that affect TNF-alpha signaling include adalimumab, etanercept, and infliximab (Table 5.1). These work by binding to TNF-alpha, resulting in attenuation of the downstream effects of the cytokine.

Etanercept

Etanercept was approved for the treatment of psoriatic arthritis in 2002 after initially being approved for use in rheumatoid arthritis in 1998. Then in 2004, it was approved for use in moderate-to-severe plaque psoriasis. It was the first biologic approved for use in the treatment of moderate-to-severe psoriasis vulgaris.

Other Indications

Etanercept is also approved for the treatment of rheumatoid arthritis, juvenile rheumatoid arthritis, psoriatic arthritis, and ankylosing spondylitis.

Mechanism of Action

Etanercept is a recombinant molecule of the TNF-alpha p75 receptor fused to the Fc portion of human IgG1. It binds to TNF-α and prevents its interaction with in vivo TNF-alpha receptors, thereby preventing its downstream cell signaling [20].

Dosing

In adults with psoriasis, etanercept is dosed at 50 mg twice weekly for the first 3 months, followed by 50 mg weekly for maintenance.

In pediatric patients (ages 4–18 years), etanercept is dosed by weight, with pediatric patients weighing 63 kg or greater receiving a dose of 50 mg weekly, while patients weighing less than 63 kg receiving 0.8 mg/kg weekly.

Efficacy

The initial phase II trial for etanercept showed significant improvement in psoriasis severity in patients treated with just 25 mg of etanercept administered twice weekly; 30% and 56% of patients in the treatment arm achieved PASI-75 response, a reduction in Psoriasis Area Severity Index (PASI) of 75% or greater from baseline, at weeks 12 and 24, respectively [21]. A phase III trial showed that 50 mg of etanercept administered twice weekly led to a PASI-75 response rate of 49% at week 12 and 59% at week 24, 25 mg administered twice weekly led to PASI-75 response rates of 34% at week 12 and 44% at week 24, while 25 mg administered weekly led to

S. Sekhon · C. Jeon · W. Liao (✉)
Department of Dermatology, UCSF Psoriasis Center,
University of California San Francisco,
San Francisco, CA, USA
e-mail: sahil.sekhon@ucsf.edu; caljeon@hawaii.edu;
Wilson.liao@ucsf.edu

© Springer International Publishing AG, part of Springer Nature 2018
T. Bhutani et al. (eds.), *Evidence-Based Psoriasis*, Updates in Clinical Dermatology,
https://doi.org/10.1007/978-3-319-90107-7_5

Table 5.1 Clinical features of currently approved biologic medications for psoriasis in the United States

Medication	Mechanism	Dosing	Other indications	PASI-75	PASI-90	PASI-100	Safety and comments
Adalimumab	Human monoclonal antibody to TNF-alpha	80 mg subcutaneous on day 0, then 40 mg every other week starting on day 8. Available as pre-filled syringe or auto-injector pen	Rheumatoid arthritis, psoriatic arthritis, ankylosing spondylitis, Crohn's disease, ulcerative colitis, juvenile idiopathic arthritis, uveitis, hidradenitis suppurativa	Week 16: 71–79.6% [1, 2] Week 100: 83% [3]	Week 16: 45–51.3% [1, 2] Week 100: 59% [3]	Week 16: 17.6–20% [1, 2] Week 100: 33% [3]	Can be immunogenic and induce neutralizing antibodies. Possible increased risk of NMSC
Etanercept	Recombinant human TNF-alpha receptor (p75):Fc fusion protein (extracellular domain of TNF-alpha receptor)	Subcutaneous injections: Adults, 50 mg twice weekly for 3 months and then 50 mg weekly pediatrics: <63 kg, 0.8 mg/kg weekly: ≥63 kg: 50 mg weekly. Available as pre-filled syringe or auto-injector pen	Rheumatoid arthritis, juvenile idiopathic arthritis, psoriatic arthritis, ankylosing spondylitis	Week 12: 49% Week 24: 50–59% [4, 5]	Week 12: 21–22% [4, 5] Week 24: 30% [4]	N/A	Possible increased risk of NMSC
Infliximab	Chimeric mouse-human antibody to TNF-alpha	Induction: 5 mg/kg intravenously administered at weeks 0, 2, and 6 and then maintenance with 5 mg/kg every 8 weeks. Available as intravenous infusion only	Crohn's disease, ulcerative colitis, psoriatic arthritis, ankylosing spondylitis, rheumatoid arthritis	Week 10: 75.5%–87.9% [6–8] Week 50: 54.5–61% [6, 7]	Week 10: 57–57.6% [6, 8] Week 50: 34.3–45% [6, 7]	Week 10: 26% [6]	Higher rate of immunogenicity due to murine component of the antibody
Ustekinumab	Fully human monoclonal antibody to the p40 subunit of IL-12 and IL-23	90 mg for weight ≥ 100 kg, 45 mg for weight < 100 kg. Doses administered subcutaneously at weeks 0 and 4 and then every 12 weeks. Available as pre-filled syringe	Psoriatic arthritis, Crohn's disease	Week 12: 63.3–75.7% [9–11] Week 28: 69.5–78.6% [9, 10]	Week 12: 36.7–50.9% [9–11] Week 28: 44.8–55.6% [9, 10]	Week 12: 10.9–18.2% week 28: 18.6–29.5% [9, 10]	Available only as a syringe
Brodalumab	Fully human IgG2 monoclonal antibody against IL-17 receptor	210 mg administered subcutaneously at weeks 0, 1, and 2 and then every 2 weeks. Available as pre-filled syringe	N/A	Week 12: 83.3–86% [12, 13]	Week 12: 70.3% [13]	Week 12: 37–44% [12, 13]	FDA-required REMS system for black box warning for suicide risk in patients with history of suicidality. Increased risk of mucocutaneous candidiasis
Secukinumab	Monoclonal fully human IgG1-κ antibody against interleukin-17A	300 mg subcutaneous per dose. Induction: Dose administered at weeks 0, 1, 2, 3, and 4. Maintenance every 4 weeks. Available as pre-filled syringe or auto-injector pen	Psoriatic arthritis, ankylosing spondylitis	Week 12: 75.9–86.7% [14–16] Week 52: 92.5% [17]	Week 12: 54.2–60.3% [14–16] Week 52: 60–76.2% [14, 17]	Week 12: 24.1–43.1% [14–16] Week 52: 39.2–45.9% [14, 17]	Increased risk of mucocutaneous candidiasis, new onset/ exacerbation of IBD
Ixekizumab	Monoclonal humanized IgG4-κ antibody against interleukin-17A	160 mg at week 0, then 80 mg at weeks 2, 4, 6, 8, 10, and 12, and then ever 4 weeks. Available as pre-filled syringe or auto-injector pen	N/A	Week 12: 87.4–89.7% [18, 19] Week 60: 83% [18]	Week 12: 68.1–70.9% [18, 19] Week 60: 73% [18]	Week 12: 35.3–40.5% [18, 19] Week 60: 55% [18]	Increased risk of mucocutaneous candidiasis, new onset or exacerbation of IBD

NMSC non-melanoma skin cancer, *FDA* Food and Drug Administration, *REMS* Risk Evaluation and Mitigation Strategy program, *IBD* inflammatory bowel disease

PASI-75 response rates of 14% at week 12 and 25% at week 24 [4].

Another phase III trial evaluated the maintenance of treatment effect after dose reduction of etanercept [5]. Patient received 50 mg or 25 mg of etanercept or placebo twice weekly for 12 weeks, followed by receiving etanercept at a dose of 25 mg twice weekly. At week 12, PASI-75 response rates were 49% for patients receiving 50 mg twice weekly and 34% for patients receiving 25 mg twice weekly. At week 24, PASI-75 response rate was 54% in the patients that had dose reduced from 50 mg twice weekly to 25 mg twice weekly, while the group maintained on 25 mg twice weekly had PASI-75 response rate of 45%. There was no apparent decrease in efficacy after dose reduction. Another trial evaluated time to relapse after discontinuation of etanercept as well as retreatment efficacy. Patients who achieved at least PASI-50 response by week 24 were discontinued from receiving etanercept and monitored for disease relapse, defined as loss of more than 50% of the PASI improvement at week 24. On average, patients experienced relapse after 3 months, with retreatment of these patients resulting in similar PASI improvements at 12 weeks as were experienced in the first 12 weeks of treatment [22].

A phase IV study treating patients with etanercept who had lost response to treatment with adalimumab found that these patients achieved satisfactory response to etanercept therapy. These findings held true regardless of the anti-adalimumab antibody status of the patients [23].

Anti-Etanercept Antibodies

Studies have not shown a clear association between formation of anti-etanercept antibodies and reduced treatment efficacy across studies of patients being treated for psoriasis, rheumatoid arthritis, and ankylosing spondylitis [24].

Efficacy in Pediatric Patients

The initial phase III clinical trial evaluating etanercept in pediatric patients involved 211 patients between 4 and 17 years of age, with patients receiving either etanercept at a dose of 0.8 mg/kg (up to a maximum dose of 50 mg) per week or placebo for 12 weeks [25]. After 12 weeks, all patients received etanercept at the same dose for 24 weeks. At week 36, 138 patients were re-randomized to placebo or etanercept treatment to evaluate the effect of withdrawal and retreatment. At week 12, 57% of patients receiving etanercept achieved PASI-75 response. At week 36, PASI-75 response rates were 68% for patients continued on etanercept and 65% for patients who were initially on placebo treatment and started etanercept at week 12. After withdrawal at week 36, 42% of patients experienced loss of response by week 48.

The 5-year open-label extension study enrolled 182 patients from the initial study. One hundred forty patients completed participation through 96 weeks, and 69 patients completed the full 264 weeks [25]. Most commonly, subjects discontinued due to withdrawal of consent, loss to follow up, or noncompliance. PASI-75 response rates were maintained from the initial study through week 264.

Treatment with etanercept has been shown to improve quality of life of pediatric patients. At baseline, pediatric psoriasis patients have reduced quality of life, as measured by Children's Dermatology Life Quality Index (CDLQI) and Pediatric Quality of Life Inventory (PedsQL), when compared to the general pediatric population. CDLQI scores improved significantly after 12 weeks of treatment compared to placebo (52.3% versus 17.5%), and improvement from baseline in the CDLQI was greater in patients who achieved PASI-75 response compared to those with less than PASI-75 response [26].

Safety

Given that etanercept has been approved for nearly 15 years in psoriasis, and for longer in the treatment of other diseases, it has a well-known safety profile. TNF-alpha blockers are associated with an increased risk of infection, such as upper respiratory tract infections, with most infections mild in severity.

A rare but serious side effect that has been observed in patients using etanercept is demyelinating disease (this was first observed in patients taking etanercept for various inflammatory arthritides) [27–29] . This risk will be discussed in a later section of this chapter.

The most common adverse events (AEs) in pediatric patients in clinical trials were upper respiratory tract infection, headache, and nasopharyngitis, with four serious adverse events (SAEs) seen in the open-label portion of the initial phase III clinical trial. Three of these SAEs were infections and all SAEs resolved with treatment without sequelae. In the long-term, open-label study, there were 8 SAEs, with 4 events before week 96 and 4 reported after week 96. Of the SAEs, only one, a case of cellulitis, was deemed as related to the etanercept by the investigator.

Out of eight randomized placebo-controlled trials, one open-label extension study, and two meta-analyses of randomized controlled trials and long-term extension studies using etanercept, only injection site reactions were consistently significantly increased [30]. The incidence of cutaneous squamous cell carcinoma (SCC) in patients treated with etanercept is unclear, as incidence is significantly increased in one meta-analysis and not in another meta-analysis when compared to population-based skin cancer registries in Arizona and Minnesota [31, 32].

The OBSERVE-5 registry that included 2510 patients with psoriasis treated with etanercept found the cumulative incidence of SAEs over the 5 years of collection of registry data to be 22.2% with a decrease in incremental yearly incidence (meaning that fewer SAEs were reported in each subsequent year of the registry, which is consistent with long-term safety of the medication). The most commonly reported SAEs were infections (1.2% of patients reported pneumonia and 0.9% of patients reported cellulitis), followed by myocardial infarction and coronary artery disease (0.7% and 0.6% of patients, respectively) [33].

Adalimumab

Introduction
Adalimumab was first approved for the treatment of psoriasis vulgaris in 2008, after receiving approval for use in treatment of rheumatoid arthritis in 2002 and later psoriatic arthritis in 2005. Of all the psoriasis biologics, it carries the most FDA-approved disease indications, with approval for eight other diseases as below.

Other Indications
Adalimumab carries indications for rheumatoid arthritis, Crohn's disease (adult and pediatric), ulcerative colitis, psoriatic arthritis, hidradenitis suppurativa, ankylosing spondylitis, juvenile idiopathic arthritis, and noninfectious uveitis [34].

Mechanism of Action
Adalimumab is a human, recombinant IgG monoclonal antibody that binds to TNF-alpha and prevents it from interacting with TNF receptors found on cell surfaces.

Dosing
Doses are administered subcutaneously with an initial dose of 80 mg followed by 40 mg every other week starting 1 week after the initial dose. It is available to patients as both a pre-filled syringe and pen.

Efficacy
Key clinical trials for adalimumab include REVEAL and CHAMPION [1, 2]. The REVEAL trial included three treatment phases over 52 weeks. Initially, patients were randomized in a 2:1 ratio to receive either 40 mg of adalimumab every other week or placebo every other week for 16 weeks, followed by a 17-week phase where patients who achieved at least PASI-75 response in either placebo or treatment arms were started or continued on adalimumab (if initially in the placebo arm or treatment arm, respectively). Patients who did not achieve PASI-75 response were enrolled in a separate, open-label extension study with adalimumab. Patients who were initially in the treatment arm in the first phase of the study who also maintained at least PASI-75 response at week 33 were then re-randomized in a 1:1 ratio to continue treatment with adalimumab or receive placebo. Patients who were initially in the placebo arm in the first phase of the study and who achieved at least PASI-75 response were continued on adalimumab treatment. Patients at week 33 who achieved between PASI-50 and PASI-75

responses were continued in the open-label extension study, while patients who failed to achieve PASI-50 response were discontinued in the trial. At week 16, 71% of adalimumab-treated patients achieved PASI-75 response. The third phase of the study was performed to evaluate for the percentage of patients losing adequate response, defined as less than a PASI-50 response from week 0 baseline PASI score and at least a 6-point increase in PASI score relative to PASI score at week 33. Patients randomized to placebo had a significantly higher rate of loss of adequate response, 28% versus 5% in treatment group.

In the 3-year open-label study from the REVEAL study, patients who were on adalimumab from the beginning of the initial study showed good maintenance of PASI-75 response rates, with 83% PASI-75 response at week 100 and 76% PASI-75 response at week 160 [3].

The CHAMPION trial compared the efficacy of adalimumab to that of methotrexate. At week 16, 79.6% of patients in the adalimumab treatment group achieved PASI-75 response, which was significantly higher than the 35.5% of methotrexate-treated patients [2]. A subgroup analysis of patients stratified by BMI showed that adalimumab significantly improved patients' PASI scores across normal weight, overweight, and obese subgroups, as well as improved DLQI scores [35].

In a pooled post hoc analysis of PASI response data from the REVEAL, CHAMPION, and M02-528 (a phase 2 trial) clinical trials, PASI-75 response rates were significantly greater in adalimumab-treated patients overall and in patients with prior systemic treatment or failed prior treatments compared to placebo-treated patients [36]. The PASI-75 response rates between the adalimumab-treated groups were similar, indicating that adalimumab is efficacious in patients with prior exposure to systemic therapy. Other studies have shown similar results. Patients in one sub-analysis involving 282 patients from the BELIEVE trial with prior TNF-α antagonist use had PASI-75 response at week 16 of adalimumab treatment of 53.8% in patients who had not responded to other TNF antagonists and 65.7% of patients who lost

response to other TNF antagonists [37]. In the PROGRESS trial, 61% of patients who failed methotrexate in the past achieved "clear" or "minimal" scores on the physician global assessment (PGA) at week 16 of adalimumab treatment. Forty-nine percent and 48% of patients with inadequate response to etanercept and phototherapy, respectively, also achieved PGA scores of "clear" or "minimal" [38].

Anti-Adalimumab Antibodies

Adalimumab, as with various other biologic agents, can induce the formation of antibodies in vivo. In one multicenter cohort study, 80 patients being treated with adalimumab for psoriasis were followed, with 49% of patients forming anti-adalimumab antibodies [39]. The vast majority of these patients (90%) formed antibodies before week 24. Antibodies to adalimumab are neutralizing antibodies, and so the study authors concluded that the presence of antibodies against adalimumab inversely correlates with adalimumab concentration and clinical response. A systematic review of antidrug antibodies in psoriasis treatment found that antibodies against adalimumab are associated with lower serum adalimumab concentrations and lower PASI-75 response rates [25]. In addition, in rheumatoid arthritis, formation of anti-adalimumab antibodies is associated with lower serum adalimumab levels and significantly fewer treatment responders.

Safety

In the first 16 weeks of the REVEAL trial, injection site reactions occurred in 3.2% of adalimumab-treated patients. Infectious AEs reported in the initial 16 weeks of the REVEAL trial with incidence greater than 2% were upper respiratory tract infection, nasopharyngitis, and sinusitis. The SAE rate was the same in the treatment and placebo treatment group at 1.8%. Any patients who received at least one dose of adalimumab during the 52 weeks of the study were placed in the "all-adalimumab treatment group." This group had similar AE rates as the adalimumab-treated group through the first 16 weeks. Seven patients developed NMSCs, with three developing SCCs, three with BCCs, and one with an atypical endophytic epidermoid proliferation not further classified. Notably, of these seven patients, two had a history of psoralen plus UVA therapy (with an undisclosed number of total treatments), and another patient had done narrowband UVB therapy [1].

In the open-label extension of the REVEAL study, AE and SAE rates were similar to those observed in the 52-week period of the trial. No cases of lymphoma, demyelinating disorder, or lupus-like syndrome were observed through the 3 years of the extension trial.

Long-Term Safety

Across four randomized controlled trials (RCTs), one open-label extension study, and three meta-analyses of RCTs and long-term extension studies, rates of non-melanoma skin cancer (NMSC) and NMSC designated as "serious" were significantly increased when compared to the general population in the NCI survey from 1978 to 1997. When compared to the Arizona or Minnesota databases, NMSC rate was not significantly increased [40, 41]. The rate of upper respiratory tract infections was also significantly increased in patients treated with adalimumab [1]. The rates of malignancies, other than NMSC, were not significantly elevated in patients treated with adalimumab [40–42].

Infliximab

Infliximab, approved first for use in Crohn's disease in 1998, is now used for the treatment of several diseases, including gastrointestinal diseases (pediatric and adult Crohn's disease and ulcerative colitis) and rheumatologic diseases (rheumatoid arthritis, ankylosing spondylitis, psoriatic arthritis). It was approved for use in the treatment of moderate-to-severe psoriasis vulgaris in 2006. It is a chimeric IgG1 monoclonal antibody, made of human and mouse antibody components (human Fc domain and mouse variable domain).

Mechanism of Action

Infliximab works by affecting the TNF-α signaling pathway. It does this by binding to and neutralizing the activity of TNF-α [6].

Dosing

Infliximab is dosed by weight, with a dose of 5 mg/kg administered intravenously at weeks 0, 2, and 6 and then every 8 weeks thereafter.

Efficacy

Phase III clinical trials using infliximab in psoriasis showed that the medication was highly efficacious. The EXPRESS trial evaluated the response to infliximab dosed as above compared to placebo [6]. Eighty percent of patients in the infliximab-treated group achieved PASI-75 response at week 10, with maintenance of effect through week 24 with PASI-75 response of 82%. After 50 weeks, the PASI-75 response rate was 61%. Nail psoriasis also significantly improved after 10 weeks of treatment, with continued improvement from week 10 to week 24 and improvement generally maintained through week 50. Patients who had detectable levels of serum infliximab pre-infusion tended to maintain their PASI-75 response through 1 year, while patients with undetectable serum infliximab were less likely to maintain their PASI-75 response.

Another study evaluated continuous versus intermittent infliximab maintenance regimens using two doses of infliximab (3 mg/kg and 5 mg/kg) and found that continuous maintenance regimens (infliximab infusions every 8 weeks) were superior to intermittent regimens (infliximab infusions only when observed improvement from baseline PASI score decreased below 75%) [7]. This was especially true when evaluating PASI-90 response rates, where 34.3% and 25.0% of the continuously treated 5 mg/kg and 3 mg/kg infliximab groups achieved PASI-90 response, respectively, versus 10.4% and 9.5% in the intermittently treated groups at 5 mg/kg and 3 mg/kg doses, respectively. The long-term superiority of efficacy of continuous therapy over intermittent therapy was evaluated in the RESTORE2 trial [43]. Although this trial was terminated early due to serious infusion-related reactions occurring in 4% of the intermittently treated patients without formal efficacy analyses being conducted, PASI-75 response was greater in the continuously treated group after 52 weeks, with a rate of 80% versus a rate of 47% in the intermittently treated group with infliximab dosed at 5 mg/kg. It was also suggested that intermittent therapy may be less safe than continuous therapy due to the serious infusion-related reactions observed in the intermittent group.

Infliximab has been used successfully for the treatment of many cases of erythrodermic and pustular psoriasis, although controlled studies of the efficacy of this medication in the treatment of these variants of psoriasis are lacking [44].

Infliximab has also been shown to be fast acting. Patients treated with infliximab in the EXPRESS trail showed significantly greater PASI-50 response rates as early as week 2, while 40% of patients receiving 5 mg/kg of infliximab in another trial achieved PASI-50 response at week 2 with 47% of patients achieving PASI-75 response at week 4 [6, 8].

Safety

In phase III clinical trials, infliximab was generally well tolerated. In the EXPRESS trial, 82% of patients reported at least one adverse event through week 24, compared to 71% of placebo-treated patients, and 11% of patients receiving infliximab discontinuing from the study by week 24 due to adverse events. Notably, the percentage of patients experiencing infections and infusion reactions in placebo and infliximab treatment groups was similar, with 40% versus 42% of patients in the placebo and infliximab groups experiencing infections, respectively, and 2% versus 3%, respectively, experiencing infusion reactions. Lab abnormalities experienced in the infliximab treatment group but not in the placebo group included markedly abnormal increases (>150 U/L and 100% or greater increase from baseline) in aspartate aminotransferase and alanine aminotransferase (2% and 6%, respectively, at week 24). These patients were generally asymptomatic, and most were able to complete their infusions. In a prospective, observational, open-label long-term study with 660 patients, 7.7% of patients experienced infusion-related reactions or hypersensitivity, 2.3% experienced serious infections, and 2.3% experienced upper respiratory tract infections through the first 50 weeks of the study [45]. From week 50 to

week 98, adverse events occurred in 20.7% of patients, with the most commonly reported adverse events being nasopharyngitis or pharyngitis (4.2% of patients) and upper respiratory tract infections (1.6%), with 1% of patients reporting serious infection or new or worsening congestive heart failure.

Anti-Infliximab Antibodies

Anti-infliximab antibodies are associated with lower serum infliximab concentrations and decreased clinical effect. It is thought that infliximab is more immunogenic than some other biologic agents because of the murine component in the chimeric antibody [46].

Special Considerations for Patients Using TNF-Alpha Inhibitors

TNF-Alpha Inhibitor-Induced Psoriasis

In the literature for TNF-alpha inhibitors used for other diseases including inflammatory bowel disease (Crohn's disease and ulcerative colitis), rheumatoid arthritis, ankylosing spondylitis, and juvenile idiopathic arthritis, among other diseases, there have been numerous cases of patients using these agents with de novo development of psoriasis. This phenomenon is called TNF-α inhibitor-induced psoriasis. The most common culprit is infliximab, followed by adalimumab and then etanercept [47]. The most common conditions treated with TNF-alpha inhibitors with the development of psoriasis are Crohn's disease and rheumatoid arthritis, and most patients do not have a family history of psoriasis. The most common presentations of psoriasis in this condition are plaque and palmoplantar psoriasis, with the soles, palms, and scalp commonly involved. Typically patients develop psoriasis in the first 2 years of therapy with a TNF-alpha inhibitor, with most patients developing psoriasis in the first year.

Demyelinating Disease with TNF-Alpha Inhibitors

The FDA has placed a class warning label on all TNF-alpha inhibitors stating, "demyelinating disease, exacerbation or new onset, may occur,"

[20] including multiple sclerosis (MS), transverse myelitis, optic neuritis, and peripheral demyelinating diseases including Guillain-Barré syndrome. The package insert for etanercept also states that "new onset or exacerbation of seizure disorders have been reported in post-marketing experience" with etanercept. It is recommended that prescribers exercise caution when prescribing TNF-alpha inhibitors and should carefully consider prescribing TNF-alpha inhibitors in patients with preexisting or recent-onset central or peripheral nervous system demyelinating disorders. A review of TNF-inhibitors in psoriasis treatment found that in clinical trials, there was one reported case of MS in 6990 patients receiving etanercept for psoriasis treatment, zero cases of demyelinating disorders in 5204 patients treated with adalimumab, and one case of demyelinating polyneuropathy in 2322 patients treated with infliximab [48]. Outside of clinical trials, at least 19 cases of TNF-alpha inhibitor-associated demyelinating diseases have been presented in case reports and series. Although the absolute risk of developing demyelinating neurologic diseases is small with treatment of psoriasis using TNF-alpha inhibitors, it is important to assess for history of demyelinating disorders and monitor for signs and symptoms, with prompt discontinuation of therapy and possible referral to neurology if signs and symptoms develop.

IL-12 and IL-23

Ustekinumab

Intro
Ustekinumab has been approved for use in the treatment of moderate-to-severe plaque psoriasis since 2009 (Table 5.1). It is also approved for the treatment of psoriatic arthritis and Crohn's disease. It is well known that IL-12 and IL-23 are both cytokines involved in the differentiation of T cells into Th1 and Th17 cells, both of which are important in the pathogenesis of psoriasis [49, 50]. It is well known that Th17 and Th1 cells are involved in the production of pro-inflammatory cytokines including IL-17, IL-22, IL-21, IL-6, TNF-alpha, interferon gamma, and IL-2 [51–53]. IL-23 is important in maintaining survival of Th17 cells, as well as promoting their proliferation, while IL-12 is important in differentiation of Th1 cells. IL-12 also plays a role in keratinocyte pro-inflammatory responses by promoting production of interferon gamma [54].

Mechanism of Action
Ustekinumab is a fully human monoclonal antibody to the p40 subunit of IL-12 and IL-23. As a result, it affects and blocks the downstream signaling that results from binding of these cytokines to their receptors. It is able to affect both IL-12 and IL-23 signaling because both the IL-12 and IL-23 cytokines are heterodimeric proteins that have a shared subunit (the p40 subunit), while also having their own unique subunits (IL-12 has the p35 subunit, while IL-23 has the p19 subunit).

Dosing
Ustekinumab has the most convenient dosing schedule of all of the biologics. It is dosed by weight and administered subcutaneously; patients weighing less than 100 kg receive doses of 45 mg, while patients weighing 100 kg or greater receive 90 mg doses. These doses were determined by evaluation of data from phase II clinical trials that found both doses to be effective in improving psoriasis and subgroup evaluation of data from phase III clinical trials that found decreased response of patients weighing 100 kg or greater to doses of 45 mg but not to doses of 90 mg [55, 56]. Doses of ustekinumab are administered at week 0 and week 4 and then every 12 weeks thereafter.

Efficacy
The two pivotal phase III studies for ustekinumab were PHOENIX 1 and 2 [9, 10]. Both studies compared ustekinumab to placebo. Efficacy analysis was done according to intention-to-treat groups, while safety analyses were done according to actual treatment received. A third study, ACCEPT, compared ustekinumab head-to-head against etanercept [57].

PHOENIX 1 involved 766 patients randomized to receive 45 mg or 90 mg of ustekinumab at weeks 0 and 4 and then every 12 weeks or placebo at weeks 0 and 4, with crossover to treatment with ustekinumab at week 12. Ustekinumab-treated patients since week 0 who had achieved PASI-75 at weeks 28 and 40 were re-randomized at week 40 to either continue with maintenance dosing of ustekinumab or to discontinue treatment to measure loss of response. Subjects also were randomized according to weight (>90 kg and ≤90 kg) and the number of conventional systemic therapies to which subjects had inadequate response, intolerance, or contraindication (≤3 or >3). After 12 weeks 67.1% of subjects receiving 45 mg and 66.4% of subjects receiving 90 mg achieved PASI-75 response. Maximum effect was seen after 24 weeks, with PASI-75 response achieved by 76.1% of subjects receiving 45 mg of ustekinumab and 85% by subjects receiving 90 mg of ustekinumab. At week 40, more patients in the 90 mg group maintained long-term response. Ustekinumab also improved nail psoriasis, with significant improvements in Nail Psoriasis Severity Index and nail PGA's observed through 24 weeks of treatment [58]. Patients in the treatment arms also experienced improvement of their quality of life, measured with the Dermatology Life Quality Index (DLQI). Patients with treatment withdrawal at week 40 experienced worsening in their DLQI scores, while patients continued on treatment maintained their DLQI scores. In extension studies of PHOENIX 1, 68.7% of patients completed treatment through week 244, with initial clinical response well maintained through week 244; 63.4% and 72% of subjects receiving 45 mg and 90 mg, respectively, had PASI-75 response at the end of the study [59].

The PHOENIX 2 trial involved more subjects, 1230, with initial randomization into the same three groups as PHOENIX 1. The placebo group was randomized at week 12 into 45 and 90 mg dosing groups with doses administered at weeks 12 and 16 and then every 12 weeks. Partial responders in the initial active treatment groups were randomized to continue treatment with dosing every 8 weeks and every 12 weeks at their original randomized doses. Partial responders were defined as subjects who achieved between

PASI-50 and PASI-75. A higher proportion of partial responders were seen in the 45 mg treatment group versus the 90 mg treatment group (22.7% vs. 15.8%). Partial responders were more likely to have higher body weight and more severe disease. Escalation of dosing from every 12 weeks to every 8 weeks improved PASI-75 response rates in the 90 mg dose group from 33.3% to 68.8% by week 52; this effect was not observed in the 45 mg treatment group. Based on the results of this study, it was determined that it may be helpful for partial responders to be given higher and more frequent doses, at 90 mg and every 8 weeks. Patients who achieved less than PASI-50 response were discontinued at week 28. At week 12, 66.7% of patients treated with 45 mg of ustekinumab and 75.7% in the 90 mg treatment group achieved PASI-75 response. Sixty-eight percent and 73.5% of patients in the 45 mg and 90 mg treatment groups, respectively, achieved a PGA of clear (0) or minimal (1). Maximum response was seen after 20 weeks, with 74.9% and 83.5% of patients in the 45 mg and 90 mg treatment groups achieving PASI-75 response. PASI-75 responders at week 28 maintained their PASI response through week 52, and patients without dosing adjustments maintained PASI-75 through week 244. Patients who required dosing adjustments also usually experienced improved response after dose adjustments were made [60].

In the ACCEPT trial, patients that received two doses of either 45 mg or 90 mg of ustekinumab at week 0 and week 4 achieved greater PASI-75 response rates measured at week 12 compared to patients treated with 50 mg of etanercept twice weekly (68% in 45 mg treated patients and 74% in 90 mg treated patients versus 57% for etanercept-treated patients).

Health-related quality of life measures (HRQoL) in PHOENIX 1 study participants showed that nearly all patients at baseline prior to beginning treatment had significantly decreased quality of life with an average DLQI > 10. At week 12, DLQI scores were significantly improved for patients treated with both 45 and 90 mg of ustekinumab. In PHOENIX 2, DLQI scores of 0 or 1 were observed in 55.3% and

56.4% of patients in the 45 mg and 90 mg treatment groups, respectively. Using the Work Limitations Questionnaire (WLQ) and visual analog scale (VAS) in subjects in PHOENIX 2, researchers found that ustekinumab significantly improved productivity VAS scores at week 12 in both 45 and 90 mg treatment groups, while significantly fewer subjects missed days of work compared to placebo and significantly improved work limitations as measured by the WLQ with maintenance of these improvements through week 24 [61]. In PHOENIX 1 at week 12, short form-36 health survey domains showed significant improvement with ustekinumab treatment, with the greatest improvements in bodily pain and social functioning domains. Regression analysis controlling for improvements in PASI and PGA scores also showed that DLQI improved significantly beyond what would be expected according to clinical measures, indicating that treatment with ustekinumab independently improved DLQI scores [62].

Anti-Ustekinumab Antibodies

Through the long-term extension study of PHOENIX 1, 5.2% of patients (39/746) developed antibodies to ustekinumab. Sixty-four percent of these antibodies were neutralizing, and titers of antibodies were ≤1:40 in 67% of the cases. No patients developed antibodies between years 3 and 5, while one patient developed antibodies between week 76 and year 3 [63]. In PHOENIX 2, it was observed that partial responders had a higher likelihood of developing neutralizing antibodies to ustekinumab when compared to PASI-75 responders (12.7% vs. 2%). The long-term extension of PHOENIX 2 showed that 5.4% of patients had developed antibodies by week 52, but that between that time point and week 264, no additional patients developed antibodies.

Safety

Adverse events in the clinical trials generally did not require adjustments to treatment. In PHOENIX 1, adverse events occurred in 54.5% of patients receiving ustekinumab and in 48.2% of subjects in the placebo treatment group. SAEs occurred in 1.2% of subjects receiving ustekinumab and 0.8%

of subjects receiving placebo. In PHOENIX 2, 53.1%, 47.9%, and 49.8% of patients in the 45 mg, 90 mg, and placebo treatment groups, respectively, experienced AEs in the placebo-controlled phase. SAEs were seen in 2%, 1.2%, and 2% of patients in the 45 mg, 90 mg, and placebo treatment groups, respectively.

The most commonly observed AEs were upper respiratory tract infection, nasopharyngitis, headache, and arthralgia, in both PHOENIX 1 and 2.

SAEs in PHOENIX 1 occurred in six patients receiving ustekinumab. SAEs that were observed were stroke, hypertension, serious infections (two patients), hospitalization for coronary artery bypass grafting, and worsening psoriasis during the screening period that later responded to ustekinumab therapy. The two serious infections were bilateral lower extremity cellulitis and herpes zoster reactivation with dissemination beyond the primary dermatome, both of which resolved with appropriate therapy. SAEs in PHOENIX 2 occurred in 13 subjects in the placebo-controlled phase, with 5 subjects in the 90 mg treatment group and 8 in the 45 mg treatment group. In the placebo crossover phase of the study, 8 subjects experienced SAEs in the 45 mg treatment group, 4 in the 90 mg treatment group, 6 in the placebo crossover to 45 mg treatment group, and 2 in the placebo crossover to 90 mg treatment group. In the dose intensification phase, 2 subjects who had dosing every 8 weeks and 6 subjects who had dosing every 12 weeks experienced SAEs. In the placebo-controlled phase, SAEs were angina, dactylitis, clavicular fracture, sciatica, nephrolithiasis, seroma of amputation stump, death due to nonischemic sudden cardiac death in a patient with underlying dilated cardiomyopathy, cellulitis, benign meningioma, alcohol withdrawal syndrome, a syndromic complex of symptoms including transient palpitations, vertigo, ventricular extrasystoles, hypertension after administration of ustekinumab, and two cases of intervertebral disc protrusion. Eight subjects in the placebo arm also experienced SAEs. One case of basal cell carcinoma was reported in the 90 mg treatment group, while one subject in the placebo group developed squamous cell carcinoma. By the end of the 52 weeks of the trial, infections (nine patients) and cardiac disorders (nine patients) were the most common serious adverse events reported.

3104 patient-years of follow-up showed that the overall rates of adverse events (AEs), serious AEs, serious infections, malignancies, and major adverse cardiovascular events were consistent over time and comparable between 45 mg and 90 mg doses [59].

In the PHOENIX 2 extension study, 60 patients receiving ustekinumab for at least 3 years were selected, and 56 patients with psoriasis who were not receiving systemic therapy were selected to receive vaccinations with the 23-valent pneumococcal vaccine and the tetanus toxoid vaccine. Serum was checked pre-vaccination and 4 weeks postvaccination to assess for antibody response, finding that there was no less of an antibody response in the ustekinumab treatment group compared to control [64].

Injection site reactions rarely occurred in subjects receiving ustekinumab. One percent of injections resulted in injection site reactions in PHOENIX 1. In the 12-week placebo-controlled periods across phase 2 and PHOENIX 1 and 2, 3.4% of patients treated with 45 mg experienced injection site reactions, while 4.0% in the 90 mg group experienced injection site reactions [65].

Long-Term Safety
In the long-term PHOENIX 1 study, rates of AEs, SAEs, major adverse cardiovascular events (MACE), infections, and malignancies were similar between 45 and 90 mg treatment groups. Of 753 subjects, 30 developed serious infections (32 cases of serious infections—13 cases in patients receiving 45 mg and 19 in patients receiving 90 mg), 14 (10 patients treated with 45 mg, 4 patients treated with 90 mg) developed non-melanoma skin cancer in a 3:1 ratio of basal cell carcinoma to squamous cell carcinoma, 15 developed other malignancies, 10 subjects developed MACE (8 patients treated with 45 mg and 2 patients treated with 90 mg), and 5 deaths were reported.

One death occurred in the 45 mg group that was thought to be cardiovascular in origin, while in the 90 mg treatment group, patients died from complications from bilateral pneumonia, perforated bowel secondary to trauma, cervical vertebral fracture secondary to a fall, and suicide. Another patient also died after the study period ended due to metastatic pancreatic cancer that was also the cause of premature discontinuation from the study. Zero cases of active tuberculosis or other infections of interest were reported through year 5 in this study. A study combining the results of five trials where ustekinumab was used to treat psoriasis showed no latent tuberculosis infection reactivation in patients receiving concomitant isoniazid prophylaxis for latent TB infection [66].

IL-17 Agents

The Th17 T-cell lineage plays a key role in the pathogenesis of psoriasis. One of the key cytokines in this pathway is IL-17 [67]. Binding of IL-17 to its receptor on keratinocytes leads to increased inflammation, including recruitment of multiple inflammatory cell types, resulting in the characteristic plaques of psoriasis [68]. There are three biologic medications currently approved for psoriasis that target the IL-17 pathway (Table 5.1).

Ixekizumab
Ixekizumab is a humanized IgG subclass 4-kappa (IgG4-κ) anti-interleukin-17A monoclonal antibody approved in 2016 for the treatment of moderate-to-severe plaque psoriasis [69]. It exerts its action through binding to IL-17A, preventing its interaction with the IL-17A receptor. There were three pivotal clinical trials for ixekizumab, UNCOVER-1, UNCOVER-2, and UNCOVER-3.

Mechanism of Action
Ixekizumab exerts its action by binding to IL-17A, preventing it from binding to its target IL-17 receptor. As a result, downstream effects of IL-17 receptor activation are attenuated and decreased expressions of several cytokines that play a key role in psoriasis pathogenesis are observed. Some

of these cytokines include interferon gamma, IL-17, IL-22, and IL-23, all of which have been implicated in the pathogenesis of psoriasis. These reductions, in part, lead to reduction in keratinocyte proliferation and epidermal thickness as well as reductions in epidermal infiltration by inflammatory dendritic and T-cells. It has also been shown that ixekizumab decreases the expression of inflammation-associated gene products [70].

Dosing

Ixekizumab is delivered subcutaneously according to the following induction and then maintenance schedule. An initial dose of 160 mg is given at week 0, followed by 80 mg every 2 weeks until week 12. After the week 12 dose, the maintenance period of therapy commences, with 80 mg doses administered every 4 weeks. Ixekizumab is available in 80 mg/mL pre-filled syringes and auto-injectors.

Efficacy

Ixekizumab's efficacy was assessed in three pivotal phase III clinical trials [18, 19, 71]. UNCOVER-1 involved three treatment arms, ixekizumab doses given every 4 weeks and every 2 weeks and a placebo group. UNCOVER-2 and UNCOVER-3 had four treatment arms, ixekizumab doses given every 4 weeks and every 2 weeks, etanercept 50 mg twice a week, and a placebo treatment group. In all of these trials, the 12-week induction period was performed, with ixekizumab-treated patients administered 160 mg of ixekizumab at week 0 followed by 80 mg given every 2 or 4 weeks, according to their randomized treatment arm. At week 12 in UNCOVER-1, patients treated with ixekizumab at either 2- or 4-week intervals had significantly greater improvement in their psoriasis when compared to the placebo-treated group. Patients treated with ixekizumab every 2 weeks had a PASI-75 response rate of 89.1% and a PASI-90 response rate of 70.9%, which were both better than the PASI-75 (82.6%) and PASI-90 (64.6%) response rate in the group of patients treated with ixekizumab every 4 weeks [18]. Similar results were seen in UNCOVER-2 in terms of PASI-75 and PASI-90 response rates in the every 2-week group, 89.7% and 70.7%, respectively, and every 4-week group, 77.5% and 59.7%, respectively. UNCOVER-3 reinforced these results, with significantly greater PASI-75 and PASI-90 response rates in the every 2-week and every 4-week treatment groups as compared to the etanercept-treated group. The every 2-week treatment group had rates of 87.3% and 68.1%, while the every 4-week treatment group had 84.2% and 65.3%, in PASI-75 and PASI-90 response, respectively. Interestingly, by week 4 in both UNCOVER-2 and UNCOVER-3, about 50% of patients achieved PASI-75 response in the ixekizumab-treated groups at both dosing frequencies.

In UNCOVER-2 and UNCOVER-3, quality of life, as measured by Dermatology Life Quality Index (DLQI), was also significantly improved in the ixekizumab treatment groups as compared to both placebo and etanercept treatment groups at week 12. DLQI improvements were also positively correlated with improved PASI response, such that patients who had PASI-90 response were more likely to have DLQI scores of 0 or 1 than patients with PASI-75 response.

Two percent of patients developed neutralizing anti-ixekizumab antibodies, while 22% of patients developed anti-ixekizumab antibodies. The presence of anti-ixekizumab antibodies did not seem to affect response to ixekizumab through at least week 60 of treatment [72].

Safety

Across the UNCOVER trials, ixekizumab was generally well tolerated. The most common adverse events reported included nasopharyngitis, upper respiratory tract infections, injection site reactions/erythema/pain, pruritus, headache, and arthralgia. The most common serious adverse event reported was cellulitis, with a rate of 0.4% across all patients exposed to ixekizumab in clinical trials.

No cases of active or reactivated tuberculosis were observed throughout the clinical research trials involving ixekizumab.

Rates of non-melanoma skin cancers and other malignancies were not significantly different than the rates that would be expected in the psoriasis population [73].

Major adverse cardiovascular events (MACE) were rare in the clinical trials, with one patient receiving ixekizumab every 4 weeks experiencing a stroke. The rate of MACE was less than 0.2% in the induction period with incidence rate less than 0.7 per 100 patient-years during the long-term component of the clinical trials.

Among patients treated with ixekizumab in the combined treatment period up through week 60, seven patients reported ulcerative colitis, with four having a prior history of UC, while four patients reported Crohn's disease. When evaluating the 4209 patients who had exposure to ixekizumab, there was in incidence rate of 1.1/1000 patient-exposure years of definite or probable Crohn's disease and 1.1/1000 patient-exposure years of definite or probable ulcerative colitis. Overall, 29 cases of suspected IBD adverse events were reported with 19 thought to be definite or probable with fewer than 1% of patients had Crohn's disease or ulcerative colitis [74].

Between the every 2-week and every 4-week dosing groups, there was a higher frequency of cases of oral candidiasis in the every 2-week group that was significantly greater when compared to placebo.

Overall frequency of serious infections was not increased in patients on ixekizumab during the induction phase (first 12 weeks of therapy) [75].

Secukinumab

The FDA approved secukinumab in 2015 for treatment of moderate-to-severe plaque psoriasis [76]. It also carries FDA approval for use in treatment of psoriatic arthritis and ankylosing spondylitis. Like ixekizumab and brodalumab, it exerts its effects by affecting the signaling of IL-17.

Mechanism of Action

Secukinumab is a fully human, IgG1κ, monoclonal antibody to IL-17A [68]. It selectively binds to IL-17A and prevents it from binding to its receptor.

Dosing

Dosing for secukinumab involves an induction phase and a maintenance phase. The induction phase consists of subcutaneous administration of 300 mg of secukinumab weekly for five doses (weeks 0, 1, 2, 3, and 4), followed by 300 mg administered every 4 weeks. Secukinumab is currently available in 150 mg/mL pre-filled syringes and auto-injectors.

Efficacy

In phase III clinical trials, secukinumab's efficacy was assessed compared to placebo, etanercept, and ustekinumab [77].

In the ERASURE and FIXTURE studies, there were four study periods: a screening period, a 12-week induction period, a 40-week maintenance period, and an 8-week follow-up period [14]. The ERASURE study randomized patients to placebo or secukinumab treatment at two doses, 300 and 150 mg, while the FIXTURE study randomized patients to treatment with placebo, etanercept 50 mg twice weekly, or secukinumab at doses of 300 mg and 150 mg. Patients in each study who were assigned to placebo treatment who did not achieve PASI-75 response at week 12 were randomized to receive either secukinumab at either 150 mg or 300 mg. In both ERASURE and FIXTURE studies, secukinumab-treated patients had significantly greater PASI-75 response rates than placebo-treated groups, with patients treated with 300 mg showing higher rates of response in all efficacy end points than patients treated with 150 mg. PASI-75 and PASI-90 response rates in the ERASURE study at week 12 were, respectively, 81.6% and 59.2% in the 300 mg-treated group and 71.6% and 39.1% in the 150 mg-treated group. 80.5% of patients receiving 300 mg maintained their PASI-75 response through week 52, while 72.4% of patients treated with 150 mg maintained PASI-75 response through 1 year. Similar PASI-75 and PASI-90 response rates and maintenance through week 52 of PASI-75 response rates were observed in patients in the FIXTURE study. At week 12, 54.2% of patients treated with 300 mg of secukinumab achieved PASI-90 response, while 77.1% of these patients achieved, PASI-75 response, with maintenance of this PASI-75 response in 84.3% of patients through week 52. 41. Nine percent of patients achieved PASI-90 response at week 12, 67.0% of patients achieved PASI-75 response at week 12, and 82.2% of these patients maintained PASI-75 response through week 52 in the group of patients treated with 150 mg of secukinumab. The PASI-75 and PASI-90 response rates were significantly better for both secukinumab treatment groups than those achieved by the group of patients treated with etanercept, as was the rate of maintenance of PASI-75 response through week 52 for both secukinumab treatment groups compared to the etanercept-treated group. The FEATURE trial proved that administration of the medication with a pre-filled syringe was just as effective as in the ERASURE and FIXTURE trials, while the JUNCTURE trial proved the same for administration of the medication with an auto-injector [15, 16, 78].

The CLEAR trial showed that PASI-90 response in secukinumab-treated patients was significantly greater than that of the group treated with ustekinumab at week 16, with 79.0% PASI-90 response versus 57.6%. One hundred percent PASI improvement at week 16 was also significantly greater in the secukinumab-treated group (44.3%) than in the ustekinumab group (28.4%) [17].

Quality of life scores were also significantly better in patient groups treated with secukinumab. In the ERASURE study, DLQI scores of 0 or 1 were observed in 58.8% of patients treated with 300 mg and 46.1% in patients treated with 150 mg of secukinumab at week 12. These DLQI scores were well maintained through week 52, with 66.3% of patients treated with 300 mg and 48.6% of patients treated with 150 mg of secukinumab having DLQI scores of 0 or 1 [14]. Similarly, in FIXTURE, DLQI scores were 0 or 1 in a significantly greater proportion of patients in the 300 mg (56.7%) and 150 mg (50.6%) secukinumab-treated groups at week 12 when compared to placebo (6.6%) and etanercept (34.5%)-treated groups. Rates of DLQI scores of 0 or 1 were maintained through week 52, with 69.7% of 300 mg secukinumab-treated patients, 56.2% of 150 mg secukinumab-treated patients, and 46.9% of etanercept-treated patients having DLQI scores of 0 or 1 [14]. In the CLEAR trial, 71.9% of patients treated with secukinumab had DLQI scores of 0 or 1 at the end of the trial,

which was significantly greater than the 57.4% of patients in the ustekinumab-treated group [77].

The SCULPTURE trial evaluated fixed interval dosing versus retreatment as needed dosing for maintenance in psoriasis [79]. The patients treated with fixed interval maintenance dosing maintained PASI-75 response better than the retreatment as needed patients, with 78.2% versus 67.7% of patients treated with 300 mg secukinumab in the fixed interval versus retreatment as needed groups, respectively. This study did not prove non-inferiority of retreatment as needed maintenance dosing, which suggests that it is better to dose secukinumab every 4 weeks and not as needed.

Secukinumab has been studied in use for palmoplantar psoriasis in the GESTURE clinical trial [80]. Efficacy was evaluated using a palmoplantar-specific IGA (ppIGA) that was based on the IGA modified version 2011 specifically applied to the palms and soles. 33.3% of patients treated with 300 mg and 22.1% of patients treated with 150 mg of secukinumab achieving a score of 0 or 1 on the ppIGA indicating either clear or almost clear/minimal severity of their palmoplantar psoriasis at week 16. DLQI scores were also significantly improved at week 16 in both treatment groups, and pain and function of the palms and soles were greatly improved with treatment. HRQoL is improved overall by 55% as measured by subject's global assessment, and 12.5% of patients reported absence of difficulty due to their palms and soles at week 16.

Secukinumab has also been shown in phase II clinical trials to be helpful in treatment of nail psoriasis [81, 82].

Development of anti-secukinumab antibodies was rare in both the ERASURE (0.3%) and FIXTURE (0.4%), and no neutralizing antibodies were formed in either trial. Antibody development did not correlate with loss of efficacy.

Safety

Incidence of adverse events in both ERASURE and FIXTURE studies showed that the most common adverse events in secukinumab-treated groups were nasopharyngitis, headache, and upper respiratory tract infection and diarrhea. There were higher rates of infection in secukinumab-treated patients compared to placebo-treated patients, with only 1% and 0.7% of patients in the ERASURE study developing serious infections in the 300 mg and 150 mg treatment groups, respectively. In FIXTURE, 1.1% and 0.6% of patients treated with 300 and 150 mg of secukinumab developed serious infections. MACE occurred in 0.7% of patients in both 300 and 150 mg treatment groups in ERASURE and 0.4% of patients treated with 150 mg of secukinumab (0 patients treated with 300 mg of secukinumab developed MACE). Very rarely, patients taking secukinumab experienced exacerbation or new onset of ulcerative colitis and Crohn's disease. Injection site reactions were rare, with only 0.7% of patients developing injection site reactions in the FIXTURE study.

Brodalumab

Brodalumab is a fully human IgG2 anti-IL-17RA monoclonal antibody. It is the newest biologic medication approved for use in moderate to severe plaque psoriasis, gaining FDA approval on February 15, 2017. Unlike other biologic medications, brodalumab is subject to additional monitoring under a Risk Evaluation and Mitigation Strategy (REMS) system that will be discussed in further detail below. The key phase III clinical trials with brodalumab in psoriasis were AMAGINE-1, AMAGINE-2, and AMAGINE-3. AMAGINE-1 evaluated two doses of brodalumab (210 and 140 mg) and a placebo group and AMAGINE-2 and AMAGINE-3 evaluated the same two doses of brodalumab, ustekinumab dosed as labeled and a placebo group.

Mechanism of Action

Brodalumab exerts its actions by binding to IL-17RA (the interleukin-17A receptor) and inhibiting the activity of several IL-17 cytokines that typically bind to this receptor. These cytokines include IL-17A, IL-17F, IL-17A/F heterodimer, IL-17C, IL-25, and IL-17E [83].

Dosing

Brodalumab is dosed according to this schedule: 210 mg is administered subcutaneously at weeks 0, 1, and 2 and then every 2 weeks. Brodalumab is available as a pre-filled syringe.

Efficacy

Through three phase III clinical trials, brodalumab exhibited excellent efficacy, with PASI-75 response rates in the 83–86% range [12]. In AMAGINE-1, patients receiving brodalumab at 210 mg and 140 mg doses achieved PASI-75 at week 12, 83.3% and 60.3%, respectively. 70.3% and 41.9% of patients treated with 210 mg of brodalumab achieved PASI-90 and PASI-100 at week 12, while rates for patients receiving 140 mg of brodalumab were 42.5% and 23.3% for PASI-90 and PASI-100 response [84]. 78.3% of patients receiving brodalumab at a dose of 210 mg achieved PASI-90 response at week 52, while PASI-100 response rate at week 52 was 67.5% [13]. In patients receiving 140 mg of brodalumab, these rates were 66.7% for PASI-90 response at week 52 and 43.9% for PASI-100 response. 75.7% of patients receiving 210 mg and 53.9% of patients receiving 140 mg of brodalumab achieved sPGA scores of clear or almost clear/minimal. These results were sustained after 52 weeks of treatment, where 83.1% and 70.2% of treatment responders maintained these clear or almost clear/minimal sPGA scores.

In both AMAGINE-2 and AMAGINE-3, brodalumab dosed at 210 mg was statistically superior to ustekinumab in proportion of patients achieving PASI-90 and PASI-100 responses as well as in sPGA scores of 0 or 1 at week 12. In AMAGINE-3, brodalumab dosed at 210 mg was also superior to ustekinumab in proportion of patients achieving PASI-75 response, in addition to the measurements above.

In AMAGINE-1, HADS scores for depression and anxiety both improved significantly for patients who scored "moderate" or "severe" at baseline, with 73% of patients improving in the depression severity and 67% of patients improving in their anxiety severity in the 210 mg of brodalumab treatment group.

Safety

In clinical trials, brodalumab was fairly well tolerated. In the 12-week randomized treatment period in the pooled trials, 57.6% of patients treated with 210 mg and 55.6% of patients treated with 140 mg experienced adverse events [85]. The most frequent adverse reactions that occurred in 1% or more of patients treated with brodalumab were arthralgia, headache, fatigue, diarrhea, oropharyngeal pain, and nausea [83]. 25.4% of patients experienced infections, with the majority of these consisting of nasopharyngitis or pharyngitis, upper respiratory tract infection, urinary tract infections, bronchitis, and influenza infections. Most of these infections did not result in treatment discontinuation. Patients treated with brodalumab did have an increased rate of non-serious skin and mucosal candida infections. One patient in the pooled trials attempted suicide and suicidal ideation or behavior occurred in 2 of 4019 patients (0.2 per 100 subject-years) that were treated with brodalumab. Suicidal ideation or behavior occurred in 34 of 4464 patients treated with brodalumab at a rate of 0.37 per 100 subject-years. Ten subjects attempted or completed suicide, of which eight had a history of depression and/or suicidal ideation or behavior. As a result, brodalumab was given a black box warning for risks in patients with a history of suicidal thoughts or behavior and mandated to be prescribed through a Risk Evaluation and Mitigation Strategy (REMS) system.

Special Monitoring (REMS System)

Brodalumab is only available through a restricted monitoring system called the REMS program, where patients, prescribers, and pharmacies must be enrolled into the REMS system. Prescribers must be certified with the program, patients must sign a patient-prescriber agreement form, and pharmacies must be certified with the program and only dispense the medication to patients who are authorized to receive the medication.

Special Considerations in Anti-IL-17 Therapy

IL-17 and Candidiasis

IL-17 appears to play a key role in mucocutaneous defense against candida infections [86, 87]. Therefore, blocking of IL-17 and its downstream effects can lead to increased candida infections, which have been seen in the treatment of psoriasis with anti-IL-17 biologics. However, most of these infections are not considered to be serious and resolve with antifungal treatment.

IL-17 and IBD

IL-17 inhibitors have been evaluated in the treatment of inflammatory bowel disease and have not been effective in treating IBD and may instead contribute to worsening of IBD [88, 89]. This phenomenon is not well studied, but it is suggested that practitioners use caution in prescribing IL-17 antagonists until the relationship of IL-17 and IBD is furthered.

Screening and Monitoring of All Biologics

Consensus guidelines do not exist for the monitoring of therapy with biologics. There have been some studies conducted to evaluate for evidence behind monitoring parameters and methods that many physicians may follow, which will be outlined below. These monitoring parameters apply to all biologics and not to any particular biologic agent. The FDA recommends that all patients on biologic therapy should be tested for tuberculosis infection with either a tuberculin skin test (TST) or with interferon gamma release assay (IGRA) [90]. Evaluation for hepatitis infection is at the provider's discretion, although the Centers for Disease Control and Prevention (CDC) recommends that individuals born between 1945 and 1965 be tested at least once for hepatitis C virus regardless of risk factors of HCV infection [91]. Any patients with risk factors should also be tested for hepatitis infections, per physician judgment, and for the concern for viral reactivation.

General laboratory monitoring with tests such as complete blood counts or basic metabolic panels can be done, but the evidence behind testing for these as part of routine screening is weak or insufficient.

Screening for human immunodeficiency virus (HIV) infection is not mandatory with biologic treatment and is up to the discretion of the clinician [92].

To summarize, the only well-established screening and monitoring testing with good supporting evidence is testing for tuberculosis infection. All other tests, including viral infection testing, complete blood counts, and complete metabolic panels, can be tested at the physician's discretion and if indicated by individual patient risk factors.

Biologics Now Off the Market

Two biologic medications previously FDA-approved for psoriasis have been withdrawn from the market. Alefacept (Amevive) blocked the binding of CD-2 on memory-effector T cells to the costimulatory molecule LFA-3, resulting in a decrease in number and activity of these T cells. It was voluntarily withdrawn from the market in 2011 due to its modest efficacy and business considerations. Efalizumab (Raptiva) was a monoclonal antibody directed against the CD11a subunit in lymphocyte function-associated antigen-1 (LFA-1). Efalizumab functioned by blocking T-cell adhesion that is mediated by LFA-1, which results in decreased T-cell activation, T-cell reactivation, and transmigration through blood vessel walls into inflamed tissues. Efalizumab was withdrawn from the market in 2009 due to several case reports of associated progressive multifocal leukoencephalopathy.

Future Biologics

As we have seen, biologics that are already available on the market have various immunologic targets, including TNF-α, IL-12, IL-23, and IL-17. Newer biologics under development have many of the same immunologic targets, including in combination (such as a biologic targeting both IL-17 and TNF-α). Other biologics in development are aimed at additional molecular targets including IL-23 p19, TBK1, IKK1ε, and RORγt. [93].

References

1. Menter A, Tyring S, Gordon K, Kimball A, Leonardi C, Langley R, et al. Adalimumab therapy for moderate to severe psoriasis: a randomized, controlled phase III trial. J Am Acad Dermatol. 2008;58(1):106–15.
2. Saurat J, Stingl G, Dubertret L, Papp K, Langley R, Ortonne J, et al. Efficacy and safety results from the randomized controlled comparative study of adalimumab vs. methotrexate vs. placebo in patients with psoriasis (CHAMPION). Br J Dermatol. 2007;158(3):558–66.
3. Gordon K, Papp K, Poulin Y, Gu Y, Rozzo S, Sasso E. Long-term efficacy and safety of adalimumab in patients with moderate to severe psoriasis treated continuously over 3 years: results from an open-label extension study for patients from REVEAL. J Am Acad Dermatol. 2012;66(2):241–51.
4. Leonardi C, Powers J, Matheson R, Goffe B, Zitnik R, Wang A, et al. Etanercept as monotherapy in patients with psoriasis. N Engl J Med. 2003;349(21):2014–22.
5. Papp K, Tyring S, Lahfa M, Prinz J, Griffiths C, Nakanishi A, et al. A global phase III randomized controlled trial of etanercept in psoriasis: safety, efficacy, and effect of dose reduction. Br J Dermatol. 2005;152(6):1304–12.
6. Reich K, Nestle F, Papp K, Ortonne J, Evans R, Guzzo C, et al. Infliximab induction and maintenance therapy for moderate-to-severe psoriasis: a phase III, multicentre, double-blind trial. Lancet. 2005;366(9494):1367–74.
7. Menter A, Feldman S, Weinstein G, Papp K, Evans R, Guzzo C, et al. A randomized comparison of continuous vs. intermittent infliximab maintenance regimens over 1 year in the treatment of moderate-to-severe plaque psoriasis. J Am Acad Dermatol. 2007;56(1):31.e1–31.e15.
8. Gottlieb A, Evans R, Li S, Dooley L, Guzzo C, Baker D, et al. Infliximab induction therapy for patients with severe plaque-type psoriasis: a randomized, double-blind, placebo-controlled trial. J Am Acad Dermatol. 2004;51(4):534–42.
9. Leonardi C, Kimball A, Papp K, Yeilding N, Guzzo C, Wang Y, et al. Efficacy and safety of ustekinumab, a human interleukin-12/23 monoclonal antibody, in patients with psoriasis: 76-week results from a randomised, double-blind, placebo-controlled trial (PHOENIX 1). Lancet. 2008;371(9625):1665–74.
10. Papp K, Langley R, Lebwohl M, Krueger G, Szapary P, Yeilding N, et al. Efficacy and safety of ustekinumab, a human interleukin-12/23 monoclonal antibody, in patients with psoriasis: 52-week results from a randomised, double-blind, placebo-controlled trial (PHOENIX 2). Lancet. 2008;371(9625):1675–84.
11. Griffiths C, Strober B, van de Kerkhof P, Ho V, Fidelus-Gort R, Yeilding N, et al. Comparison of ustekinumab and etanercept for moderate-to-severe psoriasis. N Engl J Med. 2010;362(2):118–28.
12. Lebwohl M, Strober B, Menter A, Gordon K, Weglowska J, Puig L, et al. Phase 3 studies comparing brodalumab with ustekinumab in psoriasis. N Engl J Med. 2015;373(14):1318–28.
13. Papp K, Reich K, Paul C, Blauvelt A, Baran W, Bolduc C, et al. A prospective phase III, randomized, double-blind, placebo-controlled study of brodalumab in patients with moderate-to-severe plaque psoriasis. Br J Dermatol. 2016;175(2):273–86.
14. Langley R, Elewski B, Lebwohl M, Reich K, Griffiths C, Papp K, et al. Secukinumab in plaque psoriasis—results of two phase 3 trials. N Engl J Med. 2014;371(4):326–38.
15. Blauvelt A, Prinz J, Gottlieb A, Kingo K, Sofen H, Ruer-Mulard M, et al. Secukinumab administration by pre-filled syringe: efficacy, safety and usability results from a randomized controlled trial in psoriasis (FEATURE). Br J Dermatol. 2014;172(2):484–93.
16. Paul C, Lacour J, Tedremets L, Kreutzer K, Jazayeri S, Adams S, et al. Efficacy, safety and usability of secukinumab administration by autoinjector/pen in

psoriasis: a randomized, controlled trial (JUNCTURE). J Eur Acad Dermatol Venereol. 2014;29(6):1082–90.

17. Blauvelt A, Reich K, Tsai T, Tyring S, Vanaclocha F, Kingo K, et al. Secukinumab is superior to ustekinumab in clearing skin of subjects with moderate-to-severe plaque psoriasis up to 1 year: results from the CLEAR study. J Am Acad Dermatol. 2017;76(1):60–69.e9.

18. Gordon K, Blauvelt A, Papp K, Langley R, Luger T, Ohtsuki M, et al. Phase 3 trials of ixekizumab in moderate-to-severe plaque psoriasis. N Engl J Med. 2016;375(4):345–56.

19. Griffiths C, Reich K, Lebwohl M, van de Kerkhof P, Paul C, Menter A, et al. Comparison of ixekizumab with etanercept or placebo in moderate-to-severe psoriasis (UNCOVER-2 and UNCOVER-3): results from two phase 3 randomised trials. Lancet. 2015;386(9993):541–51.

20. Enbrel [package insert]. Thousand Oaks: Immunex Corporation; 2016.

21. Gottlieb AB, Lowe NJ, Matheson RT et al. Efficacy of etanercept in patients with psoriasis. Presented at the American Academy of Dermatology, New Orleans, LA, USA, 22–27 February 2002.

22. Gordon K, Gottlieb A, Leonardi C, Elewski B, Wang A, Jahreis A, et al. Clinical response in psoriasis patients discontinued from and then reinitiated on etanercept therapy. J Dermatol Treat. 2006;17(1):9–17.

23. Bagel J, Tyring S, Rice K, Collier D, Kricorian G, Chung J, et al. Open-label study of etanercept treatment in patients with moderate to severe plaque psoriasis who lost a satisfactory response to adalimumab. Br J Dermatol. 2017;177:411.

24. Hsu L, Snodgrass B, Armstrong A. Antidrug antibodies in psoriasis: a systematic review. Br J Dermatol. 2014;170(2):261–73.

25. Paller A, Siegfried E, Langley R, Gottlieb A, Pariser D, Landells I, et al. Etanercept treatment for children and adolescents with plaque psoriasis. N Engl J Med. 2008;358(3):241–51.

26. Langley R, Paller A, Hebert A, Creamer K, Weng H, Jahreis A, et al. Patient-reported outcomes in pediatric patients with psoriasis undergoing etanercept treatment: 12-week results from a phase III randomized controlled trial. J Am Acad Dermatol. 2011;64(1):64–70.

27. Mohan N, Edwards E, Cupps T, Oliverio P, Sandberg G, Crayton H, et al. Demyelination occurring during anti-tumor necrosis factor ? Therapy for inflammatory arthritides. Arthritis Rheum. 2001;44(12):2862–9.

28. Sicotte N, Voskuhl R. Onset of multiple sclerosis associated with anti-TNF therapy. Neurology. 2001;57(10):1885–8.

29. Mercieca C, Vella N, Borg A. Demyelination during anti-TNFα therapy for ankylosing spondylitis. Mod Rheumatol. 2011;22(2):303–7.

30. Sorenson E, Koo J. Evidence-based adverse effects of biologic agents in the treatment of moderate-to-severe psoriasis: providing clarity to an opaque topic. J Dermatol Treat. 2015;26(6):493–501.

31. Pariser D, Leonardi C, Gordon K, Gottlieb A, Tyring S, Papp K, et al. Integrated safety analysis: short- and long-term safety profiles of etanercept in patients with psoriasis. J Am Acad Dermatol. 2012;67(2):245–56.

32. Papp K, Poulin Y, Bissonnette R, Bourcier M, Toth D, Rosoph L, et al. Assessment of the long-term safety and effectiveness of etanercept for the treatment of psoriasis in an adult population. J Am Acad Dermatol. 2012;66(2):e33-e45.

33. Kimball A, Rothman K, Kricorian G, Pariser D, Yamauchi P, Menter A, et al. OBSERVE-5: observational postmarketing safety surveillance registry of etanercept for the treatment of psoriasis final 5-year results. J Am Acad Dermatol. 2015;72(1):115–22.

34. Humira [package insert]. North Chicago: AbbVie Inc.; 2016.

35. Prussick R, Unnebrink K, Vandecantos WC. Efficacy of Adalimumab compared with methotrexate or placebo stratified by baseline BMI in a randomized placebo-controlled trial in patients with psoriasis. J Drugs Dermatol. 2015;14(8):864–8.

36. Papp K, Armstrong A, Reich K, Karunaratne M, Valdecantos W. Adalimumab efficacy in patients with psoriasis who received or did not respond to prior systemic therapy: a pooled post hoc analysis of results from three double-blind, placebo-controlled clinical trials. Am J Clin Dermatol. 2015;17(1):79–86.

37. Ortonne J, Chimenti S, Reich K, Gniadecki R, Sprøgel P, Unnebrink K, et al. Efficacy and safety of adalimumab in patients with psoriasis previously treated with anti-tumour necrosis factor agents: subanalysis of BELIEVE. J Eur Acad Dermatol Venereol. 2011;25(9):1012–20.

38. Strober B, Poulin Y, Kerdel F, Langley R, Gu Y, Gupta S, et al. Switching to adalimumab for psoriasis patients with a suboptimal response to etanercept, methotrexate, or phototherapy: efficacy and safety results from an open-label study. J Am Acad Dermatol. 2011;64(4):671–81.

39. Menting S, van Lümig P, de Vries A, van den Reek J, van der Kleij D, de Jong E, et al. Extent and consequences of antibody formation against adalimumab in patients with psoriasis. JAMA Dermatol. 2014;150(2):130.

40. Leonardi C, Papp K, Strober B, Reich K, Asahina A, Gu Y, et al. The long-term safety of adalimumab treatment in moderate to severe psoriasis. Am J Clin Dermatol. 2011;12(5):321–37.

41. Burmester G, Mease P, Dijkmans B, Gordon K, Lovell D, Panaccione R, et al. Adalimumab safety and mortality rates from global clinical trials of six immune-mediated inflammatory diseases. Ann Rheum Dis. 2009;68(12):1863–9.

42. Burmester G, Panaccione R, Gordon K, McIlraith M, Lacerda A. Adalimumab: long-term safety in 23 458 patients from global clinical trials in rheumatoid arthritis, juvenile idiopathic arthritis, ankylosing spondylitis, psoriatic arthritis, psoriasis and Crohn's disease. Ann Rheum Dis. 2012;72(4):517–24.

43. Reich K, Wozel G, Zheng H, van Hoogstraten H, Flint L, Barker J. Efficacy and safety of infliximab as continuous or intermittent therapy in patients with

moderate-to-severe plaque psoriasis: results of a randomized, long-term extension trial (RESTORE2). Br J Dermatol. 2013;168(6):1325–34.

44. Levin E, Debbaneh M, Koo J, Liao W. Biologic therapy in erythrodermic and pustular psoriasis. J Drugs Dermatol. 2014;13(3):342–54.

45. Shear N, Hartmann M, Toledo-Bahena M, Katsambas A, Connors L, Chang Q, et al. Long-term efficacy and safety of infliximab maintenance therapy in patients with plaque-type psoriasis in real-world practice. Br J Dermatol. 2014;171(3):631–41.

46. Harding F, Stickler M, Razo J, DuBridge R. The immunogenicity of humanized and fully human antibodies. MAbs. 2010;2(3):256–65.

47. Brown G, Wang E, Leon A, Huynh M, Wehner M, Matro R, et al. Tumor necrosis factor-α inhibitor-induced psoriasis: systematic review of clinical features, histopathological findings, and management experience. J Am Acad Dermatol. 2017;76(2):334–41.

48. Zhu T, Nakamura M, Abrouk M, Farahnik B, Koo J, Bhutani T. Demyelinating disorders secondary to TNF-inhibitor therapy for the treatment of psoriasis: a review. J Dermatol Treat. 2016;27(5):406–13.

49. Tesmer L, Lundy S, Sarkar S, Fox D. Th17 cells in human disease. Immunol Rev. 2008;223(1):87–113.

50. Murphy K, Reiner S. Decision making in the immune system: the lineage decisions of helper T cells. Nat Rev Immunol. 2002;2(12):933–44.

51. Stockinger B, Veldhoen M. Differentiation and function of Th17 T cells. Curr Opin Immunol. 2007;19(3):281–6.

52. Oppmann B, Lesley R, Blom B, Timans J, Xu Y, Hunte B, et al. Novel p19 protein engages IL-12p40 to form a cytokine, IL-23, with biological activities similar as well as distinct from IL-12. Immunity. 2000;13(5):715–25.

53. Harrington L, Hatton R, Mangan P, Turner H, Murphy T, Murphy K, et al. Interleukin 17–producing CD4+ effector T cells develop via a lineage distinct from the T helper type 1 and 2 lineages. Nat Immunol. 2005;6(11):1123–32.

54. Vignali D, Kuchroo V. IL-12 family cytokines: immunological playmakers. Nat Immunol. 2012;13(8):722–8.

55. Krueger G, Langley R, Leonardi C, Yeilding N, Guzzo C, Wang Y, et al. A human interleukin-12/23 monoclonal antibody for the treatment of psoriasis. N Engl J Med. 2007;356(6):580–92.

56. Lebwohl M, Yeilding N, Szapary P, Wang Y, Li S, Zhu Y, et al. Impact of weight on the efficacy and safety of ustekinumab in patients with moderate to severe psoriasis: rationale for dosing recommendations. J Am Acad Dermatol. 2010;63(4):571–9.

57. Griffiths CEM, Strober B, Fidelus-Gort R, Menter A. A phase 3, multicenter, randomized study comparing ustekinumab and etanercept for the treatment of moderate to severe plaque psoriasis. P3318. 2009 AAD meeting; San Francisco.

58. Rich P, Bourcier M, Sofen H, Fakharzadeh S, Wasfi Y, Wang Y, et al. Ustekinumab improves nail disease in patients with moderate-to-severe psoriasis: results from PHOENIX 1. Br J Dermatol. 2014;170(2):398–407.

59. Kimball A, Papp K, Wasfi Y, Chan D, Bissonnette R, Sofen H, et al. Long-term efficacy of ustekinumab in patients with moderate-to-severe psoriasis treated for up to 5 years in the PHOENIX 1 study. J Eur Acad Dermatol Venereol. 2012;27(12):1535–45.

60. Langley R, Lebwohl M, Krueger G, Szapary P, Wasfi Y, Chan D, et al. Long-term efficacy and safety of ustekinumab, with and without dosing adjustment, in patients with moderate-to-severe psoriasis: results from the PHOENIX 2 study through 5 years of follow-up. Br J Dermatol. 2015;172(5):1371–83.

61. Reich K, Schenkel B, Zhao N, Szapary P, Augustin M, Bourcier M, et al. Ustekinumab decreases work limitations, improves work productivity, and reduces work days missed in patients with moderate-to-severe psoriasis: results from PHOENIX 2. J Dermatol Treat. 2010;22(6):337–47.

62. Lebwohl M, Papp K, Han C, Schenkel B, Yeilding N, Wang Y, et al. Ustekinumab improves health-related quality of life in patients with moderate-to-severe psoriasis: results from the PHOENIX 1 trial. Br J Dermatol. 2010;162(1):137–46.

63. Kimball A, Gordon K, Fakharzadeh S, Yeilding N, Szapary P, Schenkel B, et al. Long-term efficacy of ustekinumab in patients with moderate-to-severe psoriasis: results from the PHOENIX 1 trial through up to 3 years. Br J Dermatol. 2012;166(4):861–72.

64. Brodmerkel C, Wadman E, Langley R, Papp K, Bourcier M, Poulin Y, et al. Immune response to pneumococcus and tetanus toxoid in patients with moderate-to-severe psoriasis following long-term ustekinumab use. J Drugs Dermatol. 2013;12(10):1122–9.

65. Lebwohl M, Leonardi C, Griffiths C, Prinz J, Szapary P, Yeilding N, et al. Long-term safety experience of ustekinumab in patients with moderate-to-severe psoriasis (Part I of II): results from analyses of general safety parameters from pooled Phase 2 and 3 clinical trials. J Am Acad Dermatol. 2012;66(5):731–41.

66. Tsai T, Ho V, Song M, Szapary P, Kato T, Wasfi Y, et al. The safety of ustekinumab treatment in patients with moderate-to-severe psoriasis and latent tuberculosis infection. Br J Dermatol. 2012;167(5):1145–52.

67. Krueger J, Fretzin S, Suárez-Fariñas M, Haslett P, Phipps K, Cameron G, et al. IL-17A is essential for cell activation and inflammatory gene circuits in subjects with psoriasis. J Allergy Clin Immunol. 2012;130(1):145–154.e9.

68. Canavan T, Elmets C, Cantrell W, Evans J, Elewski B. Anti-IL-17 medications used in the treatment of plaque psoriasis and psoriatic arthritis: a comprehensive review. Am J Clin Dermatol. 2015;17(1):33–47.

69. Taltz [package insert]. Indianapolis: Eli Lilly and Company; 2016.

70. Wang C, Suárez-Fariñas M, Nograles K, Mimoso C, Shrom D, Dow E, et al. IL-17 induces inflammation-associated gene products in blood monocytes, and treatment with ixekizumab reduces their expression in psoriasis patient blood. J Investig Dermatol. 2014;134(12):2990–3.

71. Syed Y. Ixekizumab: a review in moderate to severe plaque psoriasis. Am J Clin Dermatol. 2017;18(1):147–58.

72. Blauvelt A, Cameron G, Gordon K, et al. Ixekizumab, a novel anti-IL-17A antibody, exhibits low immunogenicity during long-term treatment in patients with psoriasis [abstract no. 3232]. J Am Acad Dermatol. 2016;74(5 Suppl 1):AB258.

73. Kimball A, Schenfeld J, Accortt N, Anthony M, Rothman K, Pariser D. Incidence rates of malignancies and hospitalized infectious events in patients with psoriasis with or without treatment and a general population in the U.S.A.: 2005-09. Br J Dermatol. 2014;170(2):366–73.

74. Reich K, Leonardi C, Langley R, Warren R, Bachelez H, Romiti R, et al. Inflammatory bowel disease among patients with psoriasis treated with ixekizumab: a presentation of adjudicated data from an integrated database of 7 randomized controlled and uncontrolled trials. J Am Acad Dermatol. 2017;76(3):441–448.e2.

75. Strober B, Leonardi C, Papp K, Mrowietz U, Ohtsuki M, Bissonnette R, et al. Short- and long-term safety outcomes with ixekizumab from 7 clinical trials in psoriasis: Etanercept comparisons and integrated data. J Am Acad Dermatol. 2017;76(3):432–440.e17.

76. Cosentyx [package insert]. East Hanover: Novartis Pharmaceuticals Corporation; 2015.

77. Thaçi D, Blauvelt A, Reich K, Tsai T, Vanaclocha F, Kingo K, et al. Secukinumab is superior to ustekinumab in clearing skin of subjects with moderate to severe plaque psoriasis: CLEAR, a randomized controlled trial. J Am Acad Dermatol. 2015;73(3):400–9.

78. Lacour J, Paul C, Jazayeri S, Papanastasiou P, Xu C, Nyirady J, et al. Secukinumab administration by autoinjector maintains reduction of plaque psoriasis severity over 52 weeks: results of the randomized controlled JUNCTURE trial. J Eur Acad Dermatol Venereol. 2017;31:847.

79. Mrowietz U, Leonardi C, Girolomoni G, Toth D, Morita A, Balki S, et al. Secukinumab retreatment-as-needed versus fixed-interval maintenance regimen for moderate to severe plaque psoriasis: a randomized, double-blind, noninferiority trial (SCULPTURE). J Am Acad Dermatol. 2015;73(1):27–36.e1.

80. Gottlieb A, Sullivan J, van Doorn M, Kubanov A, You R, Parneix A, et al. Secukinumab shows significant efficacy in palmoplantar psoriasis: results from GESTURE, a randomized controlled trial. J Am Acad Dermatol. 2017;76(1):70–80.

81. Paul C, Reich K, Gottlieb A, Mrowietz U, Philipp S, Nakayama J, et al. Secukinumab improves hand, foot and nail lesions in moderate-to-severe plaque psoriasis: subanalysis of a randomized, double-blind, placebo-controlled, regimen-finding phase 2 trial. J Eur Acad Dermatol Venereol. 2014;28(12):1670–5.

82. Sigurgeirsson B, Kircik L, Nemoto O, Mikazans I, Haemmerle S, Thurston H, et al. Secukinumab improves the signs and symptoms of moderate-to-severe plaque psoriasis in subjects with involvement of hands and/or feet: subanalysis of a randomized, double-blind, placebo-controlled, phase 2 dose-ranging study. J Eur Acad Dermatol Venereol. 2013;28(8):1127–9.

83. Siliq [package insert]. Bridgewater: Valeant Pharmaceuticals; 2017.

84. Papp K, Reich K, Leonardi C, et al. Efficacy and safety of brodalumab in patients with moderate to severe plaque psoriasis: results of AMAGINE-1, a phase 3, randomized, double-blind, placebo controlled study through week 12. In: Presented at the 73rd annual meeting of the American Academy of Dermatology; 2015 March 20–24; San Francisco, CA.

85. Farahnik B, Beroukhim K, Abrouk M, Nakamura M, Zhu T, Singh R, et al. Brodalumab for the treatment of psoriasis: a review of phase III trials. Dermatol Ther. 2016;6(2):111–24.

86. Puel A, Cypowyj S, Bustamante J, Wright J, Liu L, Lim H, et al. Chronic mucocutaneous candidiasis in humans with inborn errors of interleukin-17 immunity. Science. 2011;332(6025):65–8.

87. Gaffen S, Hernández-Santos N, Peterson A. IL-17 signaling in host defense against Candida albicans. Immunol Res. 2011;50(2–3):181–7.

88. Hueber W, Sands B, Lewitzky S, Vandemeulebroecke M, Reinisch W, Higgins P, et al. Secukinumab, a human anti-IL-17A monoclonal antibody, for moderate to severe Crohn's disease: unexpected results of a randomised, double-blind placebo-controlled trial. Gut. 2012;61(12):1693–700.

89. Mozaffari S, Nikfar S, Abdollahi M. Inflammatory bowel disease therapies discontinued between 2009 and 2014. Expert Opin Investig Drugs. 2015;24(7):949–56.

90. Huang W, Cordoro K, Taylor S, Feldman S. To test or not to test? An evidence-based assessment of the value of screening and monitoring tests when using systemic biologic agents to treat psoriasis. J Am Acad Dermatol. 2008;58(6):970–7.

91. Testing Recommendations for Hepatitis C Virus Infection | HCV | Division of Viral Hepatitis | CDC [Internet]. Cdc.gov. 2017 [cited 7 April 2017]. https://www.cdc.gov/hepatitis/hcv/guidelinesc.htm

92. Menter A, Gottlieb A, Feldman S, Van Voorhees A, Leonardi C, Gordon K, et al. Guidelines of care for the management of psoriasis and psoriatic arthritis. J Am Acad Dermatol. 2008;58(5):826–50.

93. Campa M, Menter A. A review of emerging IL-17 inhibitors in the treatment of psoriasis focusing on preclinical through phase II studies. Expert Opin Investig Drugs. 2016;25(11):1337–44.

Abigail Cline, Kayla H. Felix, Elias Oussedik, Leah A. Cardwell, and Steven R. Feldman

Introduction

Psoriasis is a complex systemic disease that has both genetic and environmental factors. The understanding of psoriasis pathophysiology has advanced from that of local keratinocyte dysfunction to a systemic disease with immune dysregulation and T-cell-mediated inflammation [1]. This improved understanding of the mechanisms causing psoriasis is reflected in improved treatment modalities. Older treatments— such as corticosteroids, cyclosporine, and methotrexate—have considerable effects beyond the immune system and have given way to more selective small-molecule inhibitors and biologic therapies [2]. Nevertheless, many psoriasis patients experience

A. Cline
Department of Internal Medicine, Medical College of Georgia, Augusta, GA, USA
e-mail: abcline@augusta.edu

K. H. Felix • E. Oussedik • L. A. Cardwell (✉)
Department of Dermatology, Wake Forest School of Medicine, Winston-Salem, NC, USA
e-mail: lcardwe@wakehealth.edu

S. R. Feldman
Department of Dermatology, Wake Forest School of Medicine, Winston-Salem, NC, USA

Department of Pathology, Wake Forest School of Medicine, Winston-Salem, NC, USA

Department of Public Health Sciences, Wake Forest School of Medicine, Winston-Salem, NC, USA
e-mail: sfeldman@wakehealth.edu

recalcitrant disease. Traditional topical therapies offer limited treatment to patients with extensive disease. Systemic therapies such as methotrexate, cyclosporine, or retinoids carry a risk for long-term toxicity and may fail to provide satisfactory improvement. Biologic agents are costly and are associated with rare adverse events (AEs) in patients [2].

To meet these growing needs, research has focused on specific inflammatory signaling pathways, causing a surge in drug development for psoriasis. In addition to biological therapies, several small-molecule inhibitors that target phosphodiesterase (PDE), Janus kinase (JAK), and rho-associated kinase 2 (ROCK-2) are in clinical trials. While biologic agents neutralize cytokines or cytokine receptors, small-molecule agents block intracellular targets such as transcriptional factors or enzymes. Due to their low molecular size, these small-molecule agents allow for oral or topical administration. Some of these new treatments are close to Food & Drug Administration (FDA) approval, bringing new hope to patients with psoriasis.

The psoriasis treatment arsenal is expanding, with a variety of topical agents, oral systemic therapies, injectable biologics, and small-molecule inhibitors. The purpose of this chapter is to review the clinical phase, efficacy, and safety of novel psoriasis treatments. We will discuss the evidence for therapeutic agents currently in clinical trials that have the potential to become available in the next few years. A literature search was performed using the National Psoriasis Foundation, PubMed, and Google Scholar to investigate new drugs in development for the treatment of psoriasis. In this chapter, therapies are organized by method of administration (topicals, orals, and injectables) and then phase of clinical trial (Tables 6.1, 6.2, and 6.3). This chapter will also review the specific drug targets and how they contribute to our present understanding of psoriasis pathogenesis.

Topical Psoriasis Medications

P-3073

P-3073, calcipotriol or calcipotriene, is a vitamin D_3 analog administered as a nail lacquer which is being studied in the treatment of nail psoriasis. Like other synthetic vitamin D3 analogs, calcipotriol decreases the proliferative capacity of CD29+ keratinocytes and enhances epidermal cell differentiation in psoriatic skin [3]. Compared to the endogenous bioactive form of vitamin D_3, calcipotriol and other synthetic analogs have a high affinity for the vitamin D_3 receptor, yet low tendency of harmful effects on calcium metabolism [4].

A phase II, randomized, double-blind, vehicle-controlled, parallel-group study assessed the efficacy of calcipotriol 0.005% solution, cyclosporine 5% solution, and vehicle control in 78 patients with fingernail psoriasis of the nail matrix or nail bed (Table 6.1). The primary outcome measure was the percentage improvement of the Nail Psoriasis Severity Index (NAPSI) score from baseline after 24 weeks of daily treatment. Calcipotriol 0.005% solution applied once daily to affected nails reduced signs of nail bed and nail matrix psoriasis and improved NAPSI score by 32% from baseline, compared to vehicle control and cyclosporine 5% solution [5]. These results are promising, especially considering the lack of available treatments for psoriatic disease of the nail bed and nail matrix. Common side effects of calcipotriol ointment include irritation at the application site, as well as other miscellaneous dermatologic reactions [6]. Hypercalcemia and hypercalciuria have also been reported with calcipotriol ointment use, most commonly in individuals who exceed the recommended dosage [7]. The calcipotriol nail solution is expected to have a similar side effect profile. This drug is currently in phase III of clinical trials.

IDP-118

IDP-118 is a combination of halobetasol propionate 0.01% and tazarotene 0.045% in a solution vehicle. Individually, the active ingredients are already approved by the FDA for separate use in the treatment of psoriasis.

A phase III, randomized, double-blind, vehicle-controlled study assessed the efficacy of IDP-118 compared to vehicle control applied daily for 8 weeks in 203 adult subjects with moderate-to-severe plaque psoriasis (Table 6.1). The primary outcome measure was the percent of patients with at least a two-grade improvement from baseline in the investigator's global assessment (IGA). At week 12, 35.8% of subjects achieved a "clear" to "almost clear" rating and at least two-grade improvement in IGA after 8 weeks of treatment compared to vehicle control (7.0%). In a phase III, randomized, double-blind, vehicle-controlled study assessing the efficacy of IDP-118 in 215 adult subjects with moderate-to-severe psoriasis, 45.3% of subjects achieved a "clear" to "almost clear" rating and at least two-grade improvement in IGA after 8 weeks of treatment compared to vehicle control (12.5%). These studies were preceded by a phase II randomized, double-blind, vehicle-controlled study comparing IDP-118 to halobetasol propionate 0.01% and tazarotene 0.045% alone in 212 subjects. Treatment success was achieved in 52.5% of subjects on the combination therapy, showing superior results compared to tazarotene alone (19%) and halobetasol propionate alone (33%) [8]. Use of topical corticosteroids and retinoids is associated with skin atrophy, erythema, and general irritation at the site of application. AEs of the combined medication have not yet been reported but are anticipated to be similar to that of the separate active ingredients. This drug is currently in phase III of clinical trials.

Table 6.1 Topical medications in psoriasis

Drug name	Mechanism of action	Reference/clinical trial identifier	Study design	Number of subjects	Regimen	Outcome measure	Results
P-3073 (calcipotriol, calcipotriene)	Vitamin D_3 analog	Dimitris; 2016	Phase II, R, DB, VC, PG	78	P-3073 0.005% QD Cyclosporine 5% QD Vehicle QD	Total NAPSI score at week 24	P-3073 0.005% QD (−6.78, −32% from baseline) Cyclosporine 5% QD (−2.42) Vehicle QD (−1.11)
IDP 118 (Halobetasol proprionate 0.01% (HP)/ Tazarotene 0.045% (Taz))	Corticosteroid/ retinoid	NCT02462070	Phase III, R, DB, VC	203	IDP-118 QD Vehicle QD for 8 weeks	Percent of patients with at least a two-grade improvement from baseline IGA at week 12	IDP-118 (35.76%) Vehicle (6.98%)
		NCT02462122	Phase III, R, DB, VC	215	IDP-118 QD Vehicle QD for 8 weeks	Percent of patients with at least a two-grade improvement from baseline IGA at week 12	IDP-118 (45.33%) Vehicle (12.51%)
		NCT02045277	Phase II, R, DB, VC	212	IDP-118 QD HP 0.01% QD Taz 0.045% QD Vehicle QD	Percent of patients with at least a two-grade improvement from baseline IGA at week 12	IDP-118 (52.5%) HP 0.01% (33%) Taz 0.045% (19%) Vehicle (10%)
M518101	Vitamin D_3 analog and PDE-4 inhibitor	NCT01989429	Phase III, R, DB, VC, PG	788	M518101 BID Daivonex BID Vehicle BID	Percent reduction in modified PASI at week 8	No results posted
		NCT01873677	Phase III, R, DB, VC, PG	537	M518101 Vehicle	IGA at week 8	No results posted
		NCT01301157	Phase II, R, DB, VC, PG	294	M518101 25ug BID M518101 50ug BID Dovonex BID Vehicle BID	IGA at week 8	No results posted
Crisaborole (AN2728 2%)	NSAID/PDE-4 inhibitor	NCT01300052	Phase II, R, DB, VC, PG	68	Crisaborole BID Vehicle BID	Percentage of subjects achieving clear/almost clear with a 2-grade or greater improvement in PGA score at day 84	Crisaborole (17.4%) Vehicle (13.6%)
CT 327	TrKA inhibitor	Roblin; 2015 NCT01465282	Phase II, R, DB, VC	160	CT 327 0.05% BID CT 327 0.1% BID CT 327 0.5% BID Vehicle BID	Percentage of subjects who had changes in IGA score at week 8	CT 327 0.05–0.5% (2.5–5%) Vehicle 10%

(continued)

Table 6.1 (continued)

Drug name	Mechanism of action	Reference/clinical trial identifier	Study design	Number of subjects	Regimen	Outcome measure	Results
LAS41004 (Bexarotene/ Betamethasone propionate)	Retinoid/ corticosteroid	NCT02180464	Phase II, R, DB, VC, PG	40	LAS41004 QD Comparator QD Control QD	Total symptom score, baseline versus day 28	No results posted
PH10 (Rose Bengal Disodium)	Unknown	NCT01247818	Phase II, R, VC, SB	99	PH-10 0.002% QD PH-10 0.005% QD PH-10 0.01% QD Vehicle QD	Percentage of subjects who showed improvement for all PSI efficacy parameters at day 28	PH-10 all concentrations (23–29%) Vehicle (no results given)
		NCT00941278	Phase II, NR, SG, OL	30	PH-10 0.001% QD	Percentage of subjects who showed improvement for all PSI efficacy parameters at day 28	PH-10 0.001% (79%)
WBI-1001 (Benvitimod)	NSAID/cytokine inhibitor	Bissonnette; 2011	Phase II, R, DB, VC	61	WBI-1001 1% BID Vehicle BID	Percentage change from baseline in PGA at week 12	WBI-1001 1% (62.8%) Vehicle (13%)
Tofacitinib	JAK inhibitor	Ports; 2013	Phase II, R, DB, VC	71	Tofacitinib 2% ointment 1 BID Vehicle 1 BID Tofacitinib 2% ointment 2 BID Vehicle 2 BID	Percentage change from baseline in the Target Plaque Severity Score at week 4	Tofacitinib 2% ointment 1 BID (−54.4%) Vehicle 1 BID (−41.5%) Tofacitinib 2% ointment 2 BID (24.2%) Vehicle 2 BID (17.2%)
		Papp; 2016	Phase II, R, DB, PG, VC	435	Tofacitinib 1% QD Tofacitinib 2% QD Tofacitinib 1% BID Tofacitinib 2% BID Vehicle QD Vehicle BID	Percentage of patients with PGA-C clear or almost clear and ≥2 grade improvement from baseline at week 8	Tofacitinib 1% QD (15%) Tofacitinib 2% QD (18.6%) Tofacitinib 1% BID (10%) Tofacitinib 2% BID (22.5%) Vehicle QD (8.1%) Vehicle BID (11.3%)

Efficacy of topical medications in subjects with plaque psoriasis

R randomized, *DB* double-blinded, *SB* single-blinded, *VC* placebo-controlled, *PG* parallel-group, *DC* dose-comparison, *QD* once-daily, *NAPSI* Nail Psoriasis Severity Index, *IGA* Investigator's Global Assessment, *PGA* Physician's Global Assessment, *PASI* improvement from baseline in the Psoriasis Area and Severity Index score, *PSI* Psoriasis Symptom Inventory, *PGA-C* Calculated Physician's Global Assessment

Table 6.2 Oral medications in psoriasis

Drug name	Mechanism of action	Reference/clinical trials identifier	Study design	Number of subjects	Regimen	Outcome measure	Results
Prurisol (Abacavir acetate)	Nucleoside reverse transcriptase inhibitor analog of guanosine	NCT02101216	Phase I, R, OL	18	Prurisol 50 mg Prurisol 100 mg Prurisol 200 mg Prurisol 350 mg Ziagen (abacavir sulfate) 300 mg	Area under the plasma concentration versus time curve of abacavir derived from Prurisol and Ziagen, 24 h after second and third dose	No results posted
XP23829	Fumaric acid	NCT02173301	Phase II, R, DB, PC, PG	200	XP23829 400 mg QD XP23829 800 mg QD XP23829 400 mg BID Placebo QD	Percent change in PASI score from baseline to week 12	XP23829 400 mg QD (−38.1%) XP23829 800 mg QD (−48.2%) XP23829 400 mg BID (−50.7%) Placebo (−25.0%)
KD-025 (SLx-2119)	ROCK 2 inhibitor	Zanin-Zhorov; 2017 NCT02317627	Phase II, NR, OL, PG	38	KD025 400 mg QD KD025 200 mg BID KD025 400 mg BID	Percent of patients achieving PASI 50 at week 12	KD025 400 mg QD (42%) KD025 200 mg BID (71%) KD025 400 mg BID (29%)
Alitretinoin	Retinoid	Irla; 2016	OL	7	Alitretinoin 30 mg QD	Percent change in PPPASI from baseline at week 24	Alitretinoin 30 mg QD (−75.4%)
		Reich; 2016 NCT01245140	Phase II, R, DB, PC	33	Alitretinoin 30 mg QD Placebo	Percent change in PPPASI from baseline at week 24	Alitretinoin 30 mg (−45.2%) Placebo (−44.6%)
Baricitinib	JAK 1 and 2 inhibitor	Papp; 2016	Phase II, R, DB, PC	271	Baricitinib 2 mg QD Baricitinib 4 mg QD Baricitinib 8 mg QD Baricitinib 10 mg QD Placebo QD	Percent of subjects achieving PASI75 at week 12	Baricitinib 2 mg QD (25%) Baricitinib 4 mg QD (25%) Baricitinib 8 mg QD (43%) Baricitinib 10 mg QD (54%) Placebo QD (17%)

Efficacy of oral medications in subjects with plaque psoriasis

R randomized, *DB* double-blinded, *OL* open-label, *PC* placebo-controlled, *PG* parallel-group, *QD* once-daily, *BID* twice daily, PGA-Physician's Global Assessment, *PASI* improvement from baseline in the Psoriasis Area and Severity Index score, *PASI50-50%* improvement from baseline in the Psoriasis Area and Severity Index score, *PPPASI* Palmo-plantar Pustulosis Psoriasis Area and Severity Index, *PASI75-75%* improvement from baseline in the Psoriasis Area and Severity Index score

Table 6.3 Injectable medications in psoriasis

Drug name	Mechanism of action	Reference/clinical trials identifier	Study design	No. of subjects	Regimen	Outcome measure	Results
Guselkumab	IgG1 monoclonal antibody against IL-23 p19	Sofen; 2014	Phase I, R, DB, PC	24	Guselkumab 10 mg SC Guselkumab 30 mg SC Guselkumab 100 mg SC Guselkumab 30 mg SC Placebo SC	Percent of subjects achieving PASI75 responses at week 12	Guselkumab 10 mg (50%) Guselkumab 30 mg (60%) Guselkumab 100 mg (60%) Guselkumab 30 mg (100%) Placebo (0%)
		Gordon; 2015	Phase II, R, DB, PC, AC	293	Guselkumab 5 mg SC Q12W Guselkumab 15 mg SC Q8W Guselkumab 50 mg SC Q12W Guselkumab 100 mg SC Q8W Guselkumab 200 mg SC Q12W Adalimumab SC Placebo SC	Percentage of subjects with an PGA score of 0 or 1 at week 16	Guselkumab 5 mg (34%) Guselkumab 15 mg (61%) Guselkumab 50 mg (79%) Guselkumab 100 mg (86%) Guselkumab 200 mg (83%) Adalimumab (58%) Placebo (7%)
		Blauvelt; 2017	Phase III, R, DB, PC, AC	837	Guselkumab 100 mg SC Placebo SC Adalimumab 80 mg SC	Percentage of subjects with an IGA score of 0 or 1 and percent of subjects achieving PASI90 at week 16	*IGA* Guselkumab (85.1%) Placebo (6.9%) Adalimumab (65.9%) *PASI90* Guselkumab (73.3%) Placebo (2.9%) Adalimumab (49.7%)
		Reich; 2017	Phase III, R, DB, PC, AC	992	Guselkumab 100 mg SC Placebo SC Adalimumab 80 mg SC	Percentage of subjects with an IGA score of 0 or 1 and percent of subjects achieving PASI90 at week 16	*IGA* Guselkumab (84.1%) Placebo (8.5%) Adalimumab (67.7%) *PASI90* Guselkumab (70.0%) Placebo (2.4%) Adalimumab (46.8%)
Tildrakizumab	Monoclonal antibody against IL-23 p19	Papp; 2015	Phase II, R, DB, PC	355	Tildrakizumab 5 mg SC Q12W Tildrakizumab 25 mg SC Q12W Tildrakizumab 100 mg SC Q12W Tildrakizumab 200 mg SC Q12W Placebo SC Q12W	Percent of subjects achieving PASI75 at week 16	Tildrakizumab 5 mg (33.3%) Tildrakizumab 25 mg (64.4%) Tildrakizumab 100 mg (66.3%) Tildrakizumab 200 mg (74.4%) Placebo (4.4%)

						Safety evaluation and percent of subjects achieving	Adverse Events
Risankizumab (BI 655066)	Monoclonal antibody against IL-23 p19	Krueger; 2015	Phase I, R, DB, PC	39	Risankizumab 0.01 mg/kg IV Risankizumab 0.05 mg/kg IV Risankizumab 0.25 mg/kg IV Risankizumab 1 mg/kg IV Risankizumab 3 mg/kg IV Risankizumab 5 mg/kg IV Risankizumab 0.25 mg/kg SC Risankizumab 1 mg/kg SC Placebo	Safety evaluation and percent of subjects achieving PASI75, PASI90, PASI100 at week 24	Risankizumab (65%) Placebo (88%) PASI75 Risankizumab (71%) Placebo (13%) PASI90 Risankizumab (48%) Placebo (0%) PASI 100 Risankizumab (29%) Placebo (0%)
		Papp; 2017 NCT02054481	Phase II, R, DB, AC	166	Risankizumab 18 mg SC Risankizumab 90 mg SC Risankizumab 180 mg SC Risankizumab 90 + 180 mg SC Ustekinumab SC	Percent of subjects achieving PASI90 at week 12	Risankizumab 18 mg (32.6%) Risankizumab 90 mg (73.2%) Risankizumab 180 mg (81%) Risankizumab 90 + 180 mg (77.1%) Ustekinumab (40%)
Abatacept	Fusion protein against CD80 and CD 86	Mease; 2011	Phase II, R, DB, PC	170	Abatacept 3 mg/kg IV Abatacept 10 mg/kg IV Abatacept 30/10 mg/kg IV (two initial doses of 30 mg/kg, followed by 10 mg/kg) Placebo IV	Percent of subjects achieving ARC20 at day 169	Abatacept 3 mg/kg (33%) Abatacept 10 mg/kg (48%) Abatacept 30/10 mg/kg (42%) Placebo (19%)
Neihulizumab (AbGn-168H)	Monoclonal antibody against CD162	NCT02223039	Phase II, R, DB	271	Neihulizumab Low Dose IV Neihulizumab High Dose IV Placebo IV	Percent of subjects achieving PASI75 at week 12	No study results posted
Clazakizumab	Monoclonal antibody against IL-6	Mease; 2016 NCT01490450	Phase II, R, DB, DC, PC	165	Clazakizumab 25 mg Q4W SC Clazakizumab 100 mg Q4W SC Clazakizumab 200 mg Q4W SC Placebo	Percent of subjects achieving ACR20 at week 16 and percent of subjects achieving PASI75 at week 24	ACR20 Clazakizumab 25 mg (46.3%) Clazakizumab 100 mg (52.4%) Clazakizumab 200 mg (39.0%) Placebo (29.3%) PASI75 Clazakizumab 25 mg (19.5%) Clazakizumab 100 mg (28.6%) Clazakizumab 200 mg (12.2%) Placebo (12.2%)

(continued)

Table 6.3 (continued)

Drug name	Mechanism of action	Reference/clinical trials identifier	Study design	No. of subjects	Regimen	Outcome measure	Results
Tregalizumab (BT-061)	Monoclonal antibody against CD4	Abufarag; 2010	Phase II, R, DB, PC, DC	55	Tregalizumab 0.5 mg IV Tregalizumab 2.5 mg IV Tregalizumab 5 mg IV Tregalizumab 10 mg IV Tregalizumab 20 mg IV Tregalizumab 12.5 mg SC Tregalizumab 25 mg SC Placebo IV Placebo SC	Percent of subjects achieving PASI50 at day 75	Tregalizumab 0.5 mg IV (50%) Tregalizumab 2.5 mg IV (50%) Tregalizumab 5 mg IV (0%) Tregalizumab 10 mg IV (35%) Tregalizumab 20 mg IV (50%) Tregalizumab 12.5 mg SC (35%) Tregalizumab 25 mg SC (60%) Placebo IV (30%) Placebo SC (25%)
Namilumab (MT203)	Monoclonal antibody against GM-CSF	NCT02129777	Phase II, R, DB, PC, PG	122	Namilumab 300 mg SC Day 1, 150 mg SC Days 15, 43 and 71 Namilumab 160 mg SC Day 1, 80 mg SC Days 15, 43 and 71 Namilumab 100 mg SC Day 1, 50 mg SC Days 15, 43 and 71 Namilumab 40 mg SC Day 1, 20 mg SC Days 15, 43 and 71 Placebo SC Day 1, 15, 43 and 71	Percent of subjects achieving PASI75 at week 12	Namilumab 300 mg (0%) Namilumab 160 mg (5.3%) Namilumab 100 mg (0%) Namilumab 40 mg (9.5%) Placebo (8.7%)
IMO-8400	Oligonucleotide-based antagonist of TLR 7, 8, and 9	Balak; 2015	Phase II, R, DB, PC	46	IMO-8400 0.075 mg/kg/week QW SC IMO-8400 0.15 mg/kg/week QW SC IMO-8400 0.3 SC mg/kg/week QW SC IMO-8400 0.6 mg/kg/week QW SC Placebo	Percent of subjects achieving PASI50 at week 12	IMO-8400 0.075 mg/kg/week QW SC (43%) IMO-8400 0.15 mg/kg/week QW SC (43%) IMO-8400 0.3 SC mg/kg/week QW SC (50%) IMO-8400 0.6 mg/kg/week QW SC (22%) Placebo (11%)

Efficacy of injectable medications in subjects with plaque psoriasis

R randomized, *DB* double-blinded, *OL* open-label, *PC* placebo-controlled, *AC* active-controlled, *PG* parallel-group, *DC* dose-comparison, *Q2W* every 2 weeks, *Q4W* every 4 weeks, *QD* once-daily, *QW* once weekly, *QOW* every other week, *BIW* twice weekly, *SC* subcutaneous injection, *IV* intravenous injection, *PGA* Investigator's Global Assessment, *ACR20* American College of Rheumatology 20% improvement criteria, *PASI90-90%* improvement from baseline in the Psoriasis Area and Severity Index score, *PASI75-75%* improvement from baseline in the Psoriasis Area and Severity Index score, *PASI50-50%* improvement from baseline in the Psoriasis Area and Severity Index score

M518101

M518101 is an ointment containing pefcalcitol, a novel vitamin D_3 analog and a phosphodiesterase-4 (PDE-4) inhibitor. It is being evaluated as a topical treatment for plaque psoriasis. There has been no efficacy or safety data published about this drug. This drug has undergone a phase II, randomized, double-blind, vehicle-controlled, and parallel group trial in 294 patients (Table 6.1). Two separate concentrations of M518101 were used, 25 ug and 50 ug. M518101 was compared against calcipotriene and the vehicle control. Patients used the topicals twice a day, and the primary outcome was improvement of IGA at week 8. No results were posted from this trial [9]. Two phase III, randomized, double-blind, vehicle-controlled trials were conducted in 537 patients and 788 patients, comparing M518101 to vehicle and comparing M518101 to vehicle and calcipotriol, respectively, but no results were posted [10, 11]. This drug is currently in phase III of clinical trials.

Crisaborole

Crisaborole (AN2728 2%) is a nonsteroidal, boron-based, small-molecule medication that was recently approved by the FDA for topical use in mild-to-moderate atopic dermatitis. This medication is a PDE-4 inhibitor that reduces the local proliferation of pro-inflammatory cytokines [12]. In a phase II, randomized, double-blind, vehicle-controlled study, crisaborole 2% ointment was compared to vehicle control in 68 patients with mild-to-moderate plaque-type psoriasis (Table 6.1). The primary outcome was the percentage of subjects achieving "clear" to "almost clear" with a two-grade or greater improvement in physician's global assessment (PGA) score at day 84. Crisaborole performed only slightly better than the vehicle control (17.4% versus 13.6%, with a 95% confidence interval—14.3 to 21.8). Adverse event incidence was comparable between the treatment and vehicle control groups [13]. Crisaborole has minimal systemic absorption, making it a safe option with low risk of systemic side effects [14].

CT327

CT327 is a topical tropomyosin receptor kinase A (TrkA) inhibitor for treatment of psoriasis-related pruritus (Fig. 6.1). TrkA contributes to inflammation, keratinocyte proliferation, plaque formation, and pruritus in psoriasis patients. A phase IIb, randomized, double-blind, vehicle-controlled trial assessed the efficacy of CT327 0.05%, CT327 0.1%, CT327 0.5%, and vehicle control in treating psoriasis-associated pruritus in 160 subjects (Table 6.1). The primary outcome was the percentage of patients who had changes in IGA score at week 8. No improvements were seen for any dose of CT327 compared to vehicle. Controlled disease was achieved by 2.5–5% and 10% of patients on CT327 and vehicle, respectively. However, 70.6% of the study population reported statistically significant reductions in pruritus and modified Psoriasis Area and Severity Index (PASI) [15]. A measurement of pruritus severity using a 100 mm Visual Analogue Scale (VAS) in patients with at least moderate pruritus at baseline (VAS $\geq$ 40 mm) was included as a predefined secondary endpoint. At week 8, mean reductions in VAS from baseline were 37.1 mm, 31.5 mm, and 36.4 mm for CT327 0.05%, 0.1%, and 0.5% groups, respectively, versus 16.1 mm for the vehicle group. Compared to vehicle, the mean reductions were statistically significant for the CT327 0.05% and 0.5% treatment groups (−21.8 mm, 95% CI [−37.5, −6.2], $p = 0.0067$ and −19.8 mm, 95% CI [−35.2, −4.4], $p = 0.0124$, respectively; CT327 0.1%: −15.9 mm, 95% CI [−31.9, 0.2], $p = 0.052$). In assessing capsaicin-mediated calcium influx in sensory neurons, a measure of pruritus signaling, CT327 inhibited capsaicin response, indicating that the drug's action is at the nerve growth factor-TrkA-transient receptor potential cation channel subfamily V member 1 (TRPV1) pathway. Overall, the medication appears to be well-tolerated, and no study participants reported reactions at the site of application. CT327 is in phase II of clinical trials [15].

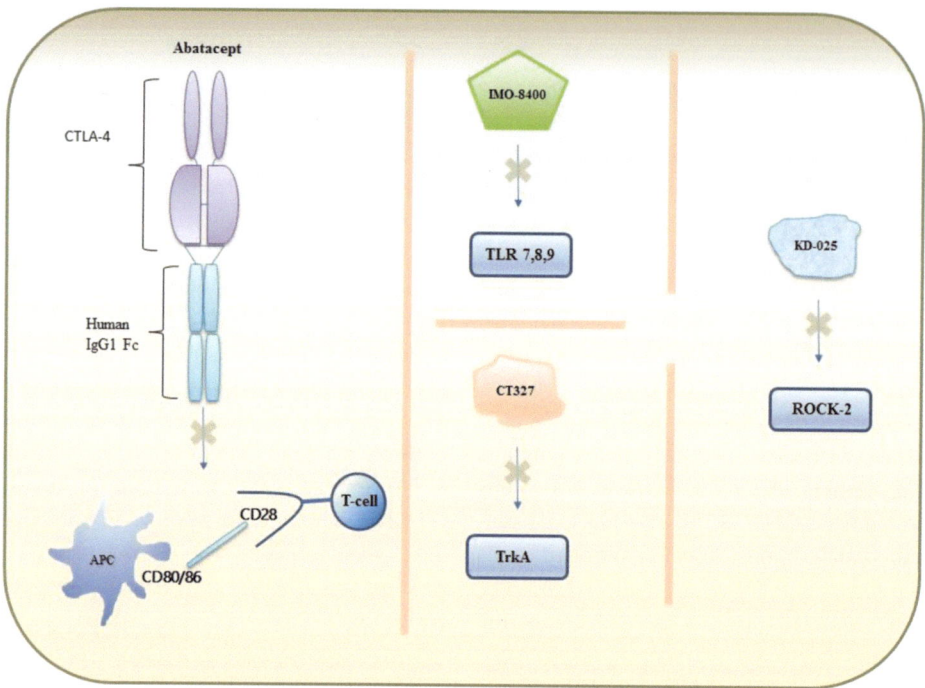

Fig. 6.1 Mechanism of action of selected future thera-peutic agents for psoriasis. Future psoriasis treatment agents target a multitude of differing molecules and recep-tors. Abatacept prevents an important pro-inflammatory cascade response between an antigen-presenting cell and a T cell. IMO-8400 is an antagonist of toll-like receptors (TLR) 7, 8, and 9. CT327 is a tropomyosin receptor kinase A (TrkA) inhibitor. KD-025 is a selective rho-associated kinase (ROCK) 2 inhibitor; it has been noted to reduce IL-17 and IL-21 levels. *APC* antigen-presenting cell, *CD* cluster of differentiation, *CTLA* cytotoxic T-lymphocyte-associated protein

LAS41004

LAS41004 is a topical medication composed of bexarotene and betamethasone dipropionate. This corticosteroid and retinoid combination is being evaluated for treatment of mild-to-moder-ate plaque psoriasis. Betamethasone dipropionate binds to the glucocorticoid receptor within the cell cytoplasm forming a complex which translo-cates into the nucleus, homodimerizes with the glucocorticoid responsive elements on DNA, and regulates the inflammatory response through stimulation or inhibition of gene transcription. Corticosteroids also modulate the activation of target cells, through second messengers and membrane-bound receptors, to reduce the inflam-matory response [16]. Bexarotene, a vitamin A derivative and selective retinoic X receptor (RXR) agonist, binds and activates RXR sub-

types and modulates cell growth, differentiation, and apoptosis [17]. A phase II, randomized, dou-ble-blind, vehicle-controlled, parallel-group trial has been conducted in 40 patients with mild-to-moderate psoriasis; however, no results have been posted (Table 6.1) [18].

PH10

PH10 is an aqueous hydrogel formulation of rose bengal (RB) disodium, a hydrophilic xanthine dye, which is being evaluated in the treatment of psoriasis. The mechanism of action of this medi-cation is unclear; studies to elucidate this infor-mation are currently underway. In a phase IIb non-randomized, single treatment group, open-label study assessing the efficacy of PH10 in 30 psoriasis subjects, 79% of subjects in the treatment group had improved Psoriasis Scoring

Index (PSI), while 83% of subjects in the treatment group had absent or mild pruritus (Table 6.1) [19]. In a more recent phase IIc randomized, single-blind, vehicle-controlled study assessing efficacy of PH10 in psoriasis, all three PH10 treatment arms (0.002% RB, 0.005% RB, and 0.01% RB) showed improved disease superior to the vehicle control arm as measured by the percentage of subjects who showed improvement for all Psoriasis Severity Index (PSI) efficacy parameters at day 28. 23–29% of subjects in the treatment arms had complete or near complete resolution of erythema, induration, and desquamation. No AEs have been reported [20, 21]. This drug is currently in phase II of clinical trials.

WBI-1001

WBI-1001, also known as benvitimod, is a non-steroidal anti-inflammatory drug which inhibits pro-inflammatory cytokines such as TNF-α and interferon (IFN)-γ [22]. A phase II, randomized, double-blind, vehicle-controlled study assessed the efficacy and safety of WBI-1001 1.0% cream compared against vehicle control in 61 patients with mild-to-moderate plaque psoriasis (Table 6.1). 62.8% of patients randomized to the treatment group had improvement in physician's global assessment (PGA) at week 12 compared to 13.0% in the placebo group. At week 12, 67.5% of subjects in the treatment arm achieved a PGA of "clear" or "almost clear" compared to 4.8% in the placebo group; mean body surface area (BSA) decreased by 79.1% in the treatment group but increased by 9.4% in the placebo group [22]. AEs were either mild or moderate, localized to the application site and included hyperpigmentation, dermatitis, folliculitis, papules, pain, and pruritus [22]. Benvitimod cream doses up to 30 mg were well-tolerated. Exposure to the medication did not result in laboratory test abnormalities or electrocardiographic changes. Benvitimod was detected in less than 5% of plasma samples in patients who received the topical drug [23].

Tofacitinib

Tofacitinib is a JAK inhibitor that is being evaluated for topical use in psoriasis, atopic dermatitis, and alopecia areata. The drug functions by competitively inhibiting the adenosine triphosphate (ATP) binding site of JAK proteins, thereby inhibiting activation of downstream signal transducer and activator of transcription (STAT) proteins which normally serve to upregulate pro-inflammatory genes. In a phase IIa, randomized, double-blind, vehicle-controlled study assessing the efficacy and safety of topical tofacitinib in patients with mild-to-moderate psoriasis, 71 patients were randomized to receive tofacitinib 2% ointment 1, vehicle ointment 1, tofacitinib 2% ointment 2, or vehicle ointment 2, each administered twice daily (BID) (Table 6.1). The only difference between vehicle ointment 1 and 2 was the presence of a penetration enhancer in the vehicle ointment 1. At week 4, there was a greater percent change from baseline target plaque severity score in the tofacitinib ointment 1 group (least squares mean = −54.4%) compared to vehicle ointment 1 (least squares mean = −41.5%). AEs were mild to moderate across treatment groups [24].

A randomized, double-blind, vehicle-controlled, parallel-group, phase IIb study assessed the efficacy of tofacitinib 1% and 2% ointment applied once daily (QD) or BID in 435 patients with mild-to-moderate plaque psoriasis. At week 8, calculated PGA of "clear" or "almost clear" was achieved in 18.6% of subjects in the tofacitinib 2% ointment QD group and 22.5% of subjects in the tofacitinib 2% ointment BID group compared to 8.1% and 11.3% in the vehicle control QD and BID groups, respectively [25]. Subjects reported rapid improvement in pruritus, even as early as day 2 of the study, with improvement lasting almost continuously through week 12. AEs were typically mild to moderate and most commonly included pruritus, psoriasis, and pain at the application site [25]. This drug is currently in phase II of clinical trials.

Oral Medications

Prurisol

Prurisol, abacavir acetate, is a nucleoside reverse transcriptase inhibitor analog of guanosine which is commonly used as therapy for human immunodeficiency virus (HIV) [26]. A phase I, randomized, open-label study evaluated the pharmacokinetics, safety, and tolerance of a single oral dose of abacavir acetate administered to healthy volunteers and the bioequivalence to abacavir sulfate (Ziagen) (Table 6.2). Patients received either Prurisol 50 mg, Prurisol 100 mg, Prurisol 200 mg, Prurisol 350 mg, or Ziagen 300 mg. The primary outcome measure was the area under the plasma concentration versus time curve (AUC) of abacavir derived from Prurisol and Ziagen 24 h after second and third dose of study drug or reference drug. No results of the trial have been posted [27]. Prurisol is currently in phase II of clinical trials for the treatment of psoriasis.

XP23829

XP23829 is a fumaric acid ester compound, a prodrug of monomethyl fumarate, with anti-inflammatory effects. A phase II, randomized, double-blind, multicenter, parallel-group, placebo-controlled study assessed the efficacy and safety of three dose levels of XP23829 in 200 subjects with moderate-to-severe chronic plaque psoriasis (Table 6.2). Patients were administered either XP23829 400 mg QD, XP23829 800 mg QD, XP23829 400 mg BID, or placebo QD for 12 weeks. The 12-week treatment period included a 3-week titration period followed by 9 weeks of treatment at the targeted dose. There was a washout phase of up to 4 weeks prior to randomization for subjects who were previously taking systemic agents for the treatment of psoriasis. The primary outcome measure was the percent change in PASI score from baseline at week 12. At week 12, the subjects experienced a 38.1%, 48.2%, 50.7%, and 25.0% decrease in PASI score from baseline in the XP23829 400 mg once daily, XP23829 800 mg once daily, XP23829 400 mg twice daily, and placebo group, respectively. Only the 800 mg once daily and 400 mg twice daily findings were statistically significant ($p < 0.001$). XP23829 was safe and generally well-tolerated. There were no deaths or life-threatening AEs. The majority of AEs were nonserious, with diarrhea being the most common. The AE rates were consistent with other drugs in the fumaric acid ester class, ranging from 22 to 40% in the XP23829 treatment groups compared with 15% for placebo [28]. This drug is currently in phase II clinical trials.

KD-025

KD-025 is a selective ROCK 2 inhibitor (Fig. 6.1). This agent reduced IL-17 and IL-21 secretion in healthy subjects [29]. In a phase II, non-randomized, open-label, dose-finding study assessing the safety, tolerability, and activity of KD-025 in 38 patients with psoriasis, subjects were randomized to receive KD-025 200 mg BID, KD-025 400 mg QD, or KD-025 400 mg BID for the 12-week study period (Table 6.2). The primary outcome measure was the percent of patients achieving PASI50. At week 12, PASI50 was achieved by 71%, 42%, and 29% of subjects in the 200 mg BID, 400 mg QD, and 400 mg BID groups, respectively [30]. This drug is currently in phase II of clinical trials for the treatment of psoriasis.

Alitretinoin

Alitretinoin is a retinoic acid which binds to and activates RARs and RXRs. Once activated, the receptors regulate gene transcription and serve to inhibit cell proliferation and induce cell differentiation [31]. This agent is being evaluated in the treatment of palmoplantar pustular psoriasis (PPP). In an open-label study assessing the efficacy of alitretinoin in the treatment of PPP, seven subjects were treated with oral alitretinoin 30 mg QD for 12 weeks. Mean Palmoplantar Pustular Psoriasis Area Severity Index (PPPASI) score was 17.5 before treatment with alitretinoin and 4.3 after treatment. One-hundred percent of subjects achieved 50% improvement in PPPASI at week 12 [32].

In a phase II, randomized, double-blind, placebo-controlled study assessing the efficacy of alitretinoin in the treatment of psoriasis, 33 subjects were randomized 2:1 to receive alitretinoin 30 mg QD or placebo for up to 24 weeks. Endpoints included PPPASI at week 24, percentage change from baseline-modified PASI (mPASI), 50% or 75% improvement in baseline PPPASI or mPASI, change in pustule count on the palms and soles, and safety, and tolerability assessments. There were no significant differences between alitretinoin 30 mg and placebo for any endpoint (−45.2% versus −44.6%, respectively) [33]. This drug is currently in phase II of clinical trials for the treatment of PPP.

Baricitinib

Baricitinib is an oral JAK 1 and 2 inhibitor. This agent binds to JAK 1 and 2, inhibits its activation, inhibits the JAK/STAT signaling pathway, and decreases production of inflammatory cytokines [34]. In a phase IIb, randomized, double-blind, placebo-controlled, dose-ranging study assessing the safety and efficacy of baricitinib in the treatment of moderate-to-severe psoriasis, 271 subjects were randomized to receive oral baricitinib 2 mg, 4 mg, 8 mg, 10 mg, or placebo QD for 12 weeks. Seventy-five percent improvement in PASI (PASI75) was achieved by week 12 in 43%, 54%, and 17% of subjects in the baricitinib 8 mg, baricitinib 10 mg, and placebo groups, respectively [35]. This drug is currently in phase II of clinical trials for the treatment of psoriasis (Table 6.2).

Injectable Medications

Guselkumab

Guselkumab is a human immunoglobulin G1 monoclonal antibody against the p19 subunit of IL-23, an important cytokine in psoriasis pathogenesis (Fig. 6.2) [36]. In a phase I, randomized, double-blind, placebo-controlled study assessing safety, tolerability, and clinical response of guselkumab in the treatment of moderate-to-severe plaque psoriasis, 24 subjects were randomized to receive subcutaneous injection of placebo, guselkumab 10 mg (G10), guselkumab 30 mg (G30), guselkumab 100 mg (G100), or guselkumab 300 mg (G300) (Table 6.3). By week 12, 100% of subjects in G300 group achieved PASI75, compared to 60% of subjects in the G30 and G100 groups, and 0% in the placebo group. These results were generally maintained through week 24. Skin biopsy of lesional and non-lesional skin noted decreased epidermal thickness, T-cell expression, and dendritic cell expression in treatment groups compared to placebo group. AE incidence was proportionally comparable in the placebo (50%, $n = 2$) and treatment groups (65%, $n = 13$). The most common AEs were infections including upper respiratory tract infections, lower respiratory tract infections, bronchitis, folliculitis, viral gastroenteritis, herpes simplex, vaginal infections, and nasopharyngitis [37].

In a phase II, randomized, dose-ranging, double-blind, placebo-controlled, active-comparator trial comparing guselkumab to adalimumab, a TNF-α inhibitor, 293 subjects were randomized to receive placebo; adalimumab; guselkumab 5 mg at weeks 0 and 4 and every 12 weeks (Q12W); 15 mg every 8 weeks (Q8W); 50 mg at week 0, 4, and Q12W; 100 mg Q8W; or 200 mg at 0,4 and Q12W over a 40-week study period. At week 16, the placebo group crossed over to the guselkumab 100 mg Q8W group. PGA score of 0 or 1 was achieved in 34% of subjects in the guselkumab 5 mg group, 61% of subjects in the guselkumab 15 mg group, 79% of subjects in the guselkumab 50 mg group, 86% of subjects in the guselkumab 100 mg group, 83% of subjects in the guselkumab 200 mg group, 7% of subjects in the placebo group, and 58% of subjects in the adalimumab group [38].

In a two-part, phase III, double-blind, placebo-controlled, active comparator study, efficacy and safety of guselkumab and adalimumab were compared. In part one, subjects were randomized to receive guselkumab 100 mg at weeks 0 and 4 and Q8W and placebo at weeks 0, 4, and 12, then switched to guselkumab at weeks 16 and 20 and then Q8W, or adalimumab 80 mg at week 0 and 40 mg at week 1 and every 2 weeks through week 47. In part two, subjects were randomized to receive guselkumab 100 mg at weeks 0 and 4 and

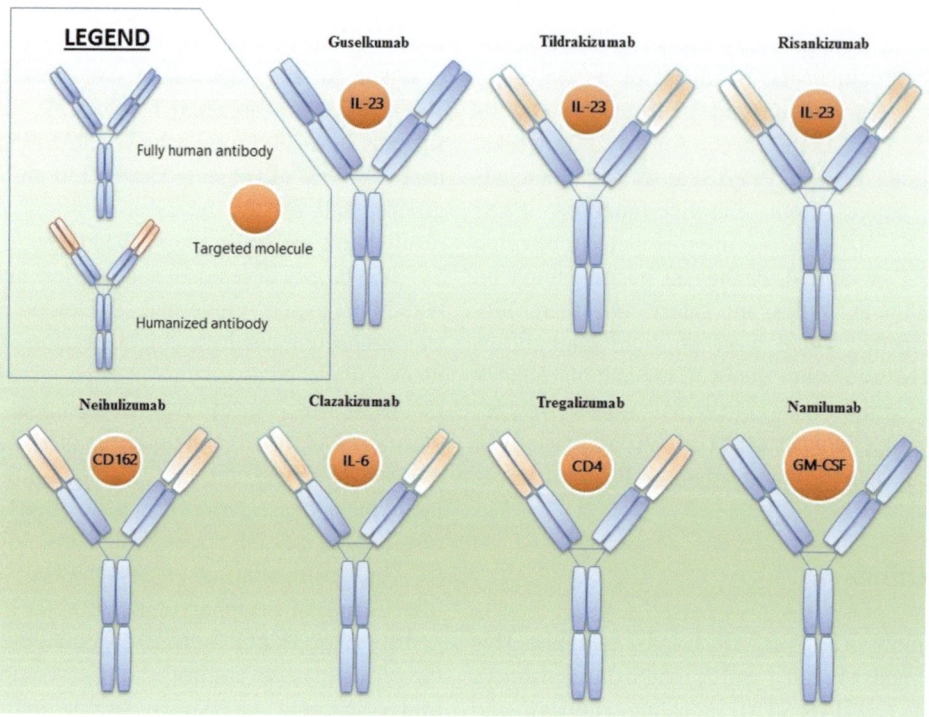

Fig. 6.2 Injectable future therapeutic antibodies for psoriasis. Future biologic antibody agents target differing molecules in the inhibition of the release of pro-inflamma- tory mediators leading to psoriasis. *CD* cluster of differentiation, *GM-CSF* granulocyte-macrophage colony-stimulating factor, *IL-23* interleukin 23

Q8W and placebo at weeks 0, 4, and 12, then switched to guselkumab at weeks 16 and 20, or adalimumab 80 mg at week 0 and 40 mg at week 1 and every 2 weeks through week 23 and then rerandomized at week 28 according to response or nonresponse to guselkumab or adalimumab. In part one, at week 16, IGA 0/1 was achieved by 85.1% of subjects in the guselkumab group compared to 6.9% of subjects in the placebo group and 65.9% of subjects in the adalimumab group, 90% improvement in PASI (PASI90) was achieved in 73.3% of subjects in the guselkumab group compared to 2.9% of subjects in the placebo group and 49.7% of subjects in the adalimumab group. In part two, at week 16, IGA 0/1 was achieved by 84.1% of subjects in the guselkumab group compared to 8.5% in the placebo group and 67.7% in the adalimumab group, PASI90 was achieved in 70.0% of the guselkumab group compared to 2.4% of the placebo group and 46.8% of the adalimumab group [39, 40]. Guselkumab was

approved by the FDA for treatment of moderate-to-severe plaque psoriasis in July 2017.

Tildrakizumab

Tildrakizumab is a high affinity, humanized, monoclonal antibody which inhibits IL-23 by targeting the IL-23p19 subunit (Fig. 6.2). In a three-part phase I randomized, placebo-controlled, sequential, rising multiple dose study, the efficacy of tildrakizumab in the treatment of moderate-to-severe psoriasis was assessed. In study parts one and three, PASI75 was achieved by day 196 in all subjects in the 3 mg/kg and 10 mg/kg groups. In part two, PASI75 was achieved by day 112 in 10 out of 15 subjects in the 3 mg/kg group and 13 out of 14 subjects in the 10 mg/kg group [41].

In a three-part, randomized, double-blind, phase IIb study, evaluating the safety and efficacy of subcutaneous tildrakizumab in the treatment of moderate-to-severe psoriasis, 355 subjects were randomized to receive subcutaneous tildrakizumab 5 mg, 25 mg, 100 mg, and 200 mg or placebo at weeks 0 and 4 and Q12W through week 52 with follow-up at week 72. PASI75 was achieved by week 16 in 33.3% of subjects in the 5 mg group, 64.4% of subjects in the 25 mg group, 66.3% of subjects in the 100 mg group, and 74.4% of subjects in the 200 mg group compared to 4.4% of subjects in the placebo group. The incidence of AEs was comparable in the treatment and placebo groups; the most commonly reported AEs were nasopharyngitis and headache [42]. This drug is currently in phase III of clinical trials for the treatment of psoriasis.

Risankizumab

Risankizumab, BI 655066, is a humanized monoclonal antibody which binds to the p19 subunit of IL-23 preventing IL-23 receptor activation (Fig. 6.2). A phase I, single-rising-dose, randomized, double-blind, placebo-controlled, first-in-human, proof-of-concept study was completed to assess the clinical and biological effects of risankizumab in patients with moderate-to-severe psoriasis. Subjects were randomized to receive risankizumab IV 0.01 mg/kg, 0.05 mg/kg, 0.25 mg/kg, 1 mg/kg, 3 mg/kg, 5 mg/kg, risankizumab SC 0.25 mg/kg, 1 mg/kg, or placebo. PASI75, PASI90, and 100% improvement in baseline PASI (PASI100) was achieved at week 12 by 87%, 58%, and 16% of subjects in the risankizumab groups, respectively. At week 24, the proportion of risankizumab-treated patients achieving PASI75, PASI90, and PASI100 were 71% versus 13% in the placebo group ($p = 0.009$), 48% versus 0% in the placebo group ($p = 0.024$), and 29% versus 0% in the placebo group ($p = 0.190$), respectively. AE incidence was comparable in treatment and placebo groups (65% versus 88%, respectively). The most frequently reported AEs were mild-to-moderate upper respiratory tract infections, mild nasopharyngitis, and mild-to-moderate headache. The severity of the AEs did not appear related to the dose of risanki-

zumab. While four serious AEs occurred in the risankizumab groups, these events were not considered treatment-related [43].

In a phase II, randomized, double-blind, active-controlled study comparing the efficacy of risankizumab and ustekinumab in the treatment of moderate-to-severe psoriasis, 166 subjects were randomized to receive risankizumab 18 mg at week 0; risankizumab 90 mg at week 0, 4, and 16; risankizumab 180 mg at week 0, 4, and 16; or ustekinumab 45 mg or 90 mg, based on body weight, at weeks 0, 4, and 16 (Table 6.3). PASI90 was achieved at week 12 in 77% of subjects in risankizumab 90 mg and 180 mg groups pooled, compared to 40% of subjects in the ustekinumab group. Serious AEs occurred in the 18 mg risankizumab group (12% of subjects), the 90 mg risankizumab group (15% of subjects), and the ustekinumab group (8% of subjects) [44]. This drug is currently in phase III of clinical trials for the treatment of psoriasis.

Abatacept

Abatacept is a soluble fusion protein which inhibits full activation of T cells by binding to CD80 and CD86 on antigen presenting cells preventing their interaction with CD28 on T cells. This fusion protein is composed of the extracellular domain of human cytotoxic T-lymphocyte-associated antigen 4 (CTLA-4) and the modified Fc portion of the human immunoglobulin G1 (Fig. 6.1). In a randomized, double-blind, placebo-controlled, phase II study assessing the safety and efficacy of abatacept in the treatment of psoriatic arthritis, subjects were randomized to receive two doses of abatacept 30 mg/kg, followed by 10 mg/kg, abatacept 10 mg/kg, abatacept 3 mg/kg, or placebo at day 1, 15, and 29 and every 28 days. The primary endpoint was the American College of Rheumatology 20% criteria for improvement (ACR20); IGA and PASI were assessed as secondary endpoints. IGA of "clear" or "almost clear" was achieved by day 169 in 21% of subjects in the 30/10 mg/kg abatacept group, 25% of subjects in the 10 mg/kg abatacept group, 38% of subjects in the 3 mg/kg abatacept group, and 26% of subjects in the placebo group, while PASI50 was achieved at day 169 in 35%, 29%, 43%, and 14% of subjects, respectively [45]. Though these results are promising, it should be noted that abatacept treatment has resulted in psoriasis onset or exacerbation in some cases [46–50]. This drug is currently in phase III of clinical trials for the treatment of psoriatic arthritis (Table 6.3).

Neihulizumab

Neihulizumab, AbGn-168H, is a humanized monoclonal antibody which targets CD162 (also known as P-selectin glycoprotein ligand 1) which is expressed on activated T lymphocytes (Fig. 6.2). Apoptosis of activated T cells is induced, leading to reduction of T-cell-mediated immune responses. This drug is being studied in the treatment of graft versus host disease and psoriasis [51, 52]. A phase II, randomized, double-blind, placebo-controlled, multiple-dose, multi-center study in 271 subjects with moderate-to-severe chronic plaque psoriasis investigated the efficacy, safety, tolerability, and pharmacokinetics of multiple doses of neihulizumab administered intravenously (Table 6.3). No study results have been posted [53].

Clazakizumab

Clazakizumab is a monoclonal antibody with high affinity for IL-6, a cytokine which is increased in patients with psoriasis (Fig. 6.2) [51, 54]. In a phase IIb, randomized, double-blind, placebo-controlled, dose-ranging study assessing the efficacy of clazakizumab in the treatment of psoriatic arthritis, 165 subjects were randomized to receive subcutaneous placebo, clazakizumab 25 mg every 4 weeks (Q4W), clazakizumab 100 mg Q4W, or clazakizumab 200 mg Q4W with or without methotrexate. Primary endpoint was ACR20 at week 16. At week 16, the ACR20 response rate was significantly higher with clazakizumab 100 mg versus placebo (52.4% versus 29.3%; $p = 0.039$). ACR20 response rates at week 16 were 46.3% with clazakizumab 25 mg ($p = 0.101$ versus placebo) and 39.0% with clazakizumab 200 mg ($p = 0.178$ versus placebo). PASI75 at week 24 was evaluated as a secondary endpoint. This endpoint was achieved in 19.5% of subjects in the clazakizumab 25 mg group, 28.6% of subjects in the clazakizumab 100 mg group, 12.2% of subjects in the clazakizumab 200 mg group, and 12.2% of subjects in the placebo group [54]. This drug is currently in phase II of clinical trials for the treatment of psoriasis.

Tregalizumab

Tregalizumab is a humanized agonistic monoclonal antibody which selectively activates naturally occurring regulatory T cells (Tregs) by binding to a unique epitope of CD4 on Tregs with low nanomolar affinity, thereby inducing activation of Ick, a CD4-associated kinase, and phosphorylation of the ZAP70, the T-cell receptor-associated kinase which in turn induces signaling events that activate Treg suppressive functions (Fig. 6.2). Upon activation, Tregs are responsible for downregulating excessive immune responses and inflammation by suppressing cytokine secretion from T cells.

In a phase II, randomized, double-blind, placebo-controlled trial assessing the efficacy of tregalizumab in patients with moderate-to-severe psoriasis, 55 subjects were randomized to receive a single dose of tregalizumab or placebo at doses ranging from 0.5–20 mg intravenous (IV) injection to 12.5–25 mg subcutaneous (SC) injection. The primary outcome was the percent of subjects achieving PASI50 at day 75. PASI50 was achieved in 37% of subjects in the treatment group, compared to 29% of subjects in the placebo group. Two subjects in the treatment group achieved PASI75. Tregalizumab was well-tolerated, with the mean number of AEs comparable between the treatment and placebo groups. The majority of AEs were mild to moderate; six subjects experienced serious AEs. The most commonly reported AEs were headache and erythema [55]. This drug is currently in phase II of clinical trials for the treatment of psoriasis.

Namilumab

Namilumab, MT203, is a human monoclonal antibody against granulocyte macrophage colony-stimulating factor (GM-CSF), with efficacy in the treatment of rheumatoid arthritis (Fig. 6.2) [56]. This agent binds to GM-CSF, a pro-inflammatory cytokine, and prevents it from binding to its associated receptor to initiate signaling processes. GM-CSF-mediated inflammation is thereby inhibited [57].

A recent phase II, randomized, double-blind, placebo-controlled, parallel group study evaluated the efficacy for namilumab in moderate-to-severe plaque psoriasis, as measured by PASI75 response rate at week 12 (Table 6.3). One hundred twenty-two participants with moderate-to-severe chronic plaque psoriasis were randomly assigned to five treatment groups: namilumab 300 mg followed by 150 mg days 15, 43, and 71; namilumab 160 mg followed by 80 mg days 15, 43, and 71; namilumab 100 mg followed by 50 mg days 15, 43, and 71; namilumab 40 mg followed by 20 mg days 15, 43, and 71; and placebo. The primary outcome measure was the percent of subjects achieving PASI75 at week 12. Only namilumab 40 mg followed by 20 mg were superior to placebo (9.5% versus 8.7%) although this was not statistically significant ($p = 0.162$) [58].

IMO-8400

IMO-8400 is an oligonucleotide-based antagonist of toll-like receptors (TLR) 7, 8, and 9 (Fig. 6.1). TLRs are proteins involved in the innate immune system; they recognize typical molecules of pathogens and activate immune cell responses accordingly. TLR 1 and 2 are expressed by keratinocytes in the epidermis; their expression is upregulated in psoriatic lesions. TLR 7 and 8 signaling is involved in psoriasis exacerbations [59, 60].

A phase II, randomized, double-blind, placebo-controlled, proof-of-concept study assessed the safety, tolerability, and clinical activity of IMO-8400 in patients with moderate-to-severe psoriasis (Table 6.3). Forty-six subjects were randomized to receive IMO-8400 0.075 mg/kg/week, IMO-8400 0.15 mg/kg/week, IMO-8400 0.3 mg/kg/week, IMO-8400 0.6 mg/kg/week, or placebo for 12 weeks with follow-up at 18 weeks. Improvements in baseline PASI of 50% to 92% was achieved in 38% of subjects in the IMO-8400 groups compared to 11% of subjects in the placebo group. There were no serious AEs, treatment-related severe AEs, or drug discontinuations due to treatment-related AEs [60]. This drug is currently in phase II of clinical trials for the treatment of psoriasis.

Conclusion

Our understanding of the immunological factors behind psoriasis pathogenesis has led to the development of multiple medications with a variety of action mechanisms. This surge in immunology-related research has enhanced our understanding of psoriasis but also has the potential to build on the knowledge base pertaining to other immune-mediated conditions. Novel medications which modulate the immune system will benefit dermatology patients but may have some utility in the treatment of immune-mediated conditions across medical specialties. In the near future, ongoing psoriasis research will bring greater understanding to the progression of psoriasis and other chronic inflammatory diseases. As newer targets such as small-molecule agents undergo investigation, clinicians will have more tools for manipulating immune processes. However, it is too early to know the efficacy and safety of many of these agents. With so many options to choose from, treatment algorithms will be necessary. Patient and clinician preferences will need to be taken into account. Additionally, as more treatment options become available, the need for head-to-head studies will increase, as well as studies investigating therapies in psoriasis patients with comorbidities. It will remain critical for clinicians to be aware of the limitations of drug safety when selecting these cutting edge treatments.

References

1. Nestle FO, Kaplan DH, Barker J Psoriasis. N Engl J Med [Internet]. 2009 [cited 2017 May 8];361:496–509. http://www.ncbi.nlm.nih.gov/pubmed/19641206

2. Menter A, Gottlieb A, Feldman SR, Van Voorhees AS, Leonardi CL, Gordon KB, et al. Guidelines of care for the management of psoriasis and psoriatic arthritis: Section 1. Overview of psoriasis and guidelines of care for the treatment of psoriasis with biologics. J Am Acad Dermatol [Internet]. 2008 [cited 2017 May 8];58:826–50. http://linkinghub.elsevier.com/retrieve/pii/S0190962208002739

3. Jensen AM, Lladó MB, Skov L, Hansen ER, Larsen JK, Baadsgaard O. Calcipotriol inhibits the proliferation of hyperproliferative CD29 positive keratinocytes in psoriatic epidermis in the absence of an effect on the function and number of antigen-presenting cells. Br J Dermatol [Internet]. 1998 [cited 2017 Apr 27];139:984–91. http://www.ncbi.nlm.nih.gov/pubmed/9990360

4. Kragballe K. Treatment of psoriasis with calcipotriol and other vitamin D analogues. J Am Acad Dermatol [Internet]. 1992 [cited 2017 Apr 27];27:1001–8. http://www.ncbi.nlm.nih.gov/pubmed/1479078

5. Dimitris R, Palmieri R, Caserini M, Iorizzo M. Phase-2 controlled study to assess the efficacy of two new nail solutions in the treatment of nail psoriasis. J Am Acad Dermatol [Internet]. Elsevier; 2016 [cited 2017 Apr 28];74:AB137. http://linkinghub.elsevier.com/retrieve/pii/S0190962216006708

6. Scott LJ, Dunn CJ, Goa KL. Calcipotriol ointment. A review of its use in the management of psoriasis. Am J Clin Dermatol [Internet]. 2001 [cited 2017 Apr 27];2:95–120. http://www.ncbi.nlm.nih.gov/pubmed/11705309

7. Georgiou S, Tsambaos D. Hypercalcaemia and hypercalciuria after topical treatment of psoriasis with excessive amounts of calcipotriol. Acta Derm Venereol [Internet]. 1999 [cited 2017 Apr 25];79:86. http://www.ncbi.nlm.nih.gov/pubmed/10086871

8. Valeant Pharmaceuticals Announces Results of Second Phase 3 Study for Psoriasis Treatment IDP-118 – Valeant [Internet]. [cited 2017 Apr 28]. http://ir.valeant.com/news-releases/2017/01-10-2017-110212002

9. Study to Investigate the Efficacy and the Safety of M518101 in Plaque Psoriasis Patients—Full Text View—ClinicalTrials.gov-NCT01301157 [Internet]. [cited 2017 May 8]. https://clinicaltrials.gov/ct2/show/NCT01301157

10. Study to Evaluate the Efficacy and Safety of M518101 in Subjects With Plaque Psoriasis—Full Text View—ClinicalTrials.gov-NCT01873677 [Internet]. [cited 2017 May 8]. https://clinicaltrials.gov/ct2/show/NCT01873677

11. Efficacy Study Comparing Topical M518101 and Vitamin D3 in Adult Psoriasis Patients—Full Text View—ClinicalTrials.gov-NCT01989429 [Internet]. [cited 2017 May 8]. https://clinicaltrials.gov/ct2/show/NCT01989429

12. Boguniewicz M, Paller AS, Tom WL, Lebwohl MG, Blumenthal RL, Call RS, et al. Efficacy and safety of crisaborole topical ointment, 2%, a novel, nonsteroidal, topical, anti-inflammatory, phosphodiesterase inhibitor in 2 Phase 3 studies in children and adults with mild-to-moderate atopic dermatitis. J Allergy Clin Immunol [Internet]. 2016 [cited 2017 Apr 28];137:AB397. http://linkinghub.elsevier.com/retrieve/pii/S0091674915030444

13. AN2728 Topical Ointment to Treat Mild-to-Moderate Plaque-Type Psoriasis—Study Results—ClinicalTrials.gov-NCT01300052 [Internet]. [cited 2017 May 10]. https://clinicaltrials.gov/ct2/show/results/NCT01300052?sect=X40156#othr

14. Paller AS, Tom WL, Lebwohl MG, Blumenthal RL, Boguniewicz M, Call RS, et al. Efficacy and safety of crisaborole ointment, a novel, nonsteroidal phosphodiesterase 4 (PDE4) inhibitor for the topical treatment of atopic dermatitis (AD) in children and adults. J Am Acad Dermatol [Internet]. 2016 [cited 2017 Apr 28];75:494–503.e6. http://www.ncbi.nlm.nih.gov/pubmed/27417017

15. Roblin D, Yosipovitch G, Boyce B, Robinson J, Sandy J, Mainero V, et al. Topical TrkA Kinase Inhibitor CT327 is an effective, novel therapy for the treatment of pruritus due to psoriasis: results from experimental studies, and efficacy and safety of CT327 in a Phase 2b clinical trial in patients with psoriasis. Acta Derm Venereol [Internet]. 2015 [cited 2017 Apr 27];95:542–8. http://www.ncbi.nlm.nih.gov/pubmed/25594427

16. Uva L, Miguel D, Pinheiro C, Antunes J, Cruz D, Ferreira J, et al. Mechanisms of action of topical corticosteroids in psoriasis. Int J Endocrinol [Internet]. 2012 [cited 2017 Apr 28];2012:1–16. http://www.ncbi.nlm.nih.gov/pubmed/23213332

17. Lowe MN, Plosker GL. Bexarotene. Am J Clin Dermatol [Internet]. Springer International Publishing; 2000 [cited 2017 Apr 26];1:245–50. http://link.springer.com/10.2165/00128071-200001040-00006

18. A Intra-individual Comparison to Investigate the Efficacy and the Safety of LAS41004 Formulation in Mild to Moderate Psoriasis—Full Text View—ClinicalTrials.gov-NCT02180464 [Internet]. [cited 2017 May 8]. https://clinicaltrials.gov/ct2/show/NCT02180464

19. An Efficacy and Safety Study of PH-10 Aqueous Hydrogel for the Treatment of Plaque Psoriasis—Full Text View—ClinicalTrials.gov-NCT00941278 [Internet]. [cited 2017 May 8]. https://clinicaltrials.gov/ct2/show/NCT00941278

20. PH-10 For Psoriasis [Internet]. [cited 2017 Apr 28]. http://www.provectusbio.com/ph-10-for-psoriasis

21. Randomized Study of PH-10 for Psoriasis—Full Text View—ClinicalTrials.gov-NCT01247818 [Internet]. [cited 2017 May 8]. https://clinicaltrials.gov/ct2/show/NCT01247818

22. Bissonnette R, Bolduc C, Maari C, Nigen S, Webster JM, Tang L, et al. Efficacy and safety of topical WBI-1001 in patients with mild to moderate psoriasis: results from a randomized double-blind placebo-controlled, phase II trial. J Eur Acad

Dermatol Venereol [Internet]. Blackwell Publishing Ltd; 2011 [cited 2017 Apr 26];26. http://doi.wiley.com/10.1111/j.1468-3083.2011.04332.x

23. Zhao L, Chen X, Cai L, Zhang C, Wang Q, Jing S, et al. Randomized, double-blind, placebo-controlled, multiple-dose study of the safety, tolerability and pharmacokinetics of benvitimod, a candidate drug for the treatment of psoriasis. J Clin Pharm Ther [Internet]. 2014 [cited 2017 Apr 26];39:418–23. http://www.ncbi.nlm.nih.gov/pubmed/24673513

24. Ports WC, Khan S, Lan S, Lamba M, Bolduc C, Bissonnette R, et al. A randomized phase 2a efficacy and safety trial of the topical Janus kinase inhibitor tofacitinib in the treatment of chronic plaque psoriasis. Br J Dermatol [Internet]. 2013 [cited 2017 Apr 27];169:137–45. http://doi.wiley.com/10.1111/bjd.12266

25. Papp KA, Bissonnette R, Gooderham M, Feldman SR, Iversen L, Soung J, et al. Treatment of plaque psoriasis with an ointment formulation of the Janus kinase inhibitor, tofacitinib: a Phase 2b randomized clinical trial. BMC Dermatol [Internet]. 2016 [cited 2017 Apr 27];16:15. http://www.ncbi.nlm.nih.gov/pubmed/27716172

26. NCI Thesaurus-Abacavir [Internet]. [cited 2017 Apr 29]. https://ncit.nci.nih.gov/ncit-browser/ConceptReport.jsp?dictionary=NCI_Thesaurus&version=17.03d&ns=NCI_Thesaurus&code=C61523&key=n785246928&b=1&n=null

27. Bioequivalence and Pharmacokinetic Study of Prurisol™ and Abacavir Sulfate in Healthy Volunteers—Full Text View—ClinicalTrials.gov-NCT02101216 [Internet]. [cited 2017 May 8]. https://clinicaltrials.gov/ct2/show/NCT02101216

28. XenoPort Announces Positive Phase 2 Study Results for XP23829 as a Potential Treatment for Patients with Psoriasis|Business Wire [Internet]. [cited 2017 May 8]. http://www.businesswire.com/news/home/20150915005703/en/XenoPort-Announces-Positive-Phase-2-Study-Results

29. Zanin-Zhorov A, Weiss JM, Nyuydzefe MS, Chen W, Scher JU, Mo R, et al. Selective oral ROCK2 inhibitor down-regulates IL-21 and IL-17 secretion in human T cells via STAT3-dependent mechanism. Proc Natl Acad Sci [Internet]. 2014 [cited 2017 Apr 29];111:16814–9. http://www.ncbi.nlm.nih.gov/pubmed/25385601

30. Zanin-Zhorov A, Weiss JM, Trzeciak A, Chen W, Zhang J, Nyuydzefe MS, et al. Cutting edge: selective oral ROCK2 inhibitor reduces clinical scores in patients with psoriasis vulgaris and normalizes skin pathology via concurrent regulation of IL-17 and IL-10. J Immunol [Internet]. 2017 [cited 2017 Apr 29]. http://www.jimmunol.org/content/early/2017/04/06/jimmunol.1602142

31. NCI Thesaurus-Alitretinoin [Internet]. [cited 2017 Apr 29]. https://ncit.nci.nih.gov/ncitbrowser/pages/concept_details.jsf

32. Irla N, Navarini AA, Yawalkar N. Alitretinoin abrogates innate inflammation in palmoplantar pustular psoriasis. Br J Dermatol [Internet].

Blackwell Publishing Ltd; 2012 [cited 2017 Apr 29];167:1170–4. http://doi.wiley.com/10.1111/j.1365-2133.2012.11063.x

33. Reich K, Graff O, Mehta N. Oral alitretinoin treatment in patients with palmoplantar pustulosis inadequately responding to standard topical treatment: a randomized phase II study. Br J Dermatol [Internet]. 2016 [cited 2017 Apr 29];174:1277–81. http://www.ncbi.nlm.nih.gov/pubmed/26800106

34. NCI Thesaurus-Baricitinib [Internet]. [cited 2017 Apr 29]. https://ncit.nci.nih.gov/ncitbrowser/pages/concept_details.jsf

35. Papp KA, Menter MA, Raman M, Disch D, Schlichting DE, Gaich C, et al. A randomized phase 2b trial of baricitinib, an oral Janus kinase (JAK) 1/JAK2 inhibitor, in patients with moderate-to-severe psoriasis. Br J Dermatol [Internet]. 2016 [cited 2017 Apr 29];174:1266–76. http://www.ncbi.nlm.nih.gov/pubmed/26800231

36. Nawas Z, Hatch M, Ramos E, Liu M, Tong Y, Peranteau A, et al. A review of guselkumab, an IL-23 inhibitor, for moderate-to-severe plaque psoriasis. Skin Ther Lett [Internet]. 2017 [cited 2017 Apr 28];22:8–10. http://www.ncbi.nlm.nih.gov/pubmed/28329405

37. Sofen H, Smith S, Matheson RT, Leonardi CL, Calderon C, Brodmerkel C, et al. Guselkumab (an IL-23-specific mAb) demonstrates clinical and molecular response in patients with moderate-to-severe psoriasis. J Allergy Clin Immunol [Internet]. 2014 [cited 2017 Apr 28];133:1032–40. http://www.ncbi.nlm.nih.gov/pubmed/24679469.

38. Gordon KB, Duffin KC, Bissonnette R, Prinz JC, Wasfi Y, Li S, et al. A Phase 2 trial of guselkumab versus adalimumab for plaque psoriasis. N Engl J Med [Internet]. Massachusetts Medical Society; 2015 [cited 2017 Apr 28];373:136–44. http://www.nejm.org/doi/abs/10.1056/NEJMoa1501646

39. Blauvelt A, Papp KA, Griffiths CEM, Randazzo B, Wasfi Y, Shen Y-K, et al. Efficacy and safety of guselkumab, an anti-interleukin-23 monoclonal antibody, compared with adalimumab for the continuous treatment of patients with moderate to severe psoriasis: results from the phase III, double-blinded, placebo- and active comparator-controlled VOYAGE 1 trial. J Am Acad Dermatol [Internet]. 2017 [cited 2017 Apr 28];76:405–17. http://www.ncbi.nlm.nih.gov/pubmed/28057360

40. Reich K, Armstrong AW, Foley P, Song M, Wasfi Y, Randazzo B, et al. Efficacy and safety of guselkumab, an anti-interleukin-23 monoclonal antibody, compared with adalimumab for the treatment of patients with moderate to severe psoriasis with randomized withdrawal and retreatment: results from the phase III, double-blind, placebo- and active comparator-controlled VOYAGE 2 trial. J Am Acad Dermatol [Internet]. 2017 [cited 2017 Apr 28];76:418–31. http://linkinghub.elsevier.com/retrieve/pii/S0190962216311586

41. Kopp T, Riedl E, Bangert C, Bowman EP, Greisenegger E, Horowitz A, et al. Clinical improvement in psoriasis with specific targeting of interleukin-23. Nature

[Internet]. 2015 [cited 2017 Apr 28];521:222–6. http://www.ncbi.nlm.nih.gov/pubmed/25754330

42. Papp K, Thaçi D, Reich K, Riedl E, Langley RG, Krueger JG, et al. Tildrakizumab (MK-3222), an anti-interleukin-23p19 monoclonal antibody, improves psoriasis in a phase IIb randomized placebo-controlled trial. Br J Dermatol [Internet]. 2015 [cited 2017 Apr 28];173:930–9. http://doi.wiley.com/10.1111/bjd.13932

43. Krueger JG, Ferris LK, Menter A, Wagner F, White A, Visvanathan S, et al. Anti-IL-23A mAb BI 655066 for treatment of moderate-to-severe psoriasis: safety, efficacy, pharmacokinetics, and biomarker results of a single-rising-dose, randomized, double-blind, placebo-controlled trial. J Allergy Clin Immunol [Internet]. 2015 [cited 2017 Apr 29];136:116–124.e7. http://www.ncbi.nlm.nih.gov/pubmed/25769911

44. Papp KA, Blauvelt A, Bukhalo M, Gooderham M, Krueger JG, Lacour J-P, et al. Risankizumab versus Ustekinumab for Moderate-to-Severe Plaque Psoriasis. N. Engl. J. Med. [Internet]. Massachusetts Medical Society; 2017 [cited 2017 Apr 29];376:1551–60. http://www.nejm.org/doi/10.1056/NEJMoa1607017

45. Mease P, Genovese MC, Gladstein G, Kivitz AJ, Ritchlin C, Tak PP, et al. Abatacept in the treatment of patients with psoriatic arthritis: results of a six-month, multicenter, randomized, double-blind, placebo-controlled, phase II trial. Arthritis Rheum. [Internet]. Wiley Subscription Services, Inc., A Wiley Company; 2011 [cited 2017 Apr 29];63:939–48. http://doi.wiley.com/10.1002/art.30176

46. Silverman D, Oliver A. Abatacept-induced psoriasis. Cutis [Internet]. 2011 [cited 2017 Apr 29];88:117–8. http://www.ncbi.nlm.nih.gov/pubmed/22017062

47. Brigant F, Clavel G, Chatelain D, Lok C, Chaby G. Letter: a case of generalized guttate psoriasis induced by etanercept with relapse after abatacept. Dermatol Online J [Internet]. 2011 [cited 2017 Apr 29];17:11. http://www.ncbi.nlm.nih.gov/pubmed/21696691

48. Florent A, Albert C, Giacchero D, Roux C, Euller-Ziegler L. Reactivation of cutaneous psoriasis during abatacept therapy for spondyloarthropathy. Joint Bone Spine [Internet]. 2010 [cited 2017 Apr 29];77:626–7. http://linkinghub.elsevier.com/retrieve/pii/S1297319X10002460

49. Jost C, Hermann J, Caelen LE-S, Graninger W. New onset psoriasis in a patient receiving abatacept for rheumatoid arthritis. BMJ Case Rep [Internet]. 2009 [cited 2017 Apr 29];2009:bcr0920080845.http://casereports.bmj.com/cgi/doi/10.1136/bcr.09.2008.0845

50. Sibilia J, Westhovens R. Safety of T-cell co-stimulation modulation with abatacept in patients with rheumatoid arthritis. Clin Exp Rheumatol [Internet]. [cited 2017 Apr 29];25:S46–56. http://www.ncbi.nlm.nih.gov/pubmed/17977488

51. Lubrano E, Perrotta FM. Beyond TNF inhibitors: new pathways and emerging treatments for psoriatic arthritis. Drugs [Internet]. Springer International Publishing; 2016 [cited 2017 Apr 28];76:663–73. http://link.springer.com/10.1007/s40265-016-0557-4

52. NCI Thesaurus-Neihulizumab [Internet]. [cited 2017 Apr 29]. https://ncit.nci.nih.gov/ncit-browser/ConceptReport.jsp?dictionary=NCI_Thesaurus&code=C121711&ns=NCI_Thesaurus

53. A Study of Multiple Doses of AbGn-168H by Intravenous Infusion in Patients With Moderate to Severe Chronic Plaque Psoriasis—Full Text View—ClinicalTrials.gov-NCT02223039 [Internet]. [cited 2017 May 8]. https://clinicaltrials.gov/ct2/show/NCT02223039

54. Mease PJ, Gottlieb AB, Berman A, Drescher E, Xing J, Wong R, et al. The efficacy and safety of clazakizumab, an anti-interleukin-6 monoclonal antibody, in a Phase IIb study of adults with active psoriatic arthritis. Arthritis Rheumatol [Internet]. 2016 [cited 2017 Apr 28];68:2163–73. http://doi.wiley.com/10.1002/art.39700

55. Abufarag A, Aigner S, Czeloth N, Dalken B, Koch H, Niemann G, Uherek C, Osterroth F, Wartenberg-Demand A, Haefeli W, Schopf R, Enk A. Selective activation of naturally occurring regulatory T cells (Tregs) by the monoclonal antibody BT-061 as a novel therapeutic opportunity in psoriasis: early clinical results after single doses [Internet]. [cited 2017 Apr 29]. http://www.biotest.de/shared/data/pdf/bio-therapeutics/esdr_2010.pdf

56. Huizinga TWJ, Batalov A, Stoilov R, Lloyd E, Wagner T, Saurigny D, et al. Phase 1b randomized, double-blind study of namilumab, an anti-granulocyte macrophage colony-stimulating factor monoclonal antibody, in mild-to-moderate rheumatoid arthritis. Arthritis Res Ther [Internet]. 2017 [cited 2017 Apr 29];19:53. http://arthritis-research.biomedcentral.com/articles/10.1186/s13075-017-1267-3

57. NCI Thesaurus-Namilumab [Internet]. [cited 2017 Apr 29]. https://ncit.nci.nih.gov/ncitbrowser/pages/concept_details.jsf

58. Efficacy and Safety of Namilumab (MT203) for Plaque Psoriasis—Study Results—ClinicalTrials.gov-NCT02129777 [Internet]. [cited 2017 May 8]. https://clinicaltrials.gov/ct2/show/results/NCT02129777?sect=X01256#all

59. Hari A, Flach TL, Shi Y, Mydlarski PR. Toll-like receptors: role in dermatological disease. Mediators Inflamm [Internet]. Hindawi Publishing Corporation; 2010 [cited 2017 Apr 29];2010:437246. http://www.ncbi.nlm.nih.gov/pubmed/20847936

60. Balak DMW, Van Doorn A, Rissmann R, Sullivan T, Burggraaf J, Arbeit RD. Results from a randomized, double-blind, placebo-controlled, monotherapy trial of IMO-8400 demonstrate clinical proof- of-concept for Toll-like receptor 7, 8 and 9 antagonism in psoriasis. [cited 2017 Apr 29]; http://www.iderapharma.com/wp-content/uploads/2015/11/imo-8400_psoriasis_aad_poster-final.pdf

Combination Therapy

Mio Nakamura, Caleb Jeon, and John Koo

Introduction

Psoriasis is a chronic inflammatory skin disease with a remitting and relapsing course. Long-term remission can be difficult to achieve regardless of severity of psoriasis. Using two or more therapies with varying mechanisms of action and safety profiles is often necessary to maintain adequate disease control while minimizing toxicity of treatments. Some psoriasis therapies can be safely and effectively used concomitantly. Two or more therapies can also be used as part of rotational therapy or sequential therapy. *Rotational therapy* was first described by Weinstein and White in 1993 and proposes rotating available psoriasis treatments every 2 to 3 years, which minimize cumulative toxicity by long periods off each treatment [1]. *Sequential therapy*, first described by Koo, recognizes that some psoriasis therapies are better suited for rapid clearance, while others are more appropriate for long-term maintenance. By using

these therapies in a deliberate sequence, therapeutic outcome can be optimized [2].

Choosing a combination regimen that maximizes safety and efficacy, while at the same time considers patient usability and compliance, can be difficult. This chapter will review various combination therapy strategies for the treatment of psoriasis.

Rationale for Combination Therapy

Because psoriasis is a chronic disease with episodic flares, both acutely acting treatment options and long-term maintenance agents are needed for adequate disease control [3]. Unfortunately, some of the most effective, rapid-acting psoriasis therapies, such as class I superpotent topical steroids, cyclosporine, and infliximab, are also among the most toxic. On the other hand, treatment options with low safety profiles, such as topical vitamin D, acitretin, and apremilast, tend to be less powerful in terms of efficacy and onset of action [4]. In combination therapy, one agent can be used to treat psoriasis acutely, and the safer of the two agents can be used as maintenance treatment [5]. The use of two or more agents with varying mechanisms of action may also increase the overall efficacy of psoriasis therapy in an additive or synergist manner, which may be required for patients with severe, recalcitrant disease. Another benefit to combination therapy is that it can allow for use of lower doses

M. Nakamura (✉) · J. Koo
Department of Dermatology, Psoriasis and Skin Treatment Center, University of California San Francisco, San Francisco, CA, USA
e-mail: mionak@med.umich.edu; john.koo2@ucsf.edu

C. Jeon
Department of Dermatology, UCSF Psoriasis Center, University of California San Francisco, San Francisco, CA, USA
e-mail: caljeon@hawaii.edu

© Springer International Publishing AG, part of Springer Nature 2018
T. Bhutani et al. (eds.), *Evidence-Based Psoriasis*, Updates in Clinical Dermatology,
https://doi.org/10.1007/978-3-319-90107-7_7

of each agent to minimize toxicity [5]. When utilizing combination therapy, caution should be taken to avoid overlapping side effect profiles, such as immunosuppression that can increase risk of malignancy or infection.

Presently, numerous treatment options are available for the treatment of psoriasis including topical agents, phototherapy, oral systemic agents, and biologics, with many more therapeutic agents in the pipeline. With the increasing number of available therapies, there are many opportunities to combine various therapies. It is crucial for clinicians to carefully consider the fine balance between safety and efficacy when combining various therapeutic agents and utilize strategies such as rotational therapy and sequential therapy when appropriate.

Rotational Therapy

When the concept of rotational therapy was first introduced in 1993, psoriasis therapies were limited to topical therapies, phototherapy, methotrexate, and etretinate. Because of cumulative toxicities such as skin cancer with psoralen-ultraviolet A (PUVA), hepatic fibrosis with methotrexate, and hepatotoxicity with etretinate, it was suggested to use each of these monotherapies for 2–3 years before switching to another form of treatment. It may take 4–6 years before returning to the initial treatment. The purpose was to decrease the cumulative, long-term toxicity of each of these therapies [1]. It is thought that the patient can reverse or partially recover from some of side effects during the time off of a given medication [5].

Sequential Therapy

Sequential therapy was first described in 1999 and involves the use of specific therapeutic agents in a deliberate sequence. The sequence is designed to maximize the rate of initial improvement, minimize long-term toxicity, and improve the overall outcome [2]. In the armamentarium of psoriasis therapies, some agents are effective at producing rapid clearing of psoriasis, while oth-

Table 7.1 Sequential therapy for treatment of psoriasis consists of three phases

Phase 1	Clearing	Initiation of a very efficacious, rapidly acting agent, which may have more long-term risks
Phase 2	Transition	Introduction of the maintenance agent and tapering of the rapidly acting agent
Phase 3	Maintenance	Stabilization with maintenance agent with less efficacy but better long-term safety profile

ers are better suited for maintenance therapy. Therefore, sequential therapy consists of three distinct phases (Table 7.1):

Phase 1: The clearing phase involving the use of a very efficacious, rapidly acting agent, which may have more long-term risks.
Phase 2: The transitional phase involving introduction of the maintenance agent and tapering of the rapidly acting agent.
Phase 3: The maintenance phase involving the maintenance agent with less efficacy but better long-term safety profile.

The transitional phase is likely to be the most challenging, as tapering off of the rapidly acting agent requires prevention of breakthrough flares. A careful, individualized tapering regimen is required while waiting for the maintenance agent to fully take effect. Depending on the maintenance agent, this can easily take 2–3 months, such as with acitretin or apremilast. Sequential therapy can be applied to systemic agents [2], as well as topical agents [6].

The concept of sequential therapy involves a strategy of pairing two specific treatment modalities in order to transition from one agent to another. The purpose of sequential therapy is to get the patient on a safe, long-term maintenance regimen after achieving clearance or near clearance using a rapid-acting and effective but more toxic agent. This differs from rotational therapy and combination therapy, which does not involve such specific design.

Combination Therapy with Topical Agents.

Although topical corticosteroid therapy is a mainstay treatment for psoriasis, long-term monotherapy with a topical corticosteroid may not be feasible due to local adverse effects such as skin atrophy, striae formation, and tachyphylaxis [7]. On the other hand, steroid-sparing agents, such as calcipotriene and tazarotene, can be used long-term without such ill effects. Although nonsteroid agents have low cumulative toxicity potential, their efficacy and onset of action may not be as optimal compared to superpotent topical steroids. By utilizing combination techniques, safety and efficacy of topical steroid and nonsteroid agents, respectively, can be used to the clinician's advantage.

Topical Corticosteroids and Topical Vitamin D Analogues

Studies of superpotent topical corticosteroids in combination with topical calcipotriene have found greater improvement of psoriasis and fewer local side effects compared to when each agent is used alone [8]. In a multicenter trial of subjects with chronic plaque psoriasis, subjects were treated with calcipotriene ointment twice daily, halobetasol ointment twice daily, or combination of calcipotriene once daily and halobetasol once daily for 2 weeks [9]. It was found that the combination of calcipotriene and halobetasol is more effective than either agent alone. Furthermore, the number of cutaneous adverse effects observed during the 2 weeks was the lowest in the combination therapy group compared to the monotherapy groups. Interestingly, skin irritation commonly observed with calcipotriene was mitigated by use of halobetasol. The combination of halobetasol and calcipotriene was also shown to be safe and effective for long-term maintenance by using calcipotriene twice daily on weekdays and halobetasol twice daily on weekends [10].

Similarly, sequential therapy using clobetasol ointment or spray twice daily for 2 or 4 weeks, respectively, in the clearing phase, followed by calcipotriene, calcipotriol, or calcitriol twice daily on weekdays and clobetasol twice daily on weekends in the maintenance phase, has been shown to be effective [11–15]. In another study by Koo et al., both clobetasol foam and calcipotriene ointment were applied twice daily for 2 weeks, followed by calcipotriene twice daily on weekdays and clobetasol twice daily on weekends [16]. This combination therapy was more effective than either monotherapy alone. Furthermore, the results of this study support that there is no degradation of either agent when calcipotriene is applied immediately after clobetasol foam [6]. Rotational therapy using augmented betamethasone and calcipotriene alternating weekly is also shown to be more effective than topical corticosteroid alone [17].

Topical Corticosteroids and Tazarotene

The efficacy of combination therapy of superpotent topical corticosteroids and the topical vitamin A derivative tazarotene has been well studied [18–22]. In a double-blind, randomized, parallel-group study by Lebwohl et al., patients were treated with an initial open-label treatment phase consisting of tazarotene 0.1% gel plus clobetasol propionate 0.05% ointment for 6 weeks. The frequency of application of both medications was slowly weaned off over these 6 weeks. In the subsequent double-blind maintenance phase, patients were randomized to receive one of three maintenance regimens for 20 weeks: tazarotene/clobetasol, tazarotene/vehicle, and vehicle. The combination of tazarotene and clobetasol during the initial treatment phase showed marked global improvement of psoriasis, and the maintenance regimen of tazarotene/clobetasol was superior to tazarotene/vehicle and vehicle [18].

The combination of topical corticosteroid and tazarotene is also shown to be superior compared to calcipotriene monotherapy [19, 20]. In a multicenter, investigator-blinded, parallel-group study, 120 adult patients with chronic, stable plaque psoriasis were randomly treated for up to 8 weeks with either mometasone 0.1% cream in the morning plus tazarotene 0.1% gel in the evening or calcipotriene 0.005% ointment twice daily [19]. After 2 weeks of treatment, 45% of patients in the combined tazarotene/mometasone group achieved at least 75% global improvement of psoriasis compared with only 26% of patients in the calcipotriene group. The significantly greater reduction in trunk scaling, erythema, plaque elevation, and body surface area involvement in the combination group was maintained to the 4-week posttreatment observational period.

The addition of a topical corticosteroid to tazarotene appears to reduce erythema of psoriasis and enhance the speed of efficacy while also reducing tazarotene's local side effects of irritation [23]. Furthermore, the use of tazarotene with a topical corticosteroid can be beneficial to reduce overall exposure to the steroids and, therefore, steroid-induced epidermal atrophy in normal skin [24].

Topical Vitamin D Analogues and Tazarotene

Calcipotriene and tazarotene appear to be compatible and may have synergistic effects as combination therapy [25, 26]. A prospective, open-label, right-left comparison study evaluated the efficacy of combination treatment with calcipotriene ointment and tazarotene gel compared to clobetasol ointment for 2 weeks, followed by a 4-week observation phase. The nonsteroid combination of twice-daily calcipotriene ointment and once-daily tazarotene gel was comparable to twice-daily application of clobetasol ointment in reducing psoriatic scaling, plaque elevation, and overall lesional severity over a 2-week period [27]. However, improvement in erythema was better with clobetasol compared to the nonsteroid combination therapy. This study was limited by a small sample size of 15 patients.

Combination Therapy with Topical Agents and Phototherapy

UVB and Topical Corticosteroids

There is no convincing evidence that the concomitant use of topical corticosteroids is beneficial in patients receiving ultraviolet B (UVB) phototherapy for psoriasis [28]. A prospective, randomized,

double-blind, placebo-controlled trial compared the efficacy of topical corticosteroid plus UVB to placebo plus UVB. Although there was a trend toward a slightly more rapid response in the topical corticosteroid-treated group, there was no significant difference in patients' early response to therapy, number of treatments, and UVB dose required to achieve clearing. However, patients in the topical corticosteroid-treated group remained in remission longer than did patients in the control group (183 vs. 116 days) [29]. Other studies show that topical corticosteroids do not decrease the number of phototherapy treatments required to clear psoriasis and that the use of a topical corticosteroid in conjunction with UVB leads to a faster relapse rate than UVB alone [30, 31].

UVB and Topical Vitamin D Analogues

A number of studies have suggested that the combination of a topical vitamin D analogues (calcipotriene, calcipotriol, calcitriol) and UVB phototherapy is beneficial in patients with psoriasis [32–40]. An analysis of two right-left comparison studies showed that in both treatment series, the therapeutic effect of the combination of calcipotriol plus UVB was enhanced compared to either therapy alone at the end of the 2-week treatment period [36]. However, no differences between the two sides were observed after 8 weeks. Another study showed that UVB plus calcipotriene is superior to UVB plus mineral oil starting at week 1, peaking at weeks 3 to 6, and maintained for 12 weeks [35]. In these studies, the combination of topical vitamin D plus UVB had a similar adverse event profile with either treatment alone. UVB does not alter the tolerability or safety of the topical vitamin D but may cause irritation and burning sensation if applied immediately before phototherapy [36]. If the topical vitamin D agent is applied immediately prior to phototherapy, it should be applied in a thin layer to avoid blocking of UV light [41]. Alternatively, it can be applied after administration of phototherapy or at night.

A limited number of studies have shown no benefit of combining topical vitamin D and UVB phototherapy. An 8-week, right-left comparison study by Kragballe showed no benefit of adding broadband UVB to topical application of calcipotriol [42]. Another study by Brands et al. showed that adding calcipotriol ointment does not improve efficacy of low-dose narrowband UVB (NB-UVB) [43].

UVB and Tazarotene

The combination of tazarotene and UVB phototherapy has been well described in the literature and demonstrates beneficial effects including quicker time to clearance of psoriasis with less number of UVB treatments and lower cumulative UVB dose [44–47]. In a multicenter, investigator-masked, randomized study of 54 patients with psoriasis, a 2-week pretreatment with tazarotene 0.1% gel once daily was followed by tazarotene plus UVB therapy three times per week for 10 weeks [44]. This combination regimen was more effective than UVB therapy alone or in combination with vehicle gel in reducing plaque elevation, scaling, and erythema.

Multiple other studies have supported the efficacy of this combination therapy, which is well tolerated without observed phototoxicity [44–47]. However, one study by Hecker et al. found that pretreatment with tazarotene 0.1% gel three times per week for 2 weeks prior to initiating phototherapy significantly reduced the mean minimal erythema dose (MED) of UVB from 56.25 to 42.50 mJ/cm^2 [48]. Although a thin layer of tazarotene applied prior to phototherapy has no significant effect on the mean MED for UVB, the dose of UVB should be reduced by 50–75% of the MED to avoid potential burn or tan [48]. Alternatively, tazarotene can be applied after phototherapy sessions or at night [44].

UVB and Tar/Anthralin

The Goeckerman regimen is one of the oldest, yet most effective treatments for psoriasis [49]. The Goeckerman regimen involves the combination of coal tar plus UVB phototherapy. A study by Lowe et al. found that topical tar enhances the effects of suberythemogenic phototherapy compared to erythemogenic phototherapy using higher doses of UVB, suggesting that a lower cumulative dose of UVB is required when used in conjunction with tar [50]. Furthermore, the risk of phototoxic reaction is lower when suberythemogenic phototherapy is used in conjunction with tar. Studies have shown that nearly 100% of patients who undergo Goeckerman achieve PASI-75 over 12 weeks or less [49], which can be maintained for 8 months to 1 year [51]. Unfortunately, given the extensive resources required by medical facilities to conduct the Goeckerman regimen, combined with the time commitment required for patients (all-day treatments for approximately 4–6 weeks), Goeckerman therapy is rarely available today [52]. An alternative to the Goeckerman regimen is the use of liquor carbonis detergens (LCD) or gold tar at home in conjunction with outpatient NB-UVB, which is shown to be more effective than NB-UVB alone [53]. It should be clarified that the tar is applied after UVB treatments, as tar can block the effective transmission of light if applied prior to UVB treatments [54].

The combination of short contact anthralin and UVB has been tested as an alternative to the Goeckerman regimen, which involves the application of anthralin for 10 to 30 minutes daily in addition to UVB phototherapy. This combination has been studied in limited number and appears to have little benefit compared to UVB treatments alone [55, 56].

PUVA and Topical Corticosteroids

Overall, studies suggest that the combination of PUVA and topical corticosteroids results in more rapid clearing of psoriasis compared to PUVA alone [28, 57–60]. However, some of these studies suggest a quicker time to relapse in patients treated with PUVA plus topical corticosteroid [57].

PUVA and Topical Vitamin D Analogues

The combination of PUVA plus topical vitamin D appears to be more efficacious compared to PUVA alone [61–63]. In a systematic review of 11 randomized controlled trials involving a total of 756 patients with plaque psoriasis, the rate ratio of marked improvement in patients receiving PUVA plus calcipotriene versus those receiving PUVA alone was found to be 1.2 (1.0 = benefit) [63]. Calcipotriene should be applied after PUVA treatment as, unlike UVB, UVA can inactivate vitamin D [41].

PUVA and Tazarotene

Although studies are limited, topical retinoid tazarotene appears to enhance the efficacy of PUVA [64]. In a single-center, right-left comparison study, 12 patients were treated with tazarotene versus placebo prior to bath PUVA four times per week. The tazarotene plus PUVA-treated side was superior to placebo versus PUVA after 3 weeks [64]. Tazarotene remains chemically stable with application of UVA; however, there may be reduced threshold for immediate skin pigment darkening caused by UVA. Therefore, it is recommended that UV doses be reduced by at least one third if tazarotene is added to an established phototherapy regimen [48].

Excimer Laser and Topical Agents

In a 12-week, single-center study, 30 patients with moderate to severe psoriasis received treatments with the 308-nm excimer laser twice weekly combined with clobetasol propionate 0.05% spray twice daily for 4 weeks, followed by calcitriol ointment twice daily for the next 4 weeks. At 12 weeks, 83% of patients achieved 75% improvement of better in the Psoriasis Area and Severity Index (PASI-75) [65–67]. Another study by Dong et al. showed superior efficacy of excimer laser in combination with a topical corticosteroid flumetasone ointment compared to excimer laser monotherapy [68]. Some studies have also shown that excimer laser can be safely combined with calcipotriol or dithranol with additive benefit [69].

Combination Therapy with Topical Agents and Oral Systemic Agents

In the real-world, clinical setting, topical agents are often used in conjunction with oral systemic agents to treat resistant areas or to minimize toxic exposure and adverse effects of systemic agents [4]. Only a few of these combinations have been studied formally.

Retinoids and Topical Corticosteroids

There is evidence to suggest that acitretin in combination with topical corticosteroids is a safe and effective long-term treatment options for psoriasis. In a 3-year follow-up study of patients treated with etretinate who had initial improvement, more than 40% of these patients showed prolonged clearance on acitretin plus a topical corticosteroid [70].

Retinoids and Topical Vitamin D Analogues

The combination of an oral retinoid plus topical vitamin D appears to have better efficacy than oral retinoid monotherapy. In a multicenter, randomized, double-blind placebo-controlled study, 76 patients were treated with acitretin plus calcipotriol ointment twice daily and 59 patients were treated with acitretin plus vehicle. The dose of acitretin was adjusted as needed every 2 weeks. The proportion of patients receiving acitretin plus calcipotriol combination who reached clear or marked improvement was statistically higher compared to the acitretin plus vehicle group. Furthermore, the cumulative dose of acitretin was lower in the combination group. No additional adverse events were reported with the addition of calcipotriol [71]. Other studies have found similar results [63, 72].

Cyclosporine and Topical Vitamin D Analogues

Some studies have shown the effectiveness of the combination of cyclosporine plus topical vitamin D [63, 73, 74]. In a multicenter, placebo-controlled study, patients with severe psoriasis were treated with low-dose cyclosporine (2 mg/kg/day) combined with calcipotriol or vehicle for 6 weeks. Complete clearing or PASI-90 occurred in 50% of patients in the cyclosporine plus calcipotriol group versus 11.8% in the cyclosporine plus vehicle group [73].

Methotrexate and Topical Vitamin D Analogues

One multicenter, double-blind, placebo-controlled study has shown the superior efficacy of the combination of methotrexate (MTX) plus calcipotriol compared to MTX plus vehicle for the treatment of psoriasis [75]. MTX plus calcipotriol resulted in lower cumulative dose of MTX and lower incidence of liver function test abnormalities. Furthermore, this study found that the addition of calcipotriol increased the time to relapse of psoriasis following discontinuation of MTX [75].

Combination Therapy with Topical Agents and Biologics

Biologic agents for the treatment of moderate to severe psoriasis have shown great efficacy; however, complete clearance of psoriasis is still difficult to achieve. In such cases, topical agents are often used in conjunction with biologic therapies to augment clearance. Although commonly used in clinical practice, only some combinations of biologics plus topical agents have been studied.

Biologics and Topical Corticosteroids

Although only a few randomized, controlled studies have evaluated the use of biologics plus topical corticosteroids, the combination appears to be safe and effective for augmenting disease clearance. The combination of etanercept in combination with clobetasol foam has been studied in a phase 3b, multicenter, randomized trial of 592 subjects, 295 receiving etanercept plus clobetasol foam and 297 receiving etanercept only. At week 12, the combination group showed increased efficacy, better patient satisfaction, and no additional adverse events compared to the etanercept mono-therapy group [76].

A phase 4, multicenter, open-label, community-based studies called the COBRA (Clobex Spray Community-Based Research Assessment) trial studied the combination of various biologic agents plus clobetasol spray [77]. The addition of clobetasol spray to a stable regimen of biologic therapy resulted in improvements in disease severity.

Biologics and Topical Vitamin D Analogues

The addition of calcipotriol to etanercept in patients who were partial responders to etanercept was found to be beneficial in a prospective study by Campione et al. In this study, 120 patients with psoriasis and psoriatic arthritis were treated with etanercept 50 mg twice weekly for 12 weeks followed by 25 mg twice weekly. Patients who did not achieve PASI-50 at week 12 received calcipotriol twice daily for 4 weeks, then once daily. The application of calcipotriol in etanercept partial responders allowed 37 out of 120 patients (31%) achieve at least PASI 50 at week 24 [78].

Biologics and Combination Topical Corticosteroid and Vitamin D Analogues

The topical calcipotriene 0.005% and beta-methasone dipropionate 0.064% combination ointment has been studied in conjunction with both etanercept and adalimumab and is shown to be a safe and effective adjunct to biologic monotherapy [79, 80]. In a single-center, open-label study, 20 patients were treated with etanercept 50 mg twice weekly for 12 weeks followed by 50 mg once weekly. Patients who experienced worsening psoriasis (increase from baseline body surface area (BSA) of greater than 2%) began treatment with calcipotriene/betamethasone ointment. Initiation of the topical combination ointment led to a stable improvement in BSA [79].

The safety and efficacy of the use of adalimumab plus topical calcipotriol/betamethasone were studied in a phase 3b, multicenter, randomized, double-blind, vehicle-controlled study of 730 patients, 366 of whom received adalimumab plus calcipotriene/betamethasone and 364 of whom received adalimumab plus vehicle. The combination of adalimumab plus calcipotriol/betamethasone resulted in more rapid and higher efficacy within the first 4 weeks. There was no statistical difference in the PASI-75 response at week 16 [80].

Combination Phototherapy

A limited number of studies have evaluated the safety and efficacy of combining UVB and PUVA for treatment of psoriasis, and the benefits of this combination therapy are unclear. In a bilateral comparison study, Momtaz and Parrish evaluated 42 adult patients with severe psoriasis who failed either UVB or PUVA alone and were subsequently treated with combination of UVB and PUVA three times per week. All patients tolerated treatments well and cleared in less than half the number of treatments and in less than half of the mean UVB dose and mean cumulative PUVA dose [81]. In another bilateral comparison study, 12 patients were treated with bath PUVA followed by NB-UVB. The side receiving the combination treatment achieved more rapid clearance and required lower cumulative dose of UVA compared to the side receiving bath PUVA alone [82].

On the contrary, other studies have not found a significant difference in effectiveness of this combination therapy, including number of treatments and doses of UVB and PUVA required for clearance [83, 84].

Combination with Phototherapy and Oral Systemic Agents

UVB/PUVA and Retinoid (Re-UVB/Re-PUVA)

The use of the oral retinoid acitretin in combination with UVB and PUVA for the treatment of psoriasis has been well studied [85]. The combinations, termed Re-UVB (retinoid plus UVB) and Re-PUVA (retinoid plus PUVA), appear to have synergistic effects, reducing the number of treatments and cumulative UV and acitretin doses required for clearance. Furthermore, acitretin has tumor-suppressive effects [86] and is therefore an ideal agent to combine with phototherapy, especially PUVA, which has cutaneous carcinogenic effects after more than 200 to 250 treatments [87]. In combination with phototherapy, acitretin is typically used at a dose of 25 mg/day or less. As acitretin has photosensitizing potential, when adding acitretin to an already maximized phototherapy regimen, the dose of phototherapy should be decreased by 50% to prevent burn [88]. If acitretin is initiated first, phototherapy should be started approximately 2 weeks later per the usual dosing protocol.

In a multicenter, double-blind, randomized study, 40 patients with severe psoriasis underwent Re-UVB and 38 patients received acitretin alone for 8 weeks. Acitretin was given at a dose of 35 mg/day for the first 4 weeks, then 25 mg/day thereafter. PASI-75 was achieved by 60% of patients on Re-UVB versus 24% on acitretin alone, with a significantly lower cumulative UVB dose [89]. Side effects were similar in both groups. Other studies have found similar benefits of Re-UVB [90, 91].

A series of double-blind, randomized studies have also shown the effectiveness of Re-PUVA compared to PUVA or oral retinoid alone. Again, re-PUVA requires fewer PUVA treatment sessions and a lower cumulative dose of UVA compared to PUVA alone [92–94].

UVB and Cyclosporine

The concurrent use of phototherapy and cyclosporine is contraindicated according to cyclosporine's package insert due to increased risk of cutaneous malignancy [95]. However, many psoriasis experts agree that short-term combination therapy is acceptable, for example, as part of sequential therapy, in which psoriasis is initially cleared with cyclosporine and then maintained with UVB or PUVA. In such a case, the period of time the two therapies overlap is very short, and therefore, the risk of malignancy is theoretically negligible.

UVB/PUVA and Methotrexate

A few studies exist to evaluate the safety and efficacy of combining phototherapy with MTX, and the combination appears to work synergistically. In one study, 26 patients with severe psoriasis were treated with a 3-week course of MTX followed by combination of UVB plus MTX. When lesions cleared to less than 5% of body involvement, the MTX was stopped and UVB therapy alone was used as maintenance therapy. This protocol achieved clearance of disease in all 26 patients at relatively low doses of UVB and methotrexate [96]. A study with a similar design using PUVA plus MTX also showed similar results [97]. The long-term effects of this combination therapy, including possible increased risk of cutaneous malignancy, are not well delineated.

UVB and Apremilast

The combination use of apremilast with UVB phototherapy was officially tested in the pivotal phase 3 clinical trial for apremilast [98], and the combination appeared safe without any risk of photosensitivity. Although the data regarding the additional therapeutic benefit of adding phototherapy to apremilast has yet to be made public, in clinical practice this combination is not uncommon, and there may be synergistic benefit [99].

Combination Therapy with Phototherapy and Biologics

Overall, the combination of biologics and phototherapy appears to be well tolerated and effective in a subset of patients who have resistant disease despite treatment with a biologic agent.

Etanercept and NB-UVB

Several studies evaluated the combination of etanercept plus NB-UVB in patients who had not previously received treatment, patients who had an inadequate response with etanercept alone (50 mg once weekly or 50 mg twice weekly dosing), or patients who had an inadequate response to NB-UVB alone [100–105]. Overall, combination therapy was superior to either monotherapy, and time to clearance was reduced. In a 12-week, single-arm, open-label study, the combination of etanercept 50 mg twice weekly and NB-UVB three times weekly was evaluated in 86 patients. Impressively, PASI-75 was achieved in 84.9% of patients [101]. High adherence to the NB-UVB regimen appears to be important to achieve significant clinical improvement [103]. The addition of excimer laser to etanercept therapy has been reported to produce effective results in when etanercept plus traditional NB-UVB therapy has failed [106].

One study to date has failed to establish efficacy of combination therapy of etanercept and NB-UVB. In this head-to-head pilot study examining combination treatment of NB-UVB plus etanercept 50 mg twice weekly compared with etanercept monotherapy, combination therapy did not yield better efficacy [107]. However, this study was limited by a small sample size of 13 patients who all had a body mass index (BMI) of greater than 30. Previous studies have reported a suboptimal response to etanercept in psoriasis patients with a BMI of greater than 30 [108].

Adalimumab and NB-UVB

Two studies have evaluated the combination therapy of adalimumab plus NB-UVB in patients with psoriasis. In a 24-week, single-arm, open-label study by Bagel, 85% (17/20) of patients were clear or almost clear at 12 weeks [109]. In a half-body comparison study, Wolf et al. found overall mean PASI reduction from baseline of 86% on UV-irradiated body halves vs. 53% on non-irradiated body halves [110]. Both studies demonstrated that phototherapy significantly accelerates therapeutic response and improves the clearance of psoriatic lesions in patients treated with adalimumab.

Ustekinumab and NB-UVB

One study to date has evaluated the combination of ustekinumab plus excimer laser. This intraindividual, half-body comparison study showed that PASI-75 was achieved significantly more often on the UV-irradiated half than on the non-irradiated half at week 6 [111].

Combination Therapy with Oral Systemic Agents

Acitretin and Cyclosporine

Acitretin and cyclosporine can be used effectively in sequential therapy where cyclosporine is used as the initial rapid-acting, clearing agent and acitretin is used as the maintenance agent [2]. This combination is also ideal given that cyclosporine may increase the risk of malignancy, and acitretin appears to have anticancer effects [86].

Acitretin and Methotrexate

Although no controlled studies have been performed, the combination of acitretin and MTX is sometimes used in clinical practice. A retrospective study of 18 patients on this combination therapy has shown that it is generally effective and well tolerated [112]. The literature suggests that it is especially beneficial for treating pustular psoriasis [113–115]. Although this combination is contraindicated according to the package insert for acitretin [116], with careful monitoring of liver enzymes and abstinence from alcohol, this combination can be used safely [4].

Cyclosporine and Methotrexate

Cyclosporine and MTX have been used in combination for patients with severe psoriasis, as well as those with both psoriasis and psoriatic arthritis. In a prospective study of 20 patients and a retrospective study of 19 patients receiving combination of cyclosporine and MTX, significant improvement was observed after initiation of combination therapy, which was well-tolerated [117, 118]. Cyclosporine and MTX can also be used as part of rotational therapy using MTX as the maintenance regimen and adding cyclosporine as a short-term, occasional-clearing agent. Although this rotational regimen is not as cost-effective as MTX monotherapy, patients were able to have periods of complete clearance when cyclosporine was added to MTX therapy [119].

Apremilast and Other Oral Systemic Agents

A limited number of case reports have documented the safe and effective use of apremilast in combination with acitretin and cyclosporine [119, 120]. Apremilast has also been safely used in combination with disease-modifying antirheumatic drugs such as methotrexate in clinical trials for the treatment of psoriatic arthritis. Further studies are needed.

Combination Therapy with Oral Systemic Agents and Biologics

Acitretin and Biologics

Controlled studies evaluating the combination of acitretin plus biologics are limited. In a 24-week, randomized, controlled, investigator-blinded pilot trial, 60 patients with moderate to severe psoriasis were randomized to receive etanercept 25 mg twice weekly, acitretin 0.4 mg/kg daily, or etanercept 25 mg once weekly plus acitretin 0.4 mg/kg daily. It was found that the combination of etanercept 25 mg once weekly and acitretin 0.4 mg/kg daily is as effective as etanercept 25 mg twice weekly and more effective than acitretin alone [121]. Uncontrolled trials and reported cases in the literature also suggest that this combination is well tolerated [122–125]. Overall, it appears that acitretin can be added to decrease the dose of etanercept and maintain similar levels of efficacy [126].

Cyclosporine and Biologics

No large-scale, controlled studies have been conducted to evaluate the safety and efficacy of combining cyclosporine and biologics, but this combination may be beneficial for recalcitrant cases. In a prospective study, seven patients with refractory psoriasis were treated with cyclosporine 200 mg per day plus etanercept 50 mg weekly until their psoriasis was clear or near clear [127]. In another study, 11 patients with psoriasis and psoriatic arthritis whose cutaneous manifestations were uncontrolled on etanercept alone received cyclosporine with improvement of their psoriasis [128]. Long-term consequences of this combination are not well known. Instead of using the two agents concomitantly, this combination may be best utilized as part of sequential therapy in which cyclosporine is used as the rapid-acting clearing agent, and the biologic is used as a maintenance agent [129–131].

Methotrexate and Biologics

The combination of tumor necrosis factor-alpha (TNFa) inhibitors, including etanercept, adalimumab, and infliximab, plus MTX is often used in clinical practice, especially in patients with both psoriasis and psoriatic arthritis. The combination is well studied in patients with other disease states such as rheumatoid arthritis but is relatively limited in the psoriasis population [123, 132–140]. In a randomized, double-blind, placebo-controlled study of 239 patients per arm, PASI-75 was significantly higher at weeks 12 and 24 for the combination therapy group receiving etanercept plus MTX compared to the etanercept only group (70.2% vs. 54.3%, $P = 0.01$ and (77.3% vs. 60.3%, $P < 0.0001$, respectively). The combination was also well tolerated. The use

etanercept and MTX concomitantly can also have dose-reducing effects on MTX [138].

Studies suggest that while monotherapy with either MTX or TNFa inhibitors results in downregulation of some but not all inflammatory markers, the combination is more efficient in reducing inflammatory cell numbers in psoriatic skin than either alone [139]. There is also some data to suggest that the concomitant use of biologics and MTX may reduce antidrug antibody formation [141]. Formal studies investigating other biologic agents in combination with MTX are limited [142].

Apremilast and Biologics

Only a limited number of case reports and a retrospective study support the use of apremilast in combination with biologic agents [99, 143, 144]. Given that apremilast and biologics have completely different mechanisms of action, this combination may be safe and effective in patients with severe recalcitrant psoriasis. Further studies are needed.

References

1. Weinstein GD, White GM. An approach to the treatment of moderate to severe psoriasis with rotational therapy. J Am Acad Dermatol. 1993;28(3):454–9.
2. Koo J. Systemic sequential therapy of psoriasis: a new paradigm for improved therapeutic results. J Am Acad Dermatol. 1999;41(3 Pt 2):S25–8.
3. Emer J, Lebwohl MG. Combination, rotational, and sequential therapies. In: Koo JYM, Levin EC, Leon AWJJ, Gottlieb AB, editors. Moderate to severe psoriasis. Boca Raton: CRC Press; 2015. p. 121–38.
4. Lebwohl M, Menter A, Koo J, Feldman SR. Combination therapy to treat moderate to severe psoriasis. J Am Acad Dermatol. 2004;50(3):416–30.
5. Menter MA, See JA, Amend WJ, et al. Proceedings of the psoriasis combination and rotation therapy conference, Deer Valley, Utah, Oct. 7–9, 1994. J Am Acad Dermatol. 1996;34(2 Pt 1):315–21.
6. Koo JYM. New developments in topical sequential therapy for psoriasis. Skin Therapy Lett. 2005;10(9):1–4.
7. Horn EJ, Domm S, Katz HI, et al. Topical corticosteroids in psoriasis: strategies for improving safety. J Eur Acad Dermatol Venereol. 2010;24(2):119–24.
8. Lebwohl M. Topical application of calcipotriene and corticosteroids: combination regimens. J Am Acad Dermatol. 1997;37(3 Pt 2):S55–8.

9. Lebwohl M, Siskin SB, Epinette W, et al. A multi-center trial of calcipotriene ointment and halobetasol ointment compared with either agent alone for the treatment of psoriasis. J Am Acad Dermatol. 1996;35(2 Pt 1):268–9.

10. Lebwohl M, Yoles A, Lombardi K, Lou W. Calcipotriene ointment and halobetasol ointment in the long-term treatment of psoriasis: effects on the duration of improvement. J Am Acad Dermatol. 1998;39(3):447–50.

11. Austad J, Bjerke JR, Gjertsen BT, et al. Clobetasol propionate followed by calcipotriol is superior to calcipotriol alone in topical treatment of psoriasis. J Eur Acad Dermatol Venereol. 1998;11(1):19–24.

12. Bhutani T, Zitelli KB, Koo J. Yin-yang strategy: proposing a new, effective, repeatable, sequential therapy for psoriasis. J Drugs Dermatol. 2011;10(8):831–4.

13. Menter A, Sofen H, Smith S, et al. An open-label, multicenter study of the efficacy and safety of an AM/PM treatment regimen with clobetasol propionate spray 0.05% and calcitriol ointment 3 microg/g in the management of plaque psoriasis. Cutis. 2011;88(1):46–51.

14. Brodell RT, Bruce S, Hudson CP, et al. A multicenter, open-label study to evaluate the safety and efficacy of a sequential treatment regimen of clobetasol propionate 0.05% spray followed by Calcitriol 3 mg/g ointment in the management of plaque psoriasis. J Drugs Dermatol. 2011;10(2):158–64.

15. Hudson CP, Kempers S, Menter A, et al. An open-label, multicenter study of the efficacy and safety of a weekday/weekend treatment regimen with calcitriol ointment 3 microg/g and clobetasol propionate spray 0.05% in the management of plaque psoriasis. Cutis. 2011;88(4):201–7.

16. Koo J, Blum RR, Lebwohl M. A randomized, multicenter study of calcipotriene ointment and clobetasol propionate foam in the sequential treatment of localized plaque-type psoriasis: short- and long-term outcomes. J Am Acad Dermatol. 2006;55(4):637–41.

17. Singh S, Reddy DC, Pandey SS. Topical therapy for psoriasis with the use of augmented betamethasone and calcipotriene on alternate weeks. J Am Acad Dermatol. 2000;43(1 Pt 1):61–5.

18. Lebwohl M, Lombardi K, Tan MH. Duration of improvement in psoriasis after treatment with tazarotene 0.1% gel plus clobetasol propionate 0.05% ointment: comparison of maintenance treatments. Int J Dermatol. 2001;40(1):64–6.

19. Guenther LC, Poulin YP, Pariser DM. A comparison of tazarotene 0.1% gel once daily plus mometasone furoate 0.1% cream once daily versus calcipotriene 0.005% ointment twice daily in the treatment of plaque psoriasis. Clin Ther. 2000;22(10):1225–38.

20. Tanghetti EA. Tazarotene Stable Plaque Psoriasis Trial Study Group. An observation study evaluating the efficacy of tazarotene plus corticosteroid in treating plaque psoriasis in patients switched from treatment with calcipotriene +/− corticosteroid. Cutis. 2000;66(6 Suppl):12–8.

21. Dubertret L, Lahfa M, Altmeyer P, Prens EP, Matranga A Alternating evening applications of tazarotene 0.1% gel and corticosteroid cream in the treatment of plaque psoriasis, Poster presented at the 56th annual meeting of the American Academy of Dermatology. Orlando, FL, 27 February–4 March 1998.

22. Lebwohl MG, Breneman DL, Goffe BS, et al. Tazarotene 0.1% gel plus corticosteroid cream in the treatment of plaque psoriasis. J Am Acad Dermatol. 1998;39(4 Pt 1):590–6.

23. Lebwohl M, Poulin Y. Tazarotene in combination with topical corticosteroids. J Am Acad Dermatol. 1998;39(4 Pt 2):S139–43.

24. Kaidbey K, Kopper SC, Sefton J, Gibson JR A pilot study to determine the effect of tazarotene 0.1% gel on steroid-induced epidermal atrophy. Poster presented at the 58th annual meeting of the American Academy of Dermatology. San Francisco, CA, 10–15 March 2000.

25. Koo J, Behnam SE, Behnam SM. The efficacy of topical tazarotene monotherapy and combination therapies in psoriasis. Expert Opin Pharmacother. 2003;4(12):2347–54.

26. Hecker D, Worsley J, Yueh G, et al. In vitro compatibility of tazarotene with other topical treatments of psoriasis. J Am Acad Dermatol. 2000;42:1008–11.

27. Bowman PH, Maloney JE, Koo JY. Combination of calcipotriene (Dovonex) ointment and tazarotene (Tazorac) gel versus clobetasol ointment in the treatment of plaque psoriasis: a pilot study. J Am Acad Dermatol. 2002;46(6):907–13.

28. Meola T Jr, Soter NA, Lim HW. Are topical corticosteroids useful adjunctive therapy for the treatment of psoriasis with ultraviolet radiation? A review of the literature. Arch Dermatol. 1991;127(11):1708–13.

29. Dover JS, McEvoy MT, Rosen CF, Arndt KA, Stern RS. Are topical corticosteroids useful in phototherapy for psoriasis? J Am Acad Dermatol. 1989;20:748–54.

30. Petrozzi JW. Topical steroids and UV radiation in psoriasis. Arch Dermatol. 1983;119:207–10.

31. Horwitz SN, Johnson RA, Sefton J, Frost P. Addition of a topically applied corticosteroid to a modified Goeckerman regimen for treatment of psoriasis: effect on duration of remission. J Am Acad Dermatol. 1985;13:784–91.

32. Koo J. Calcipotriol/calcipotriene (Dovonex/Daivonex) in combination with phototherapy: a review. J Am Acad Dermatol. 1997;37(3 Pt 2):S59–61.

33. Kerscher M, Volkenandt M, Plewig G, Lehmann P. Combination phototherapy of psoriasis with calcipotriol and narrow-band UVB. Lancet. 1993;342(8876):923.

34. Kokelj F, Lavaroni G, Guadagnini A. UVB versus UVB plus calcipotriol (MC 903) therapy for psoriasis vulgaris. Acta Derm Venereol. 1995;75(5):386–7.

35. Hecker D, Lebwohl M. Topical calcipotriene in combination with UVB phototherapy for psoriasis. Int J Dermatol. 1997;36(4):302–3.

36. Molin L. Topical calcipotriol combined with phototherapy for psoriasis. The results of two randomized trials and a review of the literature. Calcipotriol-UVB Study Group. Dermatology. 1999;198(4):375–81.

37. Ring J, Kowalzick L, Christophers E, et al. Calcitriol 3 microg g⁻¹ ointment in combination with ultraviolet B phototherapy for the treatment of plaque psoriasis: results of a comparative study. Br J Dermatol. 2001;144(3):495–9.

38. Rim JH, Choe YB, Youn JI. Positive effect of using calcipotriol ointment with narrow-band ultraviolet B phototherapy in psoriatic patients. Photodermatol Photoimmunol Photomed. 2002;18(3):131–4.

39. Ozkan I, Köse O, Ozmen I, Arca E. Efficacy and safety of non-laser, targeted UVB phototherapy alone and in combination with psoralen gel or calcipotriol ointment in the treatment of localized, chronic, plaque-type psoriasis. Int J Dermatol. 2012;51(5):609–13.

40. Takahashi H, Tsuji H, Ishida-Yamamoto A, Iizuka H. Comparison of clinical effects of psoriasis treatment regimens among calcipotriol alone, narrowband ultraviolet B phototherapy alone, combination of calcipotriol and narrowband ultraviolet B phototherapy once a week, and combination of calcipotriol and narrowband ultraviolet B phototherapy more than twice a week. J Dermatol. 2013;40(6):424–7.

41. Lebwohl M, Hecker D, Martinez J, Sapadin A, Patel B. Interactions between calcipotriene and ultraviolet light. J Am Acad Dermatol. 1997;37(1):93–5.

42. Kragballe K. Combination of topical calcipotriol (MC 903) and UVB radiation for psoriasis vulgaris. Dermatologica. 1990;181(3):211–4.

43. Brands S, Brakman M, Bos JD, de Rie MA. No additional effect of calcipotriol ointment on low-dose narrow-band UVB phototherapy in psoriasis. J Am Acad Dermatol. 1999;41(6):991–5.

44. Koo JY. Tazarotene in combination with phototherapy. J Am Acad Dermatol. 1998;39(4 Pt 2):S144–8.

45. Behrens S, Grundmann-Kollmann M, Schiener R, Peter RU, Kerscher M. Combination phototherapy of psoriasis with narrow-band UVB irradiation and topical tazarotene gel. J Am Acad Dermatol. 2000;42(3):493–5.

46. Lowe NJ. Optimizing therapy: tazarotene in combination with phototherapy. Br J Dermatol. 1999;140(Suppl 54):8–11.

47. Koo JY, Lowe NJ, Lew-Kaya DA, et al. Tazarotene plus UVB phototherapy in the treatment of psoriasis. J Am Acad Dermatol. 2000;43(5 Pt 1):821–8.

48. Hecker D, Worsley J, Yueh G, Kuroda K, Lebwohl M. Interactions between tazarotene and ultraviolet light. J Am Acad Dermatol. 1999;41(6):927–30.

49. Lee E, Koo J. Modern modified 'ultra' Goeckerman therapy: a PASI assessment of a very effective therapy for psoriasis resistant to both prebiologic and biologic therapies. J Dermatolog Treat. 2005;16(2):102–7.

50. Lowe NJ, Wortzman MS, Breeding J, Koudsi H, Taylor L. Coal tar phototherapy for psoriasis reevaluated: erythemogenic versus suberythemogenic ultraviolet with a tar extract in oil and crude coal tar. J Am Acad Dermatol. 1983;8(6):781–9.

51. Menter A, Cram DL. The Goeckerman regimen in two psoriasis day care centers. J Am Acad Dermatol. 1983;9(1):59–65.

52. Gupta R, Debbaneh M, Butler D, et al. The Goeckerman regimen for the treatment of moderate to severe psoriasis. J Vis Exp. 2013;77:e50509. https://doi.org/10.3791/50509.

53. Bagel J. LCD plus NB-UVB reduces time to improvement of psoriasis vs. NB-UVB alone. J Drugs Dermatol. 2009;8(4):351–7.

54. Lebwohl M, Martinez J, Weber P, DeLuca R. Effects of topical preparations on the erythemogenicity of UVB: implications for psoriasis phototherapy. J Am Acad Dermatol. 1995;32(3):469–71.

55. Boer J, Smeenk G. Effect of short-contact anthralin therapy on ultraviolet B irradiation of psoriasis. J Am Acad Dermatol. 1986;15(2 Pt 1):198–204.

56. Lebwohl M, Berman B, France DS. Addition of short-contact anthralin therapy to an ultraviolet B phototherapy regimen: assessment of efficacy. J Am Acad Dermatol. 1985;13:780–4.

57. Morison WL, Parrish JA, Fitzpatrick TB. Controlled study of PUVA and adjunctive topical therapy in the management of psoriasis. Br J Dermatol. 1978;98(2):125–32.

58. Schmoll M, Henseler T, Christophers E. Evaluation of PUVA, topical corticosteroids and the combination of both in the treatment of psoriasis. Br J Dermatol. 1978;99(6):693–702.

59. Hanke CW, Steck WD, Roenigk HH. Combination therapy for psoriasis. Psoralens plus long-wave ultraviolet radiation with betamethasone valerate. Arch Dermatol. 1979;115(9):1074–7.

60. Gould PW, Wilson L. Psoriasis treated with clobetasol propionate and photochemotherapy. Br J Dermatol. 1978;98(2):133–6.

61. Speight EL, Farr PM. Calcipotriol improves the response of psoriasis to PUVA. Br J Dermatol. 1994;130(1):79–82.

62. Frappaz A, Thivolet J. Calcipotriol in combination with PUVA: a randomized, double-blind, placebo study in severe psoriasis. Eur J Dermatol. 1993;3:351–4.

63. Ashcroft DM, Li Wan Po A, Williams HC, Griffiths CE. Combination regimens of topical calcipotriene in chronic plaque psoriasis: systematic review of efficacy and tolerability. Arch Dermatol. 2000;136(12):1536–43.

64. Behrens S, Grundmann-Kollmann M, Peter RU, Kerscher M. Combination treatment of psoriasis with photochemotherapy and tazarotene gel, a receptor-selective topical retinoid. Br J Dermatol. 1999;141(1):177.

65. Wong JW, Nguyen TV, Bhutani T, Koo JY. Treatment of psoriasis and long-term maintenance using 308 nm excimer laser, clobetasol spray, and calcitriol ointment: a case series. J Drugs Dermatol. 2012 Aug;11(8):994–6.

66. Levin E, Debbaneh M, Malakouti M. Supraerythemogenic excimer laser in combination with clobetasol spray and calcitriol ointment for the treatment of generalized plaque psoriasis: interim results of an open label pilot study. J Dermatolog Treat. 2015;26(1):16–8.

67. Levin E, Nguyen CM, Danesh MJ, Beroukhim K, Leon A, Koo J. An open label pilot study of supraerythemogenic excimer laser in combination with clobetasol spray and calcitriol ointment for the treatment of generalized plaque psoriasis. J Dermatolog Treat. 2016;27(3):210–3.

68. Dong J, He Y, Zhang X, et al. Clinical efficacy of flumetasone/salicylic acid ointment combined with 308-nm excimer laser for treatment of psoriasis vulgaris. Photodermatol Photoimmunol Photomed. 2012;28(3):133–6.

69. Rogalski C, Grunewald S, Schetschorke M, et al. Treatment of plaque-type psoriasis with the 308 nm excimer laser in combination with dithranol or calcipotriol. Int J Hyperth. 2012;28(2):184–90.

70. Polano MK, van der Rhee HJ, van der Schroeff JG. A three-year follow-up study of psoriasis patients treated with low dosages of etretinate orally and corticosteroids topically. Acta Derm Venereol. 1982;62(4):361–4.

71. van de Kerkhof PC, Cambazard F, Hutchinson PE, et al. The effect of addition of calcipotriol ointment (50 micrograms/g) to acitretin therapy in psoriasis. Br J Dermatol. 1998;138(1):84–9.

72. Rim JH, Park JY, Choe YB, Youn JI. The efficacy of calcipotriol + acitretin combination therapy for psoriasis: comparison with acitretin monotherapy. Am J Clin Dermatol. 2003;4(7):507–10.

73. Grossman RM, Thivolet J, Claudy A, et al. A novel therapeutic approach to psoriasis with combination calcipotriol ointment and very low-dose cyclosporine: results of a multicenter placebo-controlled study. J Am Acad Dermatol. 1994;31(1):68–74.

74. Katz HI. Combined topical calcipotriene ointment 0.005% and various systemic therapies in the treatment of plaque-type psoriasis vulgaris: review of the literature and results of a survey sent to 100 dermatologists. J Am Acad Dermatol. 1997;37(3 Pt 2):S62–8.

75. de Jong EM, Mørk NJ, Seijger MM, De La Brassine M, et al. The combination of calcipotriol and methotrexate compared with methotrexate and vehicle in psoriasis: results of a multicentre placebo-controlled randomized trial. Br J Dermatol. 2003;148(2):318–25.

76. Lebwohl MG, Kircik L, Callis Duffin K, et al. A randomized study to evaluate the efficacy and safety of adding topical therapy to etanercept in patients with moderate to severe plaque psoriasis. J Am Acad Dermatol. 2013;69(3):385–92.

77. Feldman SR, Koo JY, Johnson LA, Preston NJ. Clobetasol propionate spray 0.05% add-on therapy to a stable regimen of biologic treatment in patients with moderate to very severe plaque psoriasis. Cutis. 2009;84(4 Suppl):25–32.

78. Campione E, Mazzotta A, Paternò EJ, Diluvio L, Prinz JC, Chimenti S. Effect of calcipotriol on etanercept partial responder psoriasis vulgaris and psoriatic arthritis patients. Acta Derm Venereol. 2009;89(3):288–91.

79. Kircik LH. Topical calcipotriene 0.005% and betamethasone dipropionate 0.064% maintains efficacy of etanercept after step-down dose in patients with moderate-to-severe plaque psoriasis: results of an open label trial. J Drugs Dermatol. 2011;10(8):878–82.

80. D T, Ortonne JP, Chimenti S, et al. A phase IIIb, multicentre, randomized, double-blind, vehicle-controlled study of the efficacy and safety of adalimumab with and without calcipotriol/betamethasone topical treatment in patients with moderate to severe psoriasis: the BELIEVE study. Br J Dermatol. 2010;163(2):402–11.

81. Momtaz-T K, Parrish JA. Combination of psoralens and ultraviolet A and ultraviolet B in the treatment of psoriasis vulgaris: a bilateral comparison study. J Am Acad Dermatol. 1984;10(3):481–6.

82. Calzavara-Pinton P. Narrow band UVB (311 nm) phototherapy and PUVA photochemotherapy: a combination. J Am Acad Dermatol. 1998;38:687–90.

83. Morison WL. Combination of methoxsalen and ultraviolet B (UVB) versus UVB radiation alone in treatment of psoriasis: a bilateral comparison study. Photodermatol Photoimmunol Photomed. 1995;11(1):6–8.

84. Park YK, Kim HJ, Koh YJ. Combination of photochemotherapy (PUVA) and ultraviolet B (UVB) in the treatment of psoriasis vulgaris. J Dermatol. 1988;15(1):68–71.

85. Lebwohl M. Acitretin in combination with UVB or PUVA. J Am Acad Dermatol. 1999;41(3 Pt 2):S22–4.

86. Bhutani T, Koo J. A review of the chemopreventative effects of oral retinoids for internal neoplasms. J Drugs Dermatol. 2011;10(11):1292–8.

87. Wang E, Sasaki J, Nakamura M, et al. Cuaneous carcinogenic risk of phototherapy: an updated comprehensive review. J Psoriasis Psoriatic Arth. 2015;1(1):44–51.

88. Busse K, Koo J. Introducing the delayed retinoid burn: a case report and discussion of this potential risk of retinoid-phototherapy combination management. J Am Acad Dermatol. 2011 May;64(5):1011–2.

89. Ruzicka T, Sommerburg C, Braun-Falco O, et al. Efficiency of acitretin in combination with UV-B in the treatment of severe psoriasis. Arch Dermatol. 1990;126(4):482–6.

90. Iest J, Boer J. Combined treatment of psoriasis with acitretin and UVB phototherapy compared with acitretin alone and UVB alone. Br J Dermatol. 1989;120(5):665–70.

91. Lowe NJ, Prystowsky JH, Bourget T, Edelstein J, Nychay S, Armstrong R. Acitretin plus UVB therapy for psoriasis. Comparisons with placebo plus UVB and acitretin alone. J Am Acad Dermatol. 1991;24(4):591–4.

92. Saurat JH, Geiger JM, Amblard P, et al. Randomized double-blind multicenter study comparing acitretin-PUVA, etretinate-PUVA and placebo-PUVA in the treatment of severe psoriasis. Dermatologica. 1988;177(4):218–24.

93. Lauharanta J, Geiger JM. A double-blind comparison of acitretin and etretinate in combination with bath PUVA in the treatment of extensive psoriasis. Br J Dermatol. 1989;121(1):107–12.

94. Tanew A, Guggenbichler A, Hönigsmann H, Geiger JM, Fritsch P. Photochemotherapy for severe psoriasis without or in combination with acitretin: a randomized, double-blind comparison study. J Am Acad Dermatol. 1991;25(4):682–4.

95. Neoral [package insert]. East Hanover: Novartis; 2015.

96. Paul BS, Momtaz K, Stern RS, Arndt KA, Parrish JA. Combined methotrexate--ultraviolet B therapy in the treatment of psoriasis. J Am Acad Dermatol. 1982;7(6):758–62.

97. Morison WL, Momtaz K, Parrish JA, Fitzpatrick TB. Combined methotrexate-PUVA therapy in the treatment of psoriasis. J Am Acad Dermatol. 1982;6(1):46–51.

98. Paul C, Cather J, Gooderham M, et al. Efficacy and safety of apremilast, an oral phosphodiesterase 4 inhibitor, in patients with moderate-to-severe plaque psoriasis over 52 weeks: a phase III, randomized controlled trial (ESTEEM 2). Br J Dermatol. 2015;173(6):1387–99.

99. AbuHilal M, Walsh S, Shear N. Use of Apremilast in combination with other therapies for treatment of chronic plaque psoriasis: a retrospective study. J Cutan Med Surg. 2016;20(4):313–6.

100. De Simone C, D'Agostino M, Capizzi R, et al. Combined treatment with etanercept 50 mg once weekly and narrow-band ultraviolet B phototherapy in chronic plaque psoriasis. Eur J Dermatol. 2011;21(4):568–72.

101. Kircik L, Bagel J, Korman N, et al. Utilization of narrow-band ultraviolet light B therapy and etanercept for the treatment of psoriasis (UNITE): efficacy, safety, and patient-reported outcomes. J Drugs Dermatol. 2008;7(3):245–53.

102. Wolf P, Hofer A, Legat FJ, et al. Treatment with 311-nm ultraviolet B accelerates and improves the clearance of psoriatic lesions in patients treated with etanercept. Br J Dermatol. 2009;160(1):186–9.

103. Lynde CW, Gupta AK, Guenther L, et al. A randomized study comparing the combination of nbUVB and etanercept to etanercept monotherapy in patients with psoriasis who do not exhibit an excellent response after 12 weeks of etanercept. J Dermatolog Treat. 2012;23(4):261–7.

104. Gambichler T, Tigges C, Scola N, et al. Etanercept plus narrowband ultraviolet B phototherapy of psoriasis is more effective than etanercept monotherapy at 6 weeks. Br J Dermatol. 2011;164(6):1383–6.

105. Calzavara-Pinton PG, Sala R, Arisi M, et al. Synergism between narrowband ultraviolet B phototherapy and etanercept for the treatment of plaque-type psoriasis. Br J Dermatol. 2013;169(1):130–6.

106. Park KK, Swan J, Koo J. Effective treatment of etanercept and phototherapy-resistant psoriasis using the excimer laser. Dermatol Online J. 2012;18(3):2.

107. Park KK, Wu JJ, Koo J. A randomized, 'head-to-head' pilot study comparing the effects of etanercept monotherapy vs. etanercept and narrowband ultraviolet B (NB-UVB) phototherapy in obese psoriasis patients. J Eur Acad Dermatol Venereol. 2013;27(7):899–906.

108. Strober B, Gottlieb A, Leonardi C, et al. Levels of response of psoriasis patients with different baseline characteristics treated with etanercept. J Am Acad Dermatol. 2006;54(3 Suppl):AB220.

109. Bagel J. Adalimumab plus narrowband ultraviolet B light phototherapy for the treatment of moderate to severe psoriasis. J Drugs Dermatol. 2011;10(4):366–71.

110. Wolf P, Hofer A, Weger W, et al. 311 nm ultraviolet B-accelerated response of psoriatic lesions in adalimumab-treated patients. Photodermatol Photoimmunol Photomed. 2011;27(4):86–9.

111. Wolf P, Weger W, Legat FJ, et al. Treatment with 311-nm ultraviolet B enhanced response of psoriatic lesions in ustekinumab-treated patients: a randomized intraindividual trial. Br J Dermatol. 2012;166(1):147–53.

112. Lowenthal KE, Horn PJ, Kalb RE. Concurrent use of methotrexate and acitretin revisited. J Dermatolog Treat. 2008;19(1):22–6.

113. Vanderveen EE, Ellis CN, Campbell JP, Case PC, Voorhees JJ. Methotrexate and etretinate as concurrent therapies in severe psoriasis. Arch Dermatol. 1982;118(9):660–2.

114. Rosenbaum MM, Roenigk HH. Treatment of generalized pustular psoriasis with etretinate (Ro 10-9359) and methotrexate. J Am Acad Dermatol. 1984;10(2 Pt 2):357–61.

115. Tuyp E, MacKie RM. Combination therapy for psoriasis with methotrexate and etretinate. J Am Acad Dermatol. 1986;14(1):70–3.

116. Soriatane [package insert]. Research Triangle Park; Stiefel: 2015.

117. Clark CM, Kirby B, Morris AD, et al. Combination treatment with methotrexate and cyclosporin for severe recalcitrant psoriasis. Br J Dermatol. 1999;141(2):279–82.

118. Aydin F, Canturk T, Senturk N, Turanli AY. Methotrexate and ciclosporin combination for the treatment of severe psoriasis. Clin Exp Dermatol. 2006;31(4):520–4.

119. Ellis CN, Reiter KL, Bandekar RR, Fendrick AM. Cost-effectiveness comparison of therapy for psoriasis with a methotrexate-based regimen versus a rotation regimen of modified cyclosporine and methotrexate. J Am Acad Dermatol. 2002;46(2):242–50.

120. Sasaki J, Zhu TH, Austin A, Nakamura M, Koo J. Apremilast and cyclosporine combination therapy for a patient with both psoriasis and psoriatic arthritis: a case report. J Psoriasis Psoriatic Arth. 2016;1(2):70–2.

121. Colao R, Yanofsky VR, Lebhowl MG. Successful treatment of palmoplantar psoriasis using combination acitretin and apremilast: a case report. J Psoriasis Psoriatic Arth. 2016;1(2):66–9.

122. Gisondi P, Del Giglio M, Cotena C, Girolomoni G. Combining etanercept and acitretin in the therapy of chronic plaque psoriasis: a 24-week, randomized, controlled, investigator-blinded pilot trial. Br J Dermatol. 2008;158(6):1345–9.

123. Philipp S, Wilsmann-Theis D, Weyergraf A, et al. Combination of adalimumab with traditional systemic antipsoriatic drugs—a report of 39 cases. J Dtsch Dermatol Ges. 2012;10(11):821–37.

124. Smith EC, Riddle C, Menter MA, Lebwohl M. Combining systemic retinoids with biologic agents for moderate to severe psoriasis. Int J Dermatol. 2008;47(5):514–8.

125. Conley J, Nanton J, Dhawan S, et al. Novel combination regimens: biologics and acitretin for the treatment of psoriasis—a case series. J Dermatol Treat. 2006;17:86–9.

126. Armstrong AW, Bagel J, Van Voorhees AS, Robertson AD, Yamauchi PS. Combining biologic therapies with other systemic treatments in psoriasis: evidence-based, best-practice recommendations from the medical Board of the National Psoriasis Foundation. JAMA Dermatol. 2015;151(4):432–8.

127. Lee EJ, Shin MK, Kim NI. A clinical trial of combination therapy with etanercept and low dose cyclosporine for the treatment of refractory psoriasis. Ann Dermatol. 2010;22(2):138–42.

128. D'Angelo S, Cutro MS, Lubrano E, et al. Combination therapy with ciclosporin and etanercept in patients with psoriatic arthritis. Ann Rheum Dis. 2010;69(5):934–5.

129. Yamauchi PS, Lowe NJ. Cessation of cyclosporine therapy by treatment with etanercept in patients with severe psoriasis. J Am Acad Dermatol. 2006;54(3 Suppl 2):S135–8.

130. Gattu S, Wu J, Koo J. Can adalimumab make a smooth and easy transition from cyclosporine a reality? A case series of successful transitions. Psoriasis Forum. 2009;15(2):33–5.

131. Ortiz A, Yamauchi PS. A treatment strategy for psoriasis: transitioning from systemic therapy to biologic agents. Skinmed. 2006;5:285–8.

132. Gottlieb AB, Langley RG, Strober BE, et al. A randomized, double-blind, placebo-controlled study to evaluate the addition of methotrexate to etanercept in patients with moderate to severe plaque psoriasis. Br J Dermatol. 2012;167(3):649–57.

133. Zachariae C, Mørk NJ, Reunala T, et al. The combination of etanercept and methotrexate increases the effectiveness of treatment in active psoriasis despite inadequate effect of methotrexate therapy. Acta Derm Venereol. 2008;88(5):495–501.

134. Driessen RJ, van de Kerkhof PC, de Jong EM. Etanercept combined with methotrexate for high-need psoriasis. Br J Dermatol. 2008;159(2):460–3.

135. Iyer S, Yamauchi P, Lowe NJ. Etanercept for severe psoriasis and psoriatic arthritis: observations on combination therapy. Br J Dermatol. 2002;146(1):118–21.

136. Dalaker M, Bonesrønning JH. Long-term maintenance treatment of moderate-to-severe plaque psoriasis with infliximab in combination with methotrexate or azathioprine in a retrospective cohort. J Eur Acad Dermatol Venereol. 2009;23(3):277–82.

137. van den Reek JM, van Lümig PP, Kievit W, et al. Effectiveness of adalimumab dose escalation, combination therapy of adalimumab with methotrexate, or both in patients with psoriasis in daily practice. J Dermatolog Treat. 2013;24(5):361–8.

138. Strober BE, Clarke S. Etanercept for the treatment of psoriasis: combination therapy with other modalities. J Drugs Dermatol. 2004;3(3):270–2.

139. De Groot M, Teunissen MBM, Picavet DI, et al. Adalimumab in combination with methotrexate more effectively reduces the numbers of different inflammatory cell types in lesional psoriatic skin than does single treatment with adalimumab or methotrexate. Br J Dermatol. 2008;159:1401.

140. Yamauchi PS, Lowe NJ. Etanercept therapy allows the tapering of methotrexate and sustained clinical responses in patients with moderate to severe psoriasis. Int J Dermatol. 2008;47(2):202–4.

141. Farhangian ME, Feldman SR. Immunogenicity of biologic treatments for psoriasis: therapeutic consequences and the potential value of concomitant methotrexate. Am J Clin Dermatol. 2015;16(4):285–94.

142. Heinecke GM, Luber AJ, Levitt JO, Lebwohl MG. Combination use of ustekinumab with other systemic therapies: a retrospective study in a tertiary referral center. J Drugs Dermatol. 2013 Oct;12(10):1098–102.

143. Danesh MJ, Beroukhim K, Nguyen C, Levin E, Koo J. Apremilast and adalimumab: a novel combination therapy for recalcitrant psoriasis. Dermatol Online J. 2015;21(6)

144. Rothstein BE, McQuade B, Greb JE, Goldminz AM, Gottlieb AB. Apremilast and secukinumab combined therapy in a patient with recalcitrant plaque psoriasis. J Drugs Dermatol. 2016;15(5):648–9. pii: 13030/qt5gf406zs

Kody Heubach, Leah A. Cardwell,
and Steven R. Feldman

Introduction

A host of treatment options are available for psoriasis, allowing tailored treatment regimens for patients based on disease severity and preference. Topical medications are generally prescribed to patients with limited disease involvement. However, in patients with more extensive disease, phototherapy, or systemic medications in oral or injectable formulations, may be employed. Though there are a variety of treatment options, many patients have recalcitrant disease. This recalcitrance may be due to inherent treatment inefficacy or nonadherence to treatment. Practitioners have a vested interest in patients' adherence as disease improvement is often contingent upon whether patients use the medication.

K. Heubach
Lumberton, NC, USA

L. A. Cardwell (✉)
Department of Dermatology, Wake Forest
School of Medicine, Winston-Salem, NC, USA
e-mail: lcardwe@wakehealth.edu

S. R. Feldman
Department of Dermatology, Wake Forest
School of Medicine, Winston-Salem, NC, USA

Department of Pathology, Wake Forest School
of Medicine, Winston-Salem, NC, USA

Department of Public Health Sciences, Wake Forest
School of Medicine, Winston-Salem, NC, USA
e-mail: sfeldman@wakehealth.edu

Poor adherence (Table 8.1) to medical advice is a serious issue across medical specialties, including dermatology. Nonadherence to treatment may result in over 100 billion dollars in healthcare costs annually in the United States [1]. One-third of psoriasis patients admit to not following their prescribed medication regimen [2]. Nonadherence may lead to disease exacerbation and advancement of symptoms [3]. Psoriasis patients are more likely to adhere to systemic treatment options because of ease and convenience of use, but adherence is still suboptimal [4]. Multiple factors may affect treatment adherence in psoriasis patients (Table 8.2). Strategies to improve adherence are developed in an effort to address these factors (Table 8.3).

Primary nonadherence occurs when patients fail to fill a prescribed medication. In secondary nonadherence, prescriptions are filled, but either not used as prescribed or discontinued early. In demonstrating lack of persistence, patients may have ideal primary and secondary adherence but do not follow through with refilling the medication [5, 6]. Quality of execution is represented by how often patients use the correct dose and dosing intervals [7]. Purposeful or intentional nonadherence is the process of patients actively and rationally deciding not to use the medication often after weighing the pros and cons. This decision is typically hinged on patient beliefs and cognition level. Unintentional nonadherence is unplanned and often occurs due to patients' poor understanding of how to use the medication

Table 8.1 Adherence terminology

Adherence terms	Definitions
Primary nonadherence	Failure to fill prescription
Secondary nonadherence	Failure to use the treatment as prescribed or early discontinuation of treatment
Quality of execution	Patterns of adherence, how often patients use the correct dose and dosing intervals
Early termination	Premature discontinuation of the treatment regimen
Purposeful (intentional) nonadherence	An active and rational decision not to use the medication
Accidental (unintentional) nonadherence	Unplanned nonadherence, often occurring due to poor understanding

Common terms describing adherence patterns in medicine

Table 8.2 Factors affecting adherence

- Lack of patient knowledge about psoriasis
- Lack of patient knowledge about available treatment options
- Lack of patient input regarding treatment choice
- Cost of treatment
- Chronicity of treatment
- Perceived lack of effectiveness of treatment
- Forgetfulness
- Fear of treatment side effects
- Poor physician-patient rapport

Examples of factors which influence adherence in psoriasis patients

Table 8.3 Strategies to improve adherence

Strategies	Examples
Educate the patient	• Ask the patient if they have any questions • After diagnosis of psoriasis, explain that while psoriasis is incurable, there are treatments that are effective in controlling the condition
Involve the patient	• Discuss preferred medication attributes • Ask the patient if they are comfortable with the current treatment they are using
Identify potential barriers to adherence	• Ask the patient about their daily routine • Review concomitant medications to avoid adverse drug interactions
Discuss cost	• Talk with the patient about their healthcare plan to determine if the treatment will be covered • Discuss coupons that could help the patient save on out-of-pocket costs
Use reminders	• Daily text messages • Daily emails • Automated phone call reminders • Discuss internet-based reminder applications
Use motivational techniques	• During follow-up visits, applaud the progress patients have made • Encourage patients to continue with treatment adherence to reach the goal of clearer skin
Use interactive interventions	• Encourage participation in psoriasis forums, either online or in person

Adherence strategies and implementation examples

or simply forgetting to use the medication. This process is associated with regimen complexity and lapse in memory [8].

Factors Affecting Adherence

Lack of knowledge about psoriasis may hinder patients' pursuit of dermatologic treatment. Patients may assume that since psoriasis is incurable, there must be no effective treatment [9]. They may also believe that their psoriasis will worsen regardless of whether they adhere to treatment. Patients may skip doses of an injectable medication because they believe their psoriasis is under control, not recognizing that continued use is necessary for maintenance of disease control [10]. These knowledge gaps negatively impact compliance. In some cases, physicians provide inadequate drug information to their patients regarding newly prescribed topical medications [11]. Dermatology patients have a tendency to underdose new topical treatments; this may be evidence of poor patient counseling about medication regimens [12].

Patients may have an aversion to certain treatment types, vehicles, or medication characteristics [8, 13, 14]. While some studies have attempted to categorize vehicle preferences based on demographic group, it is presumptuous to regard these preference patterns as a rule [13, 15]. Daily routines may limit patient ability to adhere to treatment. Treatment options which require frequent office visits, such as outpatient phototherapy, may be inconvenient for patients to pursue as they may not mesh well with an individual's daily routine [16].

Treatment cost is a potential barrier to adherence. Due to uncertainty regarding healthcare coverage and rising healthcare costs, patients may prioritize cost as a factor in treatment decision-making. Injectable biologics are much costlier than other psoriasis treatment options with prices ranging from $36,038 to $53,909 for a year supply in 2014. The price of commonly prescribed biologics rises by approximately 9.5% annually, adding to the financial burden of psoriasis [17]. If a medication is expensive, the patient may not purchase it, or they may limit the use of the medication once purchased [10, 18, 19]. While health insurance can lower the cost of treatments, a high co-pay may force patients to discontinue treatment due to financial constraints [20].

Psoriasis is a chronic disease, so once a treatment regimen is established, it often must be followed long term. Adherence to chronic treatment regimens may decline over time [18]. Patients may become discouraged with their psoriasis and the treatment regimen; this may lead to waning compliance. Perhaps as a function of human nature, patients may inadvertently forget to use their medication [21]. In a study evaluating the factors which contribute to nonadherence to oral hypoglycemic medications in diabetes patients, 49.6% of survey respondents cited forgetfulness as a major reason for nonadherence [22].

Patients may be fearful of the side effect profile of certain medications; this fear may lead to poor adherence [21]. In a study evaluating the barriers to treatment adherence among patients with hypertension, fear of side effects (25.4% of subjects) was the major reason for intentional nonadherence, followed by inconvenience of taking medicines outside home (17% of subjects) and fear of taking too many drugs at the same time (3.2% of subjects) [23].

Patients may be reluctant to voice treatment concerns to their practitioner. The aforementioned factors may be mediated through better communication between the patient and physician. Patient-centered communication skills can fortify the physician-patient rapport, potentially facilitating improved adherence to treatment regimens [24]. In a longitudinal study, patient satisfaction was improved by physicians' ability to provide thorough explanations and show empathy for patients [25]. Self-reported adherence to treatment regimens was lower in patients who were not satisfied with dermatologic care [26].

Measuring Adherence in Psoriasis

To determine patients' adherence to a treatment regimen, physicians may directly ask the patient about their use of the treatment. This method is unreliable as patients often overreport their adherence. Medication logs and medication weights rely on patient account and may overreport adherence. Lack of recognition of poor adherence can lead to poor treatment options, unnecessary treatment changes, and use of medications that may be more risky and costly.

The use of electronic monitoring to record patients' adherence is the most accurate adherence measure available [14, 27]. Electronic monitoring of topical and oral medication is conducted using caps that contain electronic monitors which record the opening and closing of the cap [1, 28]. The data collected by the electronic cap allows physicians to better understand the patient's adherence patterns [1]. While the information collected by the electronic monitoring cap provides the physician with a more accurate idea of the patient's adherence, it does not provide exact adherence data [28]. If the patient transfers the pills or tablets from the original bottle to a weekly pill case, but takes the medication regularly according to the prescribed schedule, the data collected by the monitor would provide a false idea of poor adherence. Some of the topical treatments prescribed to patients with psoriasis are to be used as needed, so electronic monitoring may not be effective in assessing patient's adherence to some topical regimens [28]. The electronic monitoring caps do not measure the amount of medication dispensed each time the cap is opened and cannot detect whether the patient is using too much or too little of the topical at each application [1, 28]. Such monitors are used in clinical trials and are generally not practical for use in clinical practice.

While electronic monitoring can be used as a general means of measuring adherence to topical or oral medications, new methods are being developed to measure adherence to oral methotrexate. Methotrexate is converted into methotrexate polyglutamate (MTXPG) by the addition of a glutamic acid. The serum concentration of MTXPG decreases quickly after oral administration of methotrexate, but levels remain elevated within red blood cells. The concentration of MTXPG inside of red blood cells can be measured using high-performance liquid chromatography. The red blood cell concentration of MTXPG has the potential to be an objective measure of adherence to methotrexate analogous to glycated hemoglobin in long-term blood glucose monitoring. As we enhance our understanding of MTXPG and establish concentration reference ranges, this technique may develop into a useful means of measuring methotrexate adherence [29].

Measuring a patient's adherence to clinic-administered injectable medications is uncomplicated because we have medical records which document compliance patterns. Physicians can review the electronic medical record to verify appropriate injection intervals and duration [10]. It is more difficult to measure self-injection adherence. Insurance claims analysis has been used to determine when or if a patient had their injectable drug prescription filled [30]. Adherence was considered equivalent to the proportion of days covered (PDC) and was measured as the number of days covered with the index biologic divided by a fixed time interval of 365 days. A patient was classified as adherent if the PDC value was greater than or equal to 0.80 [30]. While this method of measuring adherence to injectable drugs is novel and useful, it has its limitations. When using the PDC value as an adherence indicator, it is assumed that the patient administered the drug after having the prescription filled. If the patient does not use the prescription after having it filled, the PDC value may overestimate adherence. Another approach which may be useful in assessing adherence to injectable medications in clinical research involves the use of an electronic monitoring cap on the self-injector disposal container. This approach has

been used to document poor adherence to and patterns of adalimumab use [31]. A simple approach that can be used as an overall gauge to adherence in clinical practice is to ask patients, "Are you keeping the extra injectors that you've accumulated refrigerated like you are supposed to?" Patients who are using the medication properly will report that they do not have any extras.

Outpatient phototherapy adherence can be assessed through the review of clinic records. However, measuring adherence to home phototherapy can be challenging, and has not been extensively studied. A data-logging device containing a photosensor accurately records the on/off status of UVA and UVB phototherapy units and can be used to detect both the frequency of dosing events and the duration of administered doses. Despite some limitations, this commercially available data logger is well suited for measuring adherence to home phototherapy in clinical trials [32].

Adherence Patterns in Psoriasis

Psoriasis patients are poorly adherent to topical medications. In a European survey study conducted in 1281 patients with psoriasis, 73% of subjects reported that they did not comply with their current treatment regimen. Perceived poor efficacy and messiness of the topical medication were commonly cited reasons for nonadherence [33]. In a study assessing psoriasis treatment adherence using electronic monitoring caps, medication logs, and medication weights, adherence rates calculated using electronic monitors decreased from 84.6% to 51% during the 8-week study period and were lower than the rates calculated using medication logs and weights [27]. First-time dermatology patients tend to underdose newly prescribed topical treatments. In a prospective study assessing first-time dermatologic outpatients' adherence to topical treatments, patients used median 35% of the expected individual doses; just 1 out of 17 subjects used the expected dose [12].

Adherence to oral medication is typically better than topical treatments. Psoriasis patients reported a 21% higher adherence rate to oral medications compared to topical treatments, at 96% [34]. In a study assessing adherence to topical and oral medications in 3096 patients with atopic dermatitis, psoriasis, urticaria, or tinea, using the Morisky Medication Adherence Scale-8 (MMAS-8), the percentages for high (score 8), medium (score 6 to <8), and low (score < 6) adherence were 9.5%, 24.2%, and 66.3% in the oral medication category versus 6.9%, 17.7%, and 75.5% in the topical medication category [35]. In the psoriasis patients, the percentages for high, medium, and low adherence, according to MMAS-8, were 12.5%, 32.1%, and 55.4% in the oral medication category versus 5.6%, 18.1%, and 76.4% in the topical medication category [36].

Though injectable medications tend to have higher adherence rates than oral and topical medication, adherence to injectable drugs is not optimal. In a single-center study assessing adherence to adalimumab, etanercept, and ustekinumab in psoriasis patients using the medication possession ratio (MPR) index, 93.5% of patients had an MPR ≥8 indicating very good adherence, though etanercept had slightly lower adherence than the other biologics [19]. In a retrospective study assessing adherence to office-administered ustekinumab injections in patients with psoriasis, adherence to the 45 mg and 90 mg doses were 100% and 80%, respectively [10]. In a retrospective, claims analysis study assessing utilization patterns of biologic therapies in Medicare beneficiaries with psoriasis, 38% of patients were adherent, 46% discontinued treatment, 8% switched treatment, and 9% later restarted biologic treatment [30].

In a study assessing adherence to narrowband ultraviolet B phototherapy versus acitretin, adherence to acitretin fell from 93.6 to 54.4%, while adherence to phototherapy was more consistent, with rates starting at 2.4 uses per week and falling to 2.1 uses per week [37]. A retrospective study assessing adherence to phototherapy for vitiligo noted that out of 851 patients with psoriasis, 53% received fewer than 20 treatment sessions and approximately 33% received less than 10 treatment sessions. Psoriasis patients were considered adherent if they attended at least twice weekly for a minimum of 20 treatment sessions [38]. Psoriasis patients self-reported a 93% treatment adherence rate to phototherapy; this was higher than topical therapies (75%) but lower than biologic therapies (100%) and oral therapies (96%) [34]. A summary of adherence patterns in psoriasis and other dermatological conditions is shown in Table 8.4.

Strategies for Improving Adherence

Improving adherence is a huge challenge, complicated by the variety of factors which potentially affect adherence. Strategies to improve adherence must be diverse as psoriasis patients have variable disease severity, symptoms, and treatment preferences. Dermatologists considered good doctor-patient relationship, information from the doctor, background information, and patient's financial state to be the most important factors affecting adherence. Patients considered information from the doctor and understandable communication to be the most important determinants of adherence. Since patient communication is the common denominator between patient and physician perspective on adherence, open dialogues may be a valuable tool for improving adherence [39]. Topical medications are available in multiple vehicle options including gels, foams, lotions, solutions, creams, and ointments. Discussion of preferred topical medication vehicle engages patients in the treatment selection process and fosters a sense of patient responsibility which may in turn improve adherence [13].

Consideration of daily lifestyle is appropriate when establishing the treatment regimen as patients are more likely to adhere to regimens that seamlessly fit with their lifestyle. In a study assessing adherence to highly active antiretroviral therapy (HAART) in human immunodeficiency virus (HIV) patients, high frequency of daily routines such as eating breakfast, watching favorite television program, attending meetings, and sleeping at home was associated with higher adherence. Low frequency of activities such as having friends over to visit was associated with higher adherence [40].

Table 8.4 Adherence patterns in dermatology

Study reference	Patient characteristics	Number of subjects	Medication regimen	Study details	Findings
Balkrishnan, 2003 [1]	Psoriasis patients	10	Salicylic acid 6% gel BID	1-week, open-label pilot study	– Patients overreported adherence in self-reported patient logs – Approximately 26% of the self-reported doses were not verified by the electronic monitor
Carroll, 2004 [27]	Psoriasis patients	24	– Salicylic acid 6% gel BID + tacrolimus 0.1% ointment QD – Salicylic acid 6% gel BID + placebo	8-week, left/right controlled trial	– Mean standard deviation adherence rate was $57.8 \pm 25.5\%$, as measured by electronic monitoring medication bottle cap – Adherence rate is a predictor of change in total disease severity – In the salicylic acid + tacrolimus-treated group, a 10% decrease in adherence rate was associated with a 1-point increase in severity
Fouéré, 2005 [33]	Psoriasis patients	1281	N/A	Observation and transversal survey study	– 73% of subjects self-reported nonadherence to psoriasis treatment regimen – Lack of efficacy and messiness of treatment were the most common reasons for nonadherence
Brown, 2006 [2]	Psoriasis patients	53	N/A	1-day, survey study	– 57% of subjects self-reported adherence to topical steroid regimens; 40% of subjects self-reported nonadherence to topical steroid regimens – Self-reported adherence to topical steroids did not vary with prescribed frequency – Steroid strength had no bearing on self-reported adherence pattern
Yentzer, 2008 [37]	Moderate to severe Plaque psoriasis patients	27	– Acitretin 25 mg daily + home narrowband ultraviolet B 3 times/week	12-week, open-label study	– Mean adherence to acitretin, as measured by electronic monitoring medication bottle cap, decreased over 12-week period, slope = −0.24 – Mean adherence to home phototherapy, as measured by light-sensing data logger, remained steady over 12-week period
Storm, 2008 [12]	First-time dermatologic outpatients	17	Topical steroids	2-week prospective study	– 1 out of 17 subjects used the expected dosage of topical steroid – Median 35% of expected individual dosages of topical steroid were used
Chan, 2013 [34]	Psoriasis patients	106	N/A	1-day, survey study	– Overall self-reported rate of adherence was 85.8% – Self-reported adherence was highest for biologic treatments (100%) and lowest for topical treatments (75%) – 56.8% of patients reported that messiness of treatment affected adherence
Sandoval, 2013 [10]	Psoriasis patients on ustekinumab	45	N/A	Retrospective chart review study of psoriasis patients on clinic-administered ustekinumab	– In patients who received ≥3 doses of ustekinumab, overall adherence was 100% – Adherence to the 45 mg and 90 mg doses were 100% and 80%, respectively

Study	Population	N	Medication	Study type	Findings
Kalia, 2014 [38]	Psoriasis and vitiligo patients on phototherapy	957	N/A	Retrospective chart review study	– Of the 851 patients with psoriasis, 53% received fewer than 20 treatment sessions and were considered nonadherent – Of the 106 patients with vitiligo, 39% of subjects received fewer than 60 treatment sessions and were considered nonadherent
Furue, 2014 [35]	Patients with atopic dermatitis, urticaria, psoriasis, or tinea	3096	N/A	Retrospective survey study	– Percentages of high, medium, and low adherence as measured by MMAS-8 were 9.5, 24.2, and 66.3% for oral medication and 6.9, 17.7, and 75.5% for topical medication
Saeki, 2015 [36]	Psoriasis patients	237	N/A	Retrospective survey study	– In psoriasis patients, percentages of high, medium, and low adherence as measured by MMAS-8 were 12.5, 32.1, and 55.4% for oral medication and 5.6, 18.1, and 76.4% for topical medication
Doshi, 2016 [30]	Medicare beneficiaries with psoriasis, initiating infliximab, etanercept, adalimumab, or ustekinumab	2707	N/A	Retrospective claims analysis	– 38% of subjects were adherent to the biologic, 46% discontinued treatment, 8% switched to another biologic, and 9% later restarted biologic treatment
Hsu, 2016 [19]	Psoriasis patients on adalimumab, etanercept, or ustekinumab	247	N/A	Single-center, prospective, chart review study	– 93.5% of all patients had an MPR ≥ 0.8, indicating very good adherence – MPR for etanercept was slightly lower than that of the other studied biologics
Alinia, 2016 [28]	Mild-moderate psoriasis patients	40	Fluocinonide 0.05% ointment BID	12-month, investigator-blinded, prospective study. Subjects randomized to standard of care or Internet-reporting intervention	– The Internet-reporting intervention improved adherence—35% of the prescribed doses were taken by the control group, while 50% of prescribed doses were taken by the intervention group

Trends in treatment adherence in patients with psoriasis

QD daily, *BID* twice daily, *MMAS-8* Morisky Medication Adherence Scale-8, *MPR* medication possession ratio

Treatment cost may adversely affect adherence [18, 41]. To address this issue, physicians might consider prescribing generic medications. The generic version of a drug is typically as efficacious with a lower price [18]. Branded medication co-payments can be 3–5 times higher than that of generic medications (though prices of some generic medications have exploded recently). Triamcinolone 0.01% is 30% to 40% cheaper than other mid-potency steroids when dispensed as a 15 g or 30 g tube. Some topical steroids are cheaper to purchase in higher unit size. For instance, a 454 g jar of triamcinolone 0.01% costs $45, while ten 45 g tubes of betamethasone valerate 0.1%, a steroid of similar potency, cost $324 [42]. If physicians familiarize themselves with psoriasis treatment costs and general coverage patterns of healthcare insurance plans, they may be better informed to prescribe affordable options [20]. Assistance programs and savings coupons may be available and help lower out-of-pocket costs (though these programs may contribute to higher societal costs by removing incentives for cost-effective management) [20].

Frequent follow-up visits during clinical trials increased patients' adherence to treatment regimens. Increasing the frequency of follow-up visits, especially after initiating a new treatment, may allow practitioners to reinforce treatment regimen instructions and encourage patient compliance. Adherence to treatment during these frequent follow-up visits might be a result of "white coat compliance," defined as improved adherence preceding a clinic visit [43]. However, strong adherence early on may influence ideal adherence thereafter by establishing routine [44]. Therefore the term "frequent follow-up visit" may be a bit of a misnomer; if moving the first return visit to an earlier time encourages better adherence, better outcomes, and better long-term adherence, fewer overall visits may be needed.

Educating patients about psoriasis and treatment options may dispel misconceptions and equip patients to make informed decisions about disease management and treatment adherence. In a qualitative study assessing the unmet needs pertaining to clinician interaction and consultation structure, subjects reported limited knowledge about psoriasis [45]. A randomized trial assessed the difference between providing psoriatic arthritis and rheumatoid arthritis patients with disease-modifying antirheumatic drug (DMARD) information in groups or individually. There was a trend toward better adherence and drug continuation rates in patients counseled in groups [46]. Thus, there may be some utility in counseling patients regarding psoriasis treatment regimens in group session format.

Motivational interviewing (MI) has improved adherence in several research studies across medical specialties and may have some utility in improving psoriasis treatment adherence [18]. In a study assessing the utility of the MI intervention in improving medication adherence in patients who were either initiating or changing HAART, all participants in the intervention group self-reported taking all doses of their medication, while the control group had four subjects who missed at least one dose of medication over the 4-day study period [47]. MI intervention improved treatment adherence in acutely psychotic patients from inpatient status to 6 months after discharge. There was a 23% improvement in adherence in the MI intervention group compared to the control group which received nonspecific counseling [48]. Motivational interviewing uses five principles including expression of empathy through reflective listening, development of discrepancy between patients' goals and current behavior, avoidance of argument, adjustment to patient resistance, and support of self-efficacy and optimism. Self-efficacy is the personal belief in one's ability to succeed in specific situations and accomplish a task, in this case treatment adherence. These principles allow practitioners to build rapport with the patient and improve adherence [47]. During motivational interviewing, physicians listen to the patient's concerns about their psoriasis, restating them so the patient knows the physician was listening and shares concern. Physicians then discuss the patient's goals in psoriasis management and how nonadherence to treatment will prevent them from reaching the goal [18]. This assertion may be met with offense [47]. The technique of listening without countering the argument provides assurance that the physician will act in the patient's best interest and determine the ideal course of action. The argument presented by the patient may provide insight into reasons for nonadherence, allowing the physician to change the treatment to better fit the patient's needs. Finally, physician support of self-efficacy through acknowledgment of the patient's progress and potential motivates the patient to remain adherent [18].

A reminder approach may positively impact adherence. In our modern age of technology, the use of text message reminders may serve as a practical option for improving adherence [49]. In a study evaluating the utility of a text messaging intervention in improving adherence to psoriasis treatment regimens, self-reported adherence increased from 3.86 days per week to 6.46 days per week in the intervention group [50]. This strategy may be more effective in younger patient populations as this demographic is more accustomed to text messaging [49]. If patients desire reminders in a different format, daily emails, daily phone calls, and daily medication reminder applications are available.

Daily reminders are not limited to technology-based systems. Simple measures such as use of medication cases and storage of medication bottle in a designated area may serve as an adequate reminder system. Pill cases are convenient and increase medication adherence [51]. They typically have a compartment for each day of the week, facilitating organization of other prescriptions the patient may be taking. Patients might consider storing their pill bottles or cases in a designated, frequently visited location so that the sight of this item reminds them to use the medication [18].

To improve adherence to topical medications, physicians may engage patients in a discussion of preferred medication attributes. When patients were queried about important medication attributes, responses varied, but the ease of spreading the topical onto the skin was important to 31% of females and 11% of the males. Thirty-nine percent of full-time employed subjects preferred a non-greasy option compared to 18% of subjects who did not work full time [13]. This variability in preference underscores the importance of open dialogues during clinical encounters.

Interactive interventions are beneficial in improving adherence. In a study assessing the effect of a weekly internet discussion intervention on topical fluocinonide adherence in psoriasis, the intervention group used 50% of the prescribed doses, while the normal care group used 35% of the prescribed doses. The percentage of days with correct dosage was 34% and 20%, in the intervention and normal care groups, respectively [28]. Internet-based interventions are convenient because the patient can complete the program from the comfort of their home. These intervention programs may have a lasting effect by establishing a routine which will hopefully continue. Alternatively, the improved adherence facilitated by the intervention program may be short term, having little effect on the patient as time progresses [28]. Due to the potential short-term effect of the intervention strategy, implementation may be more beneficial early in treatment.

While adherence to oral medications for the treatment of psoriasis is higher than topical treatments, there is still room for improvement. A potential contributor to poor adherence to oral medications is patients' fear of side effects associated with the use of the medication [20]. Commonly prescribed oral medications such as methotrexate and cyclosporine may cause dangerous drug interactions; the fear of these interactions may negatively impact treatment adherence [20]. Thorough education about the drug and possible side effects could positively impact adherence. Practitioners might consider comparing risks of the side effect to some other real-world event to frame the risk in proper perspective. Providing information about what factors might increase the risk of drug-related side effects may reduce patient anxiety.

Newer oral medications, such as apremilast, target specific molecules in the inflammatory cascade to improve psoriasis and have fewer, less severe side effects than traditional oral medications [20]. In a study assessing efficacy of apremilast in the treatment of psoriasis, discontinuation rate due to side effects was approximately 5% [52]. Diarrhea and weight loss are common side effects of apremilast. While the diarrhea is probably universally frustrating (though even diarrhea might be framed as positive by saying "the diarrhea may be a sign the drug is working"), weight loss may be considered a positive attribute in some patient populations. Due to its favorable side effect profile and low discontinuation rates, apremilast may portend better adherence patterns in the oral medication category. Perceived or true suboptimal efficacy of oral medication may negatively impact treatment adherence. In such cases, treatment escalation may be a measure to improve adherence. Biologics typically require infrequent injections which may lead to missed doses. Interrupted injection schedules can lead to worsening psoriasis, perpetuating the idea that the drug is less efficacious. Frank discussions about goals of treatment and patient-perceived efficacy serve to instill realistic patient expectations. An injectable biologic may truly lack efficacy in a certain patient, so switching the patient to a different biologic agent may be beneficial in improving disease management and treatment adherence [53]. Newly developed injectable biologic agents have the potential to achieve Psoriasis Area Severity Index (PASI) 90–100. These high clearance rates might encourage improved adherence in patients who had sporadic adherence with other biologic agents [20].

Phototherapy may be administered via office unit, requiring the patients to report to the doctor's office multiple times per week for treatment. Alternatively, patients can purchase a home phototherapy unit. The latter is a convenient option as patients can administer treatment from the comfort of their homes rather than having to travel to the doctor's office for each treatment. Home-based UVB phototherapy is as effective as outpatient phototherapy with no difference in safety profile. Home phototherapy has less qual-ity-of-life burden than outpatient phototherapy, and patients reported that they preferred home phototherapy over outpatient phototherapy [16]. Psoriasis patients perceive phototherapy to be a very effective treatment for psoriasis; this perception may guide adherence patterns [54]. Patients who struggle with adherence to outpatient phototherapy may be good candidates for home phototherapy. Though home phototherapy is a practical solution, acquisition may be hindered by insurance company protocols and high co-payments.

Conclusion

The armamentarium for psoriasis has grown immensely over the years. Practitioners have a wealth of treatment options including topical medications, systemic medications, and phototherapy. Even within these categories, modern research has diversified our options. For limited disease, we might choose topical corticosteroids, topical calcineurin inhibitors, or topical vitamin D analogues. For more extensive disease, systemic medications such as small-molecule medications, biologics, methotrexate, cyclosporine, or vitamin A derivatives might be considered. However, these options are useless if patients choose not to adhere to the regimen. Studies have noted poor adherence in dermatology across treatment categories. In psoriasis management, it is important to ensure that patients adhere to the prescribed treatment regimen just as it is important to choose the best treatment regimen. Optimizing physician-patient rapport is important when discussing adherence and implementing adherence improvement strategies. Many of the electronic monitoring techniques are well suited for clinical studies in dermatology to elucidate whether disease stagnancy or worsening is due to inefficacy of treatment or nonadherence. Adherence is the cornerstone of disease management, influencing disease improvement, flaring, and stagnancy in dermatology and across medical specialties. Efforts to improve adherence may indirectly reduce the overall disease burden of psoriasis and other chronic conditions.

References

1. Balkrishnan R, Carroll CL, Camacho FT, Feldman SR. Electronic monitoring of medication adherence in skin disease: results of a pilot study. J Am Acad Dermatol. 2003;49(4):651.
2. Brown KK, Rehmus WE, Kimball AB. Determining the relative importance of patient motivations for non-adherence to topical corticosteroid therapy in psoriasis. J Am Acad Dermatol [Internet]. 2006;55:607–13. http://www.ncbi.nlm.nih.gov/pubmed/17010739
3. Carroll CL, Feldman SR, Camacho FT, Balkrishnan R. Better medication adherence results in greater improvement in severity of psoriasis. Br J Dermatol. 2004;151:895–7.
4. Storm A, Andersen SE, Benfeldt E, Serup J. One in 3 prescriptions are never redeemed: primary nonadherence in an outpatient clinic. J Am Acad Dermatol [Internet]. 2008 [cited 2017 Mar 16];59:27–33. http://www.ncbi.nlm.nih.gov/pubmed/18467003.
5. Anderson KL, Dothard EH, Huang KE, Feldman SR. Frequency of primary nonadherence to acne treatment. JAMA Dermatol [Internet]. American Medical Association; 2015 [cited 2017 Apr 15];151:623. http://archderm.jamanetwork.com/article.aspx?doi=10.1001/jamadermatol.2014.5254
6. Solomon MD, Majumdar SR. Primary non-adherence of medications: lifting the veil on prescription-filling behaviors. J Gen Intern Med [Internet]. Springer; 2010 [cited 2017 Apr 15];25:280–1. http://www.ncbi.nlm.nih.gov/pubmed/20195783
7. Schneider MP, Krummenacher I, Figueiredo H, Marquis J, Bugnon O. Adherence: a review of education, research, practice and policy in Switzerland. Pharm Pract (Granada) [Internet]. Centro de Investigaciones y Publicaciones Farmaceuticas; 2009 [cited 2017 Apr 15];7:63–73. http://www.ncbi.nlm.nih.gov/pubmed/25152780
8. Hugtenburg JG, Timmers L, Elders PJ, Vervloet M, van Dijk L. Patient preference and adherence definitions, variants, and causes of nonadherence with medication: a challenge for tailored interventions. Patient Prefer Adherence [Internet]. 2013 [cited 2017 Apr 15];7:675–82. https://www.ncbi.nlm.nih.gov/pmc/articles/PMC3711878/pdf/ppa-7-675.pdf
9. Simpson JK, Wilson M, Ahmed AA, Mizara A, Clarke A, Mcbride SR. An exploratory study to investigate health-seeking behaviour in patients with psoriasis using framework analysis. Br J Dermatol [Internet]. 2017 [cited 2017 Mar 16]; http://www.ncbi.nlm.nih.gov/pubmed/28083871
10. Sandoval LF, Huang KE, Feldman SR. Adherence to ustekinumab in psoriasis patients. J Drugs Dermatol [Internet]. 2013 [cited 2017 Mar 16];12:1090–2. http://www.ncbi.nlm.nih.gov/pubmed/24085042
11. Storm A, Benfeldt E, Andersen SE, Andersen J. Basic drug information given by physicians is deficient, and patients' knowledge low. J Dermatol Treat [Internet]. 2009 [cited 2017 Apr 12];20:190–3. http://www.ncbi.nlm.nih.gov/pubmed/19040185
12. Storm A, Benfeldt E, Andersen SE, Serup J. A prospective study of patient adherence to topical treatments: 95% of patients underdose. J Am Acad Dermatol [Internet]. 2008 [cited 2017 Apr 12];59:975–80. http://www.ncbi.nlm.nih.gov/pubmed/18817998
13. Iversen L, Jakobsen HB. Patient preferences for topical psoriasis treatments are diverse and difficult to predict. Dermatol Ther (Heidelb) [Internet]. 2016 [cited 2017 Mar 16];6:273–85. http://www.ncbi.nlm.nih.gov/pubmed/27125383
14. Tan X, Feldman SR, Chang J, Balkrishnan R. Topical drug delivery systems in dermatology: a review of patient adherence issues. Expert Opin Drug Deliv [Internet]. 2012 [cited 2017 Mar 16];9:1263–71. http://www.ncbi.nlm.nih.gov/pubmed/22861153
15. Fisher EJ, Adams BB. African American and Caucasian patients' vehicle preference for the scalp. J Am Acad Dermatol [Internet]. 2008 [cited 2017 Apr 17];58:S46–7. http://www.ncbi.nlm.nih.gov/pubmed/18191706
16. Koek MBG, Buskens E, van Weelden H, Steegmans PHA, Bruijnzeel-Koomen CAFM, Sigurdsson V. Home versus outpatient ultraviolet B phototherapy for mild to severe psoriasis: pragmatic multicentre randomised controlled non-inferiority trial (PLUTO study). BMJ [Internet]. 2009 [cited 2017 Mar 16];338:b1542. http://www.ncbi.nlm.nih.gov/pubmed/19423623.
17. Cheng J, Feldman SR. The cost of biologics for psoriasis is increasing. Drugs Context [Internet]. JUST Medical Media Limited; 2014 [cited 2017 Mar 16];3:212266. http://www.ncbi.nlm.nih.gov/pubmed/25598832
18. Aslam I, Feldman SR. Practical strategies to improve patient adherence to treatment regimens. South Med J [Internet]. 2015 [cited 2017 Mar 16];108:325–31. http://www.ncbi.nlm.nih.gov/pubmed/26079456
19. Hsu DY, Gniadecki R. Patient adherence to biologic agents in psoriasis. Dermatology [Internet]. 2016 [cited 2017 Mar 16];232:326–33. http://www.ncbi.nlm.nih.gov/pubmed/27093295
20. Hoffman MB, Hill D, Feldman SR. Current challenges and emerging drug delivery strategies for the treatment of psoriasis. Expert Opin Drug Deliv [Internet]. 2016 [cited 2017 Mar 16];13:1461–73. http://www.ncbi.nlm.nih.gov/pubmed/27164301
21. Jimmy B, Jose J. Patient medication adherence: measures in daily practice. Oman Med J [Internet]. Oman Medical Specialty Board; 2011 [cited 2017 Apr 15];26:155–9. http://www.ncbi.nlm.nih.gov/pubmed/22043406
22. Adisa R, Alutundu MB, Fakeye TO. Factors contributing to nonadherence to oral hypoglycemic medications among ambulatory type 2 diabetes patients in Southwestern Nigeria. Pharm Pract (Granada) [Internet]. 2009 [cited 2017 Apr 15];7:163–9. http://www.ncbi.nlm.nih.gov/pubmed/25143794
23. Khan MU, Shah S, Hameed T. Barriers to and determinants of medication adherence among hypertensive patients attended National Health Service

Hospital, Sunderland. J Pharm Bioallied Sci [Internet]. Medknow Publications; 2014 [cited 2017 Apr 15];6:104–8. http://www.ncbi.nlm.nih.gov/pubmed/24741278

24. Nguyen T V., Hong J, Prose NS. Compassionate care: enhancing physician–patient communication and education in dermatology: Part I: Patient-centered communication. J Am Acad Dermatol [Internet]. 2013 [cited 2017 Apr 18];68:353.e1–353.e8. http://www.sciencedirect.com/science/article/pii/S0190962212012431

25. Renzi C, Abeni D, Picardi A, Agostini E, Melchi CF, Pasquini P, et al. Factors associated with patient satisfaction with care among dermatological outpatients. Br J Dermatol [Internet]. 2001 [cited 2017 Apr 18];145:617–23. http://www.ncbi.nlm.nih.gov/pubmed/11703289

26. Renzi C, Picardi A, Abeni D, Agostini E, Baliva G, Pasquini P, et al. Association of dissatisfaction with care and psychiatric morbidity with poor treatment compliance. Arch Dermatol [Internet]. 2002 [cited 2017 Apr 18];138:337–42. http://www.ncbi.nlm.nih.gov/pubmed/11902984

27. Carroll CL, Feldman SR, Camacho FT, Manuel JC, Balkrishnan R. Adherence to topical therapy decreases during the course of an 8-week psoriasis clinical trial: commonly used methods of measuring adherence to topical therapy overestimate actual use. J Am Acad Dermatol [Internet]. 2004 [cited 2017 Mar 16];51:212–6. http://www.ncbi.nlm.nih.gov/pubmed/15280839

28. Alinia H, Moradi Tuchayi S, Smith JA, Richardson IM, Bahrami N, Jaros SC, et al. Long-term adherence to topical psoriasis treatment can be abysmal: a 1-year randomized intervention study using objective electronic adherence monitoring. Br J Dermatol [Internet]. 2016 [cited 2017 Mar 16]; http://www.ncbi.nlm.nih.gov/pubmed/27664969

29. Woolf RT, West SL, Arenas-Hernandez M, Hare N, Peters van Ton AM, Lewis CM, et al. Methotrexate polyglutamates as a marker of patient compliance and clinical response in psoriasis: a single-centre prospective study. Br J Dermatol [Internet]. 2012 [cited 2017 Mar 16];167:165–73. http://www.ncbi.nlm.nih.gov/pubmed/22309614

30. Doshi JA, Takeshita J, Pinto L, Li P, Yu X, Rao P, et al. Biologic therapy adherence, discontinuation, switching, and restarting among patients with psoriasis in the US Medicare population. J Am Acad Dermatol [Internet]. 2016 [cited 2017 Mar 16];74:1057–1065.e4. http://www.ncbi.nlm.nih.gov/pubmed/26946986

31. West C, Narahari S, O'Neill J, Davis S, Huynh M, Clark A, et al. Adherence to adalimumab in patients with moderate to severe psoriasis. Dermatol Online J [Internet]. 2013 [cited 2017 Apr 12];19:18182. http://www.ncbi.nlm.nih.gov/pubmed/24011280

32. Yelverton CB, Balkrishnan R, Feldman SR. The utility of a data-logging device for measuring adherence to home phototherapy. Photodermatol Photoimmunol Photomed [Internet]. 2006 [cited 2017 Mar 16];22:270–2. http://www.ncbi.nlm.nih.gov/pubmed/16948832

33. Fouere S, Adjadj L, Pawin H. How patients experience psoriasis: results from a European survey. J Eur Acad Dermatol Venereol [Internet]. 2005 [cited 2017 Mar 16];19:2–6. http://www.ncbi.nlm.nih.gov/pubmed/16274404

34. Chan SA, Hussain F, Lawson LG, Ormerod AD. Factors affecting adherence to treatment of psoriasis: comparing biologic therapy to other modalities. J Dermatol Treat [Internet]. 2013 [cited 2017 Mar 16];24:64–9. http://www.ncbi.nlm.nih.gov/pubmed/21797808

35. Furue M, Onozuka D, Takeuchi S, Murota H, Sugaya M, Masuda K, et al. Poor adherence to oral and topical medication in 3096 dermatological patients as assessed by the Morisky Medication Adherence Scale-8. Br J Dermatol [Internet]. Wiley-Blackwell; 2015 [cited 2017 Apr 18];172:272–5. http://www.ncbi.nlm.nih.gov/pubmed/25154923

36. Saeki H, Imafuku S, Abe M, Shintani Y, Onozuka D, Hagihara A, et al. Poor adherence to medication as assessed by the Morisky Medication Adherence Scale-8 and low satisfaction with treatment in 237 psoriasis patients. J Dermatol [Internet]. 2015 [cited 2017 Apr 18];42:367–72. http://doi.wiley.com/10.1111/1346-8138.12804

37. Yentzer BA, Yelverton CB, Pearce DJ, Camacho FT, Makhzoumi Z, Clark A, et al. Adherence to acitretin and home narrowband ultraviolet B phototherapy in patients with psoriasis. J Am Acad Dermatol [Internet]. 2008 [cited 2017 Mar 16];59:577–81. http://www.ncbi.nlm.nih.gov/pubmed/18619709

38. Kalia S, Toosi B, Bansback N, Astaneh A, Zhou Y, Shapiro J, et al. Assessing adherence with phototherapy protocols. J Am Acad Dermatol [Internet]. Elsevier; 2014 [cited 2017 Apr 19];71:1259–61. http://www.ncbi.nlm.nih.gov/pubmed/25454035

39. Szabó C, Kemény L, Csabai M. Dermatology patients' and their doctors' representations about adherence. Open Med. (Warsaw, Poland) [Internet]. De Gruyter Open; 2015 [cited 2017 Apr 19];10:216–23. http://www.ncbi.nlm.nih.gov/pubmed/28352698

40. Wagner GJ, Ryan GW. Relationship between routinization of daily behaviors and medication adherence in HIV-positive drug users. AIDS Patient Care STDS [Internet]. 2004 [cited 2017 Apr 19];18:385–93. http://www.ncbi.nlm.nih.gov/pubmed/15307927

41. Hill D, Farhangian ME, Feldman SR. Increasing adherence to topical therapy in psoriasis through use of solution medication. Dermatol Online J [Internet]. 2016 [cited 2017 Mar 16];22. http://www.ncbi.nlm.nih.gov/pubmed/27617530

42. Skojec A, Foulke G, Kirby JS. Variation in the cost of generic topical corticosteroids. JAMA Dermatol [Internet]. American Medical Association; 2015 [cited 2017 Apr 19];151:1255. http://archderm.jamanetwork.com/article.aspx?doi=10.1001/jamadermatol.2015.2394

43. Podsadecki TJ, Vrijens BC, Tousset EP, Rode RA, Hanna GJ. "White coat compliance" limits the reliability of therapeutic drug monitoring in HIV-1—infected patients. HIV Clin Trials [Internet]. 2008 [cited 2017 Apr 19];9:238–46. http://www.ncbi.nlm.nih.gov/pubmed/18753118

44. Feldman SR, Camacho FT, Krejci-Manwaring J, Carroll CL, Balkrishnan R. Adherence to topical therapy increases around the time of office visits. J Am Acad Dermatol [Internet]. 2007 [cited 2017 Apr 19];57:81–3. http://www.ncbi.nlm.nih.gov/pubmed/17498841

45. Khoury LR, Skov L, Møller T. Facing the dilemma of patient-centred psoriasis care: a qualitative study identifying patient needs in dermatological outpatient clinics. Br J Dermatol [Internet]. 2016 [cited 2017 Mar 16]; http://www.ncbi.nlm.nih.gov/pubmed/28032892

46. Homer D, Nightingale P, Jobanputra P. Providing patients with information about disease-modifying anti-rheumatic drugs: Individually or in groups? A pilot randomized controlled trial comparing adherence and satisfaction. Musculoskeletal Care [Internet]. 2009 [cited 2017 Apr 19];7:78–92. http://www.ncbi.nlm.nih.gov/pubmed/18792423

47. Diiorio C, Resnicow K, McDonnell M, Soet J, McCarty F, Yeager K. Using motivational interviewing to promote adherence to antiretroviral medications: a pilot study. J Assoc Nurses AIDS Care [Internet]. 2003 [cited 2017 Mar 16];14:52–62. http://www.ncbi.nlm.nih.gov/pubmed/12698766

48. Kemp R, Hayward P, Applewhaite G, Everitt B, David A. Compliance therapy in psychotic patients: randomised controlled trial. BMJ [Internet]. BMJ Group; 1996 [cited 2017 Apr 19];312:345–9. http://www.ncbi.nlm.nih.gov/pubmed/8611831

49. Tran N, Coffman JM, Sumino K, Cabana MD. Patient reminder systems and asthma medication adherence: a systematic review. J Asthma [Internet]. 2014 [cited 2017 Mar 16];51:536–43. http://www.ncbi.nlm.nih.gov/pubmed/24506699

50. Balato N, Megna M, Di Costanzo L, Balato A, Ayala F. Educational and motivational support service: a pilot study for mobile-phone-based interventions in patients with psoriasis. Br J Dermatol [Internet]. 2013 [cited 2017 Apr 19];168:201–5. http://www.ncbi.nlm.nih.gov/pubmed/23240729

51. Petersen ML, Wang Y, van der Laan MJ, Guzman D, Riley E, Bangsberg DR. Pillbox organizers are associated with improved adherence to HIV antiretroviral therapy and viral suppression: a marginal structural model analysis. Clin Infect Dis [Internet]. 2007 [cited 2017 Mar 16];45:908–15. http://www.ncbi.nlm.nih.gov/pubmed/17806060

52. Gooderham M, Papp K. Apremilast in the treatment of psoriasis and psoriatic arthritis. Skin Therapy Lett [Internet]. [cited 2017 Mar 16];20:1–6. http://www.ncbi.nlm.nih.gov/pubmed/26382906

53. Kerdel F, Zaiac M. An evolution in switching therapy for psoriasis patients who fail to meet treatment goals. Dermatol Ther [Internet]. 2015 [cited 2017 Apr 20];28:390–403. http://doi.wiley.com/10.1111/dth.12267

54. Nolan B V, Yentzer BA, Feldman SR. A review of home phototherapy for psoriasis. Dermatol Online J [Internet]. 2010 [cited 2017 Mar 16];16:1. http://www.ncbi.nlm.nih.gov/pubmed/20178697

Index

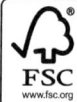